MEDIᴗAL

DESPOTISM

The health, economic and political
programme that can kill you

ROB RYDER

Patrick Quanten MD

Book cover created by Quanten Creative Solutions Limited

Email – info@quantencreative.com

ISBN: 9798865457336

This book is dedicated to historians and their pursuit of Truth, Justice, and Freedom – who have kept alive the knowledge of the true nature of human beings and suffered ridicule, injustice, and even death to set a foundation and example as mankind enters the 'end times'.

A special thank-you for Ann Leyshon for all her help and time spent for free researching the protocols put forward by the government that we knew were the real cause of excess deaths during 'the pandemic'. I was inundated with information that I was trying to piece together so as to present a credible alternative version of events at the time of the Lockdown. Trusting in Ann's understanding of disease and with us both agreeing that it was government policies killing people it was a huge help when she agreed to research these protocols so I could focus on trying to piece the book together. It turns out that the original version of 'Death by Lockdown' in the initial book 'Medical Fascism' did not need to be altered at all except to put it in the past tense. Truth, as they say, just is.

"You cannot explain phenomena you do not understand by inventing an entity that does not exist. That is not science"

- Rob Ryder

"Taking the information coming out of the official covid-19 narrative the author reconnects it to other aspects of how the medical authorities have been consistently ignoring science. He links it to the position of power the owners of the medical profession occupy within governments and within the financial system. It appears they can afford to lie and to deceive the public and not only are they getting away unscathed but they are even being rewarded for it. The author confirms that the only way this system of complete control over the population can be broken is for the population to make independent free choices. And for this to happen we all need this information."

- Patrick Quanten M.D

Contents

"Believe nothing, no matter where you read it, or who said it, no matter if I have said it, unless it agrees with your own reason and your own common sense."

– Buddha (allegedly)

I

DECLARATION

This book is an investigation into the nature of illness and infectious disease and how it relates to the people of the world in a political sense. Neither Robert Ryder nor Patrick Quanten are trying to give anyone any personal health advice and advice regarding treating their illness, as you will see in the book, illness is a very personal thing. Health issues will need personal health advice from the practitioner of your own choosing. We aim to put forward an investigation into the science of disease and how the political system works. These are our opinions based on our own research and are not to be taken as absolute truth. What you do with this information is also your own chose and we accept no responsibility for consequences of your own decision making. Life, as you will see, is about taking personal responsibility and this is something we both promote.

INTRODUCTION

I am writing this book in the middle of goings-on that are really something out of a science-fiction film.

This is a scenario that I knew was going to happen in some form for many years; I never knew exactly how but I knew it would happen. I knew when the propaganda first started coming out of China that this (the story) could well come over here and go worldwide. In fact I was warning people about this before it landed here so I was kind of prepared. When the news finally came out – "we are going into lockdown" – it felt very surreal. Obviously, there was confusion with most people, others just thought that this would be over in a couple of weeks – 'three weeks to flatten the curve' - and life would go back to 'normal' and sadly others were terrified of this invisible enemy coming to get them, coming to get all of us. I knew straight away that it wasn't going to pass over and that this was it, it was finally happening. The end battle for humanity's freedom is now underway and possibly within a year the outcome will be an absolute slavery we will never get out of or an incredible freedom which will finally give humanity the chance to see what it can really do.

Information is changing on a daily basis so I'm not even sure what the world will be like, or what new truths will be unveiled, or what the latest version of events will be by the time it is finished, so this is my best effort with the information I have at the present time to show you what is happening and why. I am not claiming my version of events is truth, but it is my truth. I have been diligent in my research but cannot say for sure that anything is absolute fact; fake news comes from all areas, especially governments and medical science, but my interpretation of the information is my own and it is for all of us to interpret as truthfully as we can regardless of what anyone else thinks, or what the crowd says, or especially what the government tells us.

There is too much information, so I have tried to put together individual pieces to show that it makes a bigger, interconnected picture. It is then up to the individual to research and put more pieces of the puzzle in and see what the end picture tells them. Whether you come to the same conclusions as me is up to you; as you will see, perceiving the world and information is a very individual thing, but I know the best place to start is from a blank page.

To find truth is like looking for a needle in a haystack; the only way to do it is to first discard the hay (untruths) and what is left over will be the needle (truth).

*The above is the introduction from the book 'Medical Fascism-How corona virus policies took away our freedoms and how to get them back' Rob Ryder March 20

LOOKING BACK

On writing the introduction for 'Medical Fascism' in March 2021 it has to be understood that it was in the middle of a level of insanity and hysteria that was new to mankind, even surpassing the insanity of two world wars. Modern technology now means information and agendas can fly round the world at record speed with no area left untouched.

In the chat with James O'Neil from Feb 6 2020, linked on the previous page, I made the comment regarding what was happening in Wuhan, China "the only thing going round the world making people ill is fear and hysteria". We also spoke about an agenda to cull elderly people and by using fear as a tool encourage people to build their own police state. If you think this sounds prophetic considering what has happened the last few years, then you need to know what made me make that statement.

In 2008, due to research and previous life experiences including traveling around North America, Mexico and South America for two years with another year spent full time in Peru, I had come to understand that the world was run by powerful big corporations. I knew though that I did not have the full picture until in 2008 when the financial crash gave me the opportunity to expand my awareness of how the world was being run. I was not happy with the official explanation of why the crash happened and began my own research on money and money creation. This research led me to more information regarding the funding of wars and what really happened at 9/11 and the collapse of the twin towers. With more research in a short space of time a picture emerged of a very organised control system which seemed to have psychological control and control on money at its heart.

In 2011 I saw an interview with medical biochemist Trevor Gunn on alternative television and immediately bought his book 'Soma Wisdom – The science of Health and Healing', now published as just 'The Science of Health and Healing'. In one read it completely changed my understanding of health, disease and the historical safety and effectiveness of vaccines to the point that we as a family walked away from modern medicine in one day and never looked back. The book introduced me to the world of the human condition, something missing from my research at that point, though I did know psychology was being used to control us.

In 2010 I had seen a talk on YouTube by Brian Gerrish of UKColumn News regarding the infiltration of society via a 'political charity' named Common Purpose. It was clear to me this was the tool being used to control and push approved narratives through public institutions and therefore control policies and public behaviour. With my time spent in Latin America and the huge, and sometimes just, influence on the people of Marxist thinking regarding oppressor and oppressed and the control of truth, it was very clear to me after listening to Brian as to what he was talking about and I coined the term, *Communism by stealth*. In simple terms it was central government control of life but sold as giving power back to the community or Communitarianism.

I soon after came across the book 'The Biology of Belief' by Bruce Lipton and this gave me the understanding I needed of how psychological manipulation works. In our book, 'A Conscious Humanity – Morality, Freedom and Natural Law '- Rob Ryder and Patrick Quanten, we go into length into the subject of the human condition, but here I will stick to the basics. Controlling what we think will in effect control our behaviour and it really is as simple as that. When you have the money and power to control the media, governments and education then you have massive power over the beliefs of the public and hence massive control over their behaviour.

In around 2010/11 I contacted the UKColumn and told them I wanted to distribute the monthly newspaper they were printing at the time before they went over to a news show. I now had a complete picture of how the world worked and had seen the game plan for the future that was to be implemented during my lifetime. The weight of the world, and my family's future, was felt on my shoulders and I decided to act. As a complete novice and going into an information war without any training I decided it would be more sensible to contact the UKColumn who had already been up and running for a good few years and had the knowledge and experience I didn't have. I decided it wasn't a good idea to go 'under the radar' as some people were doing and felt that being open and public was the way forward. I spoke with Mike Robinson of the UKColumn on the phone and asked him one simple question "what are the consequences for my family if I go public? ". His reply was simple and what I expected "what are the consequences of doing nothing?" So I started distributing the newspaper and trying my best to warn people of a global agenda to enslave humanity.

In 2014, via 'The Informed Parent' newsletter to which I subscribe, and with the help of Magda Taylor the editor, I contacted Patrick Quanten who was writing articles for the newsletter and who clearly saw things as I did but with the scientific knowledge behind him which I was lacking. In the summer of 2014 we organised an interview with UKColumn news regarding the history and science of infectious disease and vaccination. From then on Patrick made a yearly visit from Belgium to Cornwall to talk at seminars I had arranged regarding all matters of health, disease and the human condition. At the end of the book I will put information and a link to some of our interviews and work that can be found on my rumble channel. Due to censorship on YouTube I decided to back up some of the work on Rumble as for now they are not censoring information.

After spending years arranging talks and events with local people here in Cornwall I decided in about 2015 to start doing my own talks sticking to my own research areas of money, health and psychology. In Feb 2018 I did a local talk named, 'Medical Fascism – The Biggest Threat to our Children's Natural Health'. I could see clearly how allopathic thinking and Germ/Viral Theory, which was running the whole medical system, gave great power to doctors over parents as they were the only approved 'experts'. We have seen over the year's cases of forced chemotherapy and other treatments forced upon children or denied. It does though get a lot worse. The only thing an ignorant and ego driven doctor needed to say was he/she 'felt' the parent was neglecting the child and the threat of social services intervening would normally be enough to shut down any questioning of their decisions. There have been cases though where the threat has ended in children being taken off their parents just for wanting a second opinion or wanting to look into more natural treatments. In Australia recently, there was a case when a child was diagnosed with leukaemia and told to have chemotherapy. The mother just asked for a second opinion and in one day child protection services were called in and the child was taken from the mother and into 'care' so the chemotherapy could go ahead without the interference of the mother. This is the 'Medical Fascism' I was referring to and trying to warn people about.

I obviously at the time did not foresee a massive global event but I could see a national policy for pressure on parents to vaccinate children and force treatments on children going global. Modern medicine theory was in control over the nations of the world, the WHO was the self-proclaimed global expert leader on medical and health issues, and was completely controlled by allopathic thinking. My warning was to show people the need to learn natural health so as to limit contact with the medical authorities who, in my opinion, are only good for accident and emergency; though defining accident and emergency is not as easy as it sounds. Everything, especially with children, now seems to be a potential emergency, mainly due to parents and doctor's fear and ignorance.

In Feb 3 2020 I was invited to Totnes, Devon to talk about my research into the history and effectiveness of vaccines alongside Brian Gerrish who was to talk about Common Purpose and its influence of the NHS. Due to a late start Brian did not have time for his talk but the theme of what we were saying was clear regarding the lack of real science and an agenda to change the NHS. Two weeks later I went back for the follow up talk where I spoke about the psychological attack on mankind and how to take back control over our thoughts and therefore behaviour. Mike Robinson was also talking about the push for a green economy via a fake climate crisis story which would end up in total economic and financial control over humanity. By this time it was clear the happenings in Wuhan were going to go global, yet we were talking about a psychological attack and a coming financial crash and the reconstruction of the global economy via the green agenda.

When the news finally came out, "we are going into lockdown", a friend asked me "is it time to panic?" my reply was simple "no, it's time to go home for a cup of tea". It was clear that madness and hysteria was coming and the best thing to do was to 'put the kettle on...' All cultures will have something they do to calm a situation and in the British Isles no matter what the problem is' putting the kettle on' is the thing to do. It's not just the drink of sweet tea itself but the whole process which helps bring calm to any situation. After spending a few days ignoring the 'guidelines' to stay at home by going to the local beach near our home with the kids for much more than our allocated one hour, (the universe was with us as the weather was sunny and warm for that time of the year), I decided it was not 'the new normal' for me but my own normal.

I phoned up the local police station to inform them I was going out back to work and only wanted to know if they would arrest me, to which they replied "we don't know". So back to work it was driving around the empty streets and cleaning windows of houses with people mainly inside afraid to go out. Whether they were afraid of an alleged virus or not obeying the rules I'm not sure, but it was probably a bit of both. Instead of giving me the money as usual many people just opened the door and left the money on the step afraid I may pass on the invisible enemy coming to get us all. At that time I decided I was going to speak my truth from the start if asked and this lead to me losing a few jobs and some people making comments like I was betraying the country by simply going out to work. I lost a few jobs and annoyed a few people as I refused to be afraid but I had to be true to myself and it also shown me another side to so-called nice people when they feel afraid, not a pretty sight I can tell you.

During the whole lockdown me and my family never wore masks, never socially distanced, went out when we felt like it and even had a few friends round for the usual cup of tea and a chat. Sure many people distanced themselves from us, and in many places we were not welcome, but we found similar people who had the same mind-set and we just went about life as normally as we could. If we had lived back in Peru, or someplace like Australia, then I'm not sure how I would have got on as the people there who would not comply were subjected to brutal force coming from the very people claiming to be concerned for their health. The irony is not lost.

Now the hysteria has passed over and more data has come out I have decided to publish this new and more scientifically complete book. Since the publication of 'Medical Fascism' the preliminary control experiments by Dr Stephan Lanka regarding the nature of viral particles have been done and more data is out regarding the mRNA vaccine. So now I have teamed up again with former Doctor, Patrick Quanten, who will be putting the science into this new book which will explain the agenda and how science is being used against us and how it can be used to free us. I'm sure many of you will understand the need for an updated revision of the original book due to the nature of what I was saying in the first, that basically it was all a psychological operation, and now the data is out we will add more updated science to the original and leave it to be what we believe is the actual objective truth of the last few years and the alleged pandemic.

Rob Ryder August 2023

INITIAL THOUGHTS

"A dangerous virus from, once again, an obscure place, not uncommon on Chinese territory? Here we go again!

Knowing that viruses don't cause diseases, whether they are 'manufactured' or not, I wondered why they needed this 'outbreak'? I realized that it was another scare story, like the one that told us that a few birds had died somewhere in a remote village in China, which 'caused' the bird flu epidemic. I wondered what it was going to be this time.

Right from the beginning I focussed on the story, not on the content of the story. I quickly noticed that the words used in the media to cover this potentially very big danger story were the same across national borders and language barriers. Nowhere could I detect a relevant question. Everything was about building the foundation of the story. I figured out that this was not a local event that was going to be dealt with by various governments in various ways. This was unification.

Indeed, very soon we were no longer allowed to think anything else. We all needed to accept the if's and but's from the story and respond in the only possible appropriate way. Because some of us *believe something might happen* we all need to act 'to protect' them from their perceived danger. In other words, if some of us are convinced that there is going to be an air raid then we all need to live in underground shelters. I wondered how they were going to manage the control over the thoughts and actions of the unified people.

You would expect people 'to wake up' to the truth at some point. Then I discovered the really clever bit, the innovation in the whole scary story routine. They had, right from the beginning (masks are useless - everybody must wear them), ensured that there was plenty of subjects to argue about within the story and the authority's narrative. There was plenty of doubt. It created arguments, splits, anger, and it was all focussed on details that kept people's minds away from the steps the control management would follow. The authority solution to the arguments was to shame anybody who was asking questions and 'brand' them a liar, a denier, a racist, turning it up a notch by linking it to homophobia, terrorism, anti-Semitism, anti-anything, lumping it together as *conspiracy theorists*. How dare you, when we are in the middle of a war, question what our troops are doing and whether or not the war is justified? Traitor! You deserve to be shot!

They got everybody arguing over things they know nothing about, but were very scared of. Some were scared of this, and others more of another aspect of the story, but they were all scared. Scared to die or to kill someone else. Scared to lose their freedom. But who is scared enough of artificial intelligence and data control, scared enough to stop handing his or her information to the authorities? Scared enough of the authority? "But I still need to live!" Indeed, and the control of that life was put into place once they unleashed the story of a viral infection, turning it into a pandemic, onto the willing public.

The madness had taken hold of the population and I realized that almost nobody would be able to wake up from this. People would wake up to a few details but who would be able to see that the entire society structure was the problem, and not the method they were using to unify people into one thought, one feeling, one action. I feared very few people would be in a position, mental and physical, to escape the coup d'état on personal freedom. We have already been captured into a life that we no longer control. This is simply an exercise in making it clear to people that they are but slaves.

Soon I realized it was over. They control it all and they are all moving in one direction. It is slavery or nothing!

If you really want to wake up, you will need to start packing your bag. Travel light because it is a long journey back to sanity and you don't want to be lugging too much from your old life on the road to the new one. It is a journey of leaving what you know behind and embracing what you don't know as a possibility.

Follow the signs 'the natural way'!" - Patrick Quanten MD

HEALTH

What is it to be healthy?

First, we have to understand that we are all individuals. So, for example, a man of 5 feet 8 inches may weigh ten stones and have a different blood pressure and other things to a man of the same height but who weighs 14 stones. Maybe one is a runner, the other a rugby player, both physically fit for their build and lifestyle. So based on somebody's height it would be impossible to tell someone their perfect weight, blood pressure etc., as we are all different. Also, health cannot be defined by lack of symptoms, just as illness cannot be defined by the presence of symptoms. An example could be a fever; the body needs energy and vitality to produce a fever so the presence of a fever to burn up unhealthy tissues could be a sign of good health, healthy maintenance, whereas a person who cannot produce a fever could be loaded up with toxins, lacking energy and struggling to expel them.

There are basic things a human needs to be healthy, which include having the body parts/organs in good working order, clean blood, a clean and healthy environment with sunlight and fresh air, living free from enforced stress, good nutrition, and to be completely aware and in control of who you are, freely expressing yourself. The sign of good health is known as vitality, the vital force that powers our cells. This we take from the energy source that is the sun, breathing clean fresh air and being true to ourselves and expressing our true individualism. Signs of vitality are people who are creative, happy, alert, heal quickly and have a thirst for life. Lack of vitality could include depression, fatigue, low energy, slow healing and no sense of purpose. As science has shown we are all energy at our source; our physical bodies are perfect expressions of our true energetic selves. Think of that when someone asks why they have cancer and the doctor just says, 'Bad luck.'

So, health could be best described as an individual being in balance with themselves and the world they find themself in. They are living a life with purpose, following dreams and embracing the great game of life, and as we are all different – we like different foods, climates, lifestyles and have different personalities – we need to find our own personal balance. So, if health is being in balance, then sickness could be described as being out of balance, or not being or expressing your true self.

We will now delve briefly into some theories of how we go from one state to the other. Please leave any preconceived ideas at one side and start with a blank page, and go with the evidence and what feels right for you. After all, the responsibility for your health is your own. In my opinion the main things needed for health are clean water, sunshine, fresh air, family and friends and a sense of purpose. These are the very things the lockdown has taken away from people in the name of health, not a coincidence in my opinion.

SYMPTOMS OF ILLNESS

Body going wrong – Body doing right?

When we are ill we become aware of this as the body produces symptoms like fever, vomiting and rashes, etc., or just a feeling of being unwell. But what do these symptoms mean? Compare the view of your GP and, say, a homeopath.

GP, Allopathic – Body malfunctions

Trained in allopathic thinking, so symptoms like a fever, rash, headache, and inflammation are seen as the body going wrong. Very little time is spent on asking why this has come about, only that it is a discomfort to you and it needs to be fixed. Therefore, the doctor will look at his list of drugs to find one that will stop or suppress the symptom, as they see the symptom as the problem. So by taking away the discomfort (symptom) the patient feels well and believes all is fine again. Though doctors are aware that fevers are getting rid of cellular waste and toxicity, they still treat this as the problem most of the time, the body going wrong, a malfunction, part of a broken machine not knowing what it is doing. They normally get about ten minutes with patients, only enough time to look at symptoms.

Homeopath, Holistic – Body rebalances

They are trained in seeing the body, when showing symptoms of illness, as the body trying to re-establish health and view symptoms, or patterns of symptoms, as an intelligent reaction by the body to try and bring back balance, basically a clearing-out of bad stuff. Therefore, they prescribe safe remedies that aid the body with whatever symptom is being shown, going with the body, kind of giving the body a helping hand, going with the intelligence of the body and trusting that the body knows what is best. After all, it has had plenty of time to evolve and perfect these responses. They normally give the patient an hour to listen and put together a holistic view of what's going on in that particular life.

As far as comparing going with or going against the body, I will give you a quote from Trevor Gunn in his must-read book, *The Science of Health and Healing,* when talking about possible outcomes of an acute illness.

- *The individual resolves the illness and as a result their health is improved and they are stronger than they were before. They are less susceptible to those problems after the illness and more able to deal with them.*
- *The individual resolves the illness but there has been no learning as such, they are not stronger than they were before, they effectively carry on as they were before the illness, just as susceptible to succumbing to the illness as they were before.*
- *The illness is not resolved and as a result the health of the individual is worse than before and they descend into a lower level of chronic illness, more susceptible than before.*
- *The illness is not resolved and the patient is unable to react sufficiently to overcome the problem and dies."*

Inflammation

Redness – pain – swelling – heat
The first sign of an issue. It would seem that if this is happening in a particular area of the body, then that area has an issue with damaged or diseased tissue that the body is trying to heal by burning up the waste and damaged tissue to be disposed of.

Maybe we should start to see the common cold as the body telling us it's time to rest rather than something to be treated or cured. Maybe the cold is the cure after all, it certainly seems so. After buying Trevor's book over ten years ago I can honestly say the effect the simple knowledge held within the book has had on my health and that of my family is nothing short of astounding. I used to get my regular bad cold every 18 months or so; it would start as a bad cold then turn into 2/3 days in bed. What was happening was I always tried to work through the cold stage by taking suppressive over-the-counter drugs. This would keep me going for a day or two until my body just gave up. Being self-employed, this is something I needed to avoid. In trying to keep working I only made things worse and would end up in bed for a couple of days.

On reading the book it all became clear straight away, my body had reached its limit and waste was building up in my system that was over my healthy balance point. I needed to rest and let the body do its job of cleansing and rebalancing. Instead of taking a day off, not eating and going to bed to rest, I carried on which in the end made me lose three days' work instead of one when finally my body just gave up. Not long after reading the book I got hit by a heavy cold/flu. Determined not to do anything except stick it out, I suffered for three days. About a year later the same happened and I did the same; I think I had hot water with honey and lemon as my only intake for the first day. Since then I have only ever had one heavy cold that I could feel coming on beforehand so I finished work early, went to bed and got up midday the next day raring to go. KNOW THYSELF is the key.

By looking at Trevor's four outcomes on an acute illness it seems to me that acute illness is a natural and almost unavoidable part of life. The decisions we make when an acute illness comes along will decide if we heal/rebalance or go into a more chronic level of illness. Trevor brilliantly charts the direction of disease when it is not dealt with, or suppressed, and goes deeper into the body manifesting as different chronic diseases. As a foundation for understanding the intelligence of a disease process I cannot recommend this book enough. So if acute and chronic illnesses are cleansing processes initiated by the body to clear out a build-up of waste/toxicity above the normal range for the individual then what exactly is deemed *toxic* to us.

"Toxins? Make a distinction. There are things that will kill us all. These things are toxic at a level beyond the capability of the human being. It destroys the human structure at a level we have no or not enough influence on. Based on this knowledge and people's experiences authorities step in to 'protect' their people from poisons. They are instructing people on what is safe and what isn't. By claiming that responsibility they also claim the knowledge and they install fear wherever they need it."

"Every influence is caused by an interaction between the inner world and the outer environment. Some outer conditions are so powerful that our inner world does not have the capacity, the power, to adjust to it and our structure will be destroyed by it. Most outer conditions are not as powerful. On top of that we don't really know what we are capable of until we do it. This means that we should always be aware of the fact that we play a vital role in how we respond. It is this that will determine the outcome of the interaction between our inner world and the outer environment."

"So what is toxic to us? When an individual no longer has the capacity to adjust to the outside stimulus without destroying his/her structure the environment is toxic for that person. How can we adjust? We can either "ignore" the outside environment or if we don't we will have to deal with it. So, either we do not connect to it (fear mongering media news has little direct effect on me if I don't listen to the news) or we "digest" it. By not connecting we withdraw one of the essential ingredients of "the effect", and that is our participation. You can't have an interference if you don't interfere. When we do connect, or when you can't ignore it, you have to "work" with it. You are putting energy into the matter and the end result, the effect, will be determined by the disruptive power of the toxin on the one hand and by the healing power of your inner world on the other".

- Patrick Quanten MD

Now I remain conscious of how I am feeling and when I need to rest. By doing this I can honestly say I don't get ill, I know my limits and have taken total responsibility for my own health. As a family, since reading the book, we have not needed modern medicine for maintaining health or for treating illness. When normal colds and the like come along rest is certainly the cure. Fasting when a fever is present aids in detoxification, and relaxing the mind in the knowledge that the body is just doing a spring clean, all is well and it's just time to rest. There is obviously a lot more to staying in balance but best to look at the most important areas of your life, as they will have the most influence. When you have the major parts of life in balance the smaller things do not tend to affect you much, this is what we call our own life balance.

Some simple health tips are as follows.-

- Drink clean water with life-giving energy in it; we are about 70% water ourselves after all.
- Eat as much local, seasonal, natural food as you can. Food is a connection to the outside world; an exchange of information and communication. If you can't get the best food, don't worry, as Patrick Quanten says, "it's your relationship with the food that is most important." Eat when you are hungry, try not to snack, try not to eat late at night and too early in the morning. Above all, relax and enjoy your meal. The real meaning of blessing a meal is creating that energetic connection. More people now are showing how we can actually change the structure of water with our emotions. We need to literally love our food.
- Get plenty of fresh air and sunshine on your skin and enjoy being in nature; it's where you are from and we need that connection.
- Try to find a purpose or a passion in your life, whether in work or hobbies. Be excited to be alive.
- Reduce emotional stress. Do that by reducing how important a situation is, change its meaning. Change what you can and accept what you can't change.
- Reduction in the importance = reduction in the stress.

- Remember, life is just a game we have been created to play and healthy detachment helps to keep us sane. "It's just a ride"
- Most of all, find happiness in your personal relationships and social life.

Strange that these are the things that were taken away in the name of 'health'. It's almost like there was a deliberate agenda to make people ill. It's like our glorious self-proclaimed leaders did not have our best interests at heart. We as a family did all of the above as we usually do, did not follow any of the governments 'health ' advice and did not get ill once during the biggest plague mankind has ever seen.

Here is Patrick Quanten, from his book with Erik Bualda, 'Why me? Science and spirituality as inevitable bed partners:'

> "What follows is all you ever need to know about the causes of disease."

> - A yin disease is caused by either a larger than normal outer pressure on the individual, or a smaller than normal inner pressure coming from the individual.
> - A yang is caused by either a larger than normal inner pressure coming from the individual, or a smaller than normal outer pressure on the individual. (Normal = the balance point between those two forces during the creation of the individual)

It seems that life, health and disease are not as complicated as we are being led to believe. Nature seems to treat the animal kingdom well; the lion gets hurt in a hunt and goes under a bush to let the body heal, it doesn't eat and barely drinks, the body has the energy to heal and life goes on, or the wound is too severe to cope with and the lion dies. Now it is clear that in accident situations, modern medicine and all that goes with it can saves lives, but as soon as the emergency is over we should put our trust back in that which created us. That is nature and nature is what we are a part of and what we come out of. Nature is what created us, we should learn its laws and follow its guidelines; better to learn from the master itself than the ego-driven rebellious student. Every time I cut my finger I clean it, keep it dry and let air to it and within no time it is healed without leaving a mark. How that happens I don't know and it does not matter. What matters is there is clearly an intelligence within the body, body consciousness, that knows what it is doing and looks after itself whether I am aware of it or not.

The main theme of this book though is not health and life balance but a full analysis of so-called infectious disease and so-called contagious disease causing agents. For this to be done we need real a real scientific analysis to be done.

BIG QUESTIONS NEED SCIENTIFIC ANSWERS

The Germ or The Soil

"The specific disease doctrine is the grand refuge of weak, uncultured, unstable minds, such as now rule in the medical profession. There are no specific diseases; there are specific disease conditions." - Florence Nightingale

My own introduction to illness, via the book '*The Science of Health and Healing*', led to a new understanding of disease which left me wanting to understand life more. For me, as a non-trained and uneducated man, I looked to simple examples to explain this new (at least new to me) scientific idea of disease.

The flaws of germ theory regarding bacteria seemed obvious as I had my own composter in the garden. It was clear to me that the worms and microbes that we can see in the composter when I put organic waste in simply disappeared after a year when all the waste matter had been turned into healthy new soil. Seems like a perfectly good illustration of the job of bacteria.

As for viral particles, it was also clear to me that cellular debris would be a natural part of our inner system. We all know our cells are always dying and reproducing every second of the day in a process called apoptosis. We are told that the cells die and replace themselves to the extent that we have a multitude of bodies during our lifetime. So if cells were dying of natural cell death all the time then this would be cleared out via the cleansing and re-balancing system (better name then the immune system). Then if many cells were starting to die at one time, due to a build-up of toxicity and non-functioning cells dying, - a process called necrosis - then the body would have to work extra hard to clear out that extra waste. This is what we now understand as the reason we get ill, the bodies extra effort to rebalance via producing intelligent cleansing symptoms.

It's all fine me giving you simple logic which is a great way to get people to think and use common sense. What we really need though to put this issue to rest is someone who has been educated, worked and lived in this scientific world that can back up my common sense observations with actual real science. We are told after all by the self-proclaimed leaders that they are following the 'best available science'. So if all this really comes down to good science then let's see what the science really tells us.

"If I could live my life over again, I would devote it to proving that germs seek their natural habitat – diseased tissue – rather than being the cause of dead tissue."

– Dr Rudolf Virchow, the Father of Modern Pathology

A HISTORY LESSON IN GERM THEORY

Patrick Quanten MD

Physicist, Beverly Rubik Ph.D., Director of the Centre for Frontier Sciences at Temple University in Philadelphia wrote:

> Perhaps the greatest obstacle that frontier scientists are unprepared for but inevitably face is political - the tendency for human systems to resist change, to resist the impact of new discoveries, especially those that challenge the status quo of the scientific establishment ...

> 'Science' has become institutionalised and is largely regulated by an establishment community that governs and maintains itself ... In recent times there has been a narrowing of perspectives resulting in a growing dogmatism, a dogmatic scientism. There is arrogance bordering on worship of contemporary scientific concepts and models ... taught in our schools in a deadening way which only serves to perpetrate the dogma ...

> Strangely, the contemporary scientific establishment has taken on the behaviour of one of its early oppressors: the church. Priests in white lab coats work in glass-and-steel cathedral-like laboratories, under the rule of bishops and cardinals who maintain orthodoxy through mainstream 'peer review'.

This unfortunate situation within the scientific establishment, although worsening fast, has always been a feature. New ideas are readily dismissed and ridiculed and their proponents persecuted and prosecuted. Yet, only through the introduction of new discoveries can we evolve and grow with a better understanding of nature and the way it functions, which is the true field of scientific investigation. What is holding us back is a form of 'democracy' whereby the majority decides what is right or wrong, based on what is being promoted. The question that should be asked is: "Who is doing the promoting and why?"

Well, hindsight is a wonderful thing. Very often a little excursion into the past reveals that somebody somewhere has actually proven exactly that which is not being allowed to become general knowledge. To illustrate this, let's take the 'germ'-theory and explore how we got to know what we believe to be the truth.

19th Century

Louis Pasteur became famous for his demonstration that bacteria were the causes of diseases. As these germs were found in diseased tissues and not in healthy tissues, he postulated that the germs invaded the system from the outside to make it ill. The medical establishment accepted this. They were very happy with this statement and they set out to find ways to 'kill' these unseen invaders. To this day they are still pursuing the same goal, mostly unsuccessfully. On his deathbed, Louis Pasteur was reported to have said, with reference to the ideas of an eminent French physiologist, Claude Bernard: "Bernard is right ... the terrain is everything! The microbe is nothing!" Claude Bernard championed the notion the terrain was much more significant than the germs in the onset of the disease. In other words, the state the tissues were in created the disease, not the germs that were occasionally found within the diseased tissue. This notion was based on the work of a contemporary of Pasteur, named Antoine Béchamp.

Béchamp first worked in Strasbourg as a Professor of Physics and Toxicology at the Higher School of Pharmacy, later as Professor of Medical Chemistry at the University of Montpellier and, later still, as Professor of Biochemistry and Dean of the Faculty of Medicine at the University of Lille, all in France.

While labouring on problems of fermentation - the breakdown complex molecules into organic compounds via a 'ferment' -

Béchamp, at his self-made microscope, seemed to be able to visualise a host of tiny bodies in his fermenting solutions. Even before Béchamp's time other researchers had observed, but passed off as unexplainable, what they called 'scintillating corpuscles' or 'molecular granulations'. It was Béchamp who, able to ascribe strong enzymatic reactions to them, was led to coin a new word to describe them: microzymas, or 'tiny ferments'.

Among these ferments' many peculiar characteristics was one showing that microzymas were abundantly present in natural calcium carbonate, commonly known as chalk, whereas they did not exist in chemically pure calcium carbonate made in a laboratory under artificial conditions. This was the reason why chalk could easily invert cane sugar solutions, while pure calcium carbonate could not. In other words, although chemically the artificial 'pure' calcium carbonate is exactly the same as the natural calcium carbonate, only the latter has a life, which allows it to interact with its natural environment. With this knowledge it becomes easy to explain why natural vitamin C has so many health stimulating properties, which the researches have not been able to reproduce in their experiments because they used artificially made vitamin C. Once again a clear indication that the 'impurities' within the live substance are essential to its function in nature.

Béchamp went on to study microzymas located in the bodies of animals and came to the startling conclusion that the tiny forms were more basic to life than cells, long considered to be the building blocks of all living matter. Béchamp thought the microzymas to be fundamental elements responsible for the activity of cells, tissues, organs, indeed entire living organisms, from bacteria to whales, and from larks to human beings. He even found them present in life-engendering eggs, where they were responsible for the further development of the eggs.

Most incredible to Béchamp was the fact that when there occurred an event serious enough to affect the whole of an organism and disturbing its natural balance, the microzymas within the organism would begin working to disintegrate the organism, converting themselves to bacteria and other microbes, while at the same time continuing to survive. As proof of such survival, Béchamp found them in soil, swamps, chimney soot, street dust, even in air and water. These basic, and apparently eternal, elements of which we and all our animal relatives are composed, survive the remnants of living cells in our bodies. So seemingly indestructible were the microzymas that Béchamp could even find them in limestone dating back 60 million years. They are to be considered the seeds of life. Life would originate from them and be altered by them, if and when the living conditions and the balance of life changes.

He demonstrated in his laboratory that by using different solutions as an environment totally different sets of 'germs' would spontaneously arise within the solutions in spite of the fact that all solutions had been kept in the same sterile conditions. The germs, he was convinced, could not have come from an outside source but had to be originating from within each solution itself. The microzymas, which are the same basic structures for all living material, transformed themselves, through the stimulation of the various feeding grounds in which they lived, into different life-forms (in these experiments, germs) corresponding to the content of the solution itself.

He also clearly demonstrated that one sort of bacteria would develop spontaneously into another type given a change in the environmental conditions. So it was seen that the diphtheria bacteria transformed into a coccus bacteria. This is something that in the Pasteur bacteriology is impossible! Pasteur, and with him the medical establishment, promoted the idea of monomorphism, which means that every single type of bacteria stands on its own and cannot change into another type. This means that every single bacteria must be fought separately. The truth, revealed by the scientifically well executed experiments of Professor Béchamps, is called pleomorphism, whereby one form transforms into another when the environmental circumstances change.

The controversy between the two views, one scientifically proven and the other one popular is easily settled when we examine the reports that these two researches submitted to the French Academy of Science. It leads to three undisputable and striking conclusions:

1. Pasteur's reports on experiments and consequent deductions are all preceded by Béchamp's, in some cases by several years. When Pasteur proclaimed to have found the answer to a pressing question, it turns out that Béchamp had already clearly answered that question in front of the Academy. His answer invariably being opposed by Pasteur.

2. The quality control on Pasteur's experiments is very poor and allows for unaccounted interference, which is invariably completely ignored even when pointed out by his peers. In contrast, Béchamp seems to have had a more rigid and structured approach to his experiments, which allowed him to answer his contemporaries more clearly. It has been documented that Pasteur was shunned by the academic circles of his time.

3. The deductions Pasteur made from his experiments were often far beyond the scope of the actual experiment and turned out to be more speculation than science. As a consequence, Pasteur was caught out on several occasions changing his interpretation and statements as it suited his cause. Béchamp was never seen to have made a claim he had not substantiated with sound scientific proof.

The reason why Béchamp was mainly ignored by the outside world and Pasteur elevated to hero status is to be found in the different personalities and the lure of commercial success, as anticipated by investors and the industry. Again that's no different now, as we still continue to ignore the facts and figures and continue our search for the outside invader who can be blamed for an illness. This also is being perpetuated by the medical industry. Not only have we had the opportunity, right at the emergence of this dogma, to refute it once and for all, but ever since, pushed on by commercial and social rewards, we continue to ignore the reality we have discovered and, to this day, we refuse to question in real scientific terms the fundamentals on which our view of infectious diseases is based.

It has been generally accepted, even in Pasteur's time, that for a specific microorganism to be responsible for a specific disease the following conditions have to be fulfilled (Koch postulates):

1 **The said organism has to be found in each in every case of the disease.**

2 **The said organism cannot be found within any other disease or in the absence of any disease.**

3 **The said organism can be isolated from the diseased tissue in a pure culture.**

4 **Injected into a healthy system the said organism, grown in culture, always produces the disease again**.

To this day these conditions have never been met in any known infectious disease! Two hundred years of trying has resulted in not one single microorganism being proven to cause one single infectious disease and yet, we still believe they are the cause of infectious diseases. How far does one go in ignoring science as a decent way of gathering knowledge?

Independently and unaware of work done by fellow researchers other scientists have come to the same conclusion. You can check out the work of people like Claude Bernard (France), Wilhelm Reich (Austria – America), Günther Enderlein (Germany), Wilhelm von Brehmer (Germany), Harper Collins (USA), amongst many others.

And there is more!

The Universal Microscope

In February 1944 the Franklin Institute of Philadelphia (USA) published an article, 'The New Microscopes', in its prestigious journal devoted to applied science. The article included a long dissertation on the 'Universal Microscope', the brainchild of a San Diego autodidact, Royal Raymond Rife. This microscope, developed in the 1920's, overcame the greatest disadvantage of the electron microscope, which had just been put on the market by the Radio Corporation of America. Because in the electron microscope tiny living organisms are put in vacuum and are subjected to protoplasmic changes induced by a virtual hailstorm of electrons, it is unable to reveal specimens in their natural living state.

The Rife microscope has several arresting features, the most important of which are the crystal quartz out of which the entire optical system as well as the illuminating unit is made, and the extraordinary resolution it achieves. The electron microscope, while capable of attaining magnifications surpassing 500,000X at excellent resolution, was incapable of examining living things because its radiation kills them. But Rife's instrument was able to view living matter at unheard of magnifications reaching at least 60,000X also at excellent resolution.

Rife also maintained that he could select a specific frequency, or frequencies, of light which coordinated and resonated with a specimen's own chemical constituents so that a given specimen would emit its own light of a characteristic and unique colour. Specimens could easily be identified this way, by way of the frequency it emits.

With his invention Rife was able to look at living organisms. What he saw convinced him that germs could not be the cause, but are the result of disease. He demonstrated that, depending on its state, the body could convert a harmless bacterium into a lethal pathogen and that some specific bacteria introduced cancerous growths in animals and humans. Such pathogens could be instantly killed, each by a specific frequency of light. Furthermore, he noticed that cells, regarded as the irreducible building blocks of living matter, are actually composed of smaller 'cells', themselves made up of even smaller units, the real building blocks of life. This process is continuing with higher and higher magnification in a sixteen step stage by stage journey into the micro world beyond.

Thousands of still pictures and hundreds of feet of motion pictures were taken to reveal these facts.

Because he had found that microorganisms had the ability to

illuminate when stimulated by given frequencies it occurred to Rife that they might also be devitalised as a result of beaming radiations of specific frequencies upon them. To this end, he had been developing concurrently with his microscopic equipment a special frequency emitter which he continued to improve, up to at least 1953, as steady advances in electronics continued. The killing waves were projected through a tube filled with helium gas and said to be efficient in destroying micro-organisms at a distance of as much as one thousand feet. With this device he noted that when the proper mortal oscillatory rate was reached, many lethal organisms such as those that were present in tuberculosis, typhoid, leprosy, foot-and-mouth disease and others appeared to disintegrate or 'blow up'.

The next obvious step was to determine whether similar radiation would work in the bodies of cancer afflicted animals rather than in cultures. It did. And on human cancers? Indeed it worked. "The first clinical work on cancer was completed under the supervision of Milbank Johnson, M.D., which was set up under a special medical Research Committee of the University of Southern California. Sixteen cases were treated at the clinic, for many types of malignancy. After three months, fourteen of these so-called hopeless cases were signed off as clinically cured by a staff of five medical doctors and Alvin G. Foord, M.D., pathologist of the group. The treatments consisted of three minutes duration using the frequency instrument which was set on the mortal oscillatory rate for the cancer cells, at three-day intervals. It was found that the elapsed time between treatments attains better results than cases treated daily."

Once again, as was the case with Béchamp, the use of better equipment and the acceptance of the observed, in spite of it being contradictory to the established scientific knowledge, led to a significant discovery. Rife not only described what he saw, as opposed to having a guess at what he believed to be the truth, but he documented every step of his discovery with photographs and motion pictures. His contemporaries decided that it was impossible 'to see' these minute, much smaller than the cells themselves, building blocks of life as they did not have the technology themselves and refused to make use of Rife's microscope. Rife organised public shows and had many of his contemporaries witness these unbelievable changes or themselves. It had to stop! The end result is that neither you nor I have ever heard of Rife and his microscope. Furthermore, his microscope together with most of his scientific writings and evidence was thought to have been destroyed. Recently, however, some of it has been recovered in the San Diego home of John Crane, but alas in a very sorry state. To this day, no one has succeeded in rebuilding the Rife microscope to the exact specifications of the original. Many attempts are still being made in a variety of research programmes to good effect, but without reaching the accuracy and effectiveness of what Rife himself demonstrated to the world.

The consequence of Rife's discovery is that cells are not the basic building blocks of life, as believed by the medical profession and that bacteria originate from within the diseased tissue, and not, as the profession believes, invade the system from the outside. Turning our treatment attention to the environment of the bacteria, the condition of the tissue, solves the disease problem miraculously, and Rife showed that this was achieved by changing the frequency of the tissue.

Gaston Naessens

The French born biologist who lived and worked for many years in Quebec (Canada) invented a microscope in the 1950's, unaware of Rife's invention and his work, that was capable of viewing living entities far smaller than can be seen in existing light microscopes.

With his exceptional instrument, Naessens went on to discover in the blood of animals and humans, as well as in the sap of plants, a hitherto unknown, ultra-microscopic, subcellular, living and reproducing microscopic form which he christened a somatid. This particle could be cultured - grown - outside the bodies of its host. And, strangely enough, it was seen to develop in a 'form-changing' sixteen stage cycle. The first three stages - somatid, spore and double spore - are perfectly normal in healthy organisms, in fact crucial to their existence.

Even stranger, over the years the somatids were revealed to be virtually indestructible! They have resisted exposure to temperatures of 200°C and more. They have survived exposures to 50,000 rems of nuclear radiation, far more than is required to kill any living thing. They have been totally unaffected by any acid. Taken from centrifuge residues, they have been found impossible to cut with a diamond knife. The eerie implication is that these minuscule life-forms are imperishable. At the death of their host, such as ourselves, they return to the earth where they live on, maybe forever.

Naessens went on to discover that if, and when, the immune system of an animal, or human being, becomes weakened or destabilised, the normal three stage cycle goes into a thirteen more successive growth stages cycle to make up a total of sixteen separate forms, each evolving from the previous form. All of them have been clearly revealed in detail by motion pictures, and stop-frame still photography. From the double spore stage, mentioned above as the third stage in the normal cycle, it can transform into a bacterial form (4), then a double bacterial form (5), then a rod form (6), a bacterial form with double spores (7), a bacterial form with granular double spores (8), and (9) and (10) being microbial globular forms. At stage (11) this form bursts open and turns into a yeast form (12), then an ascopore form (13), with (14) and (15) being mycelial forms. Within this cycle one finds the basis of all known 'germs', having emerged from a previous less developed stage, given the right environmental conditions. In a rich, clean, environment the 15th form will burst and release somatids into the environment, whilst the outer membranes will remain as a fibrous thallus (scar-tissue). These somatids will resume the normal three-stage cycle. In simple terms, the diseased tissue develops from within itself a microorganism, specific for its environment, that will clear up the unhealthy decayed matter and disappear once this is done, leaving the tissue healthy and clean again, with the same 'life' qualities it had before it became diseased. The tissue becomes diseased from within and the tissue heals from within.

By studying the cycle, as revealed in the blood of human beings suffering from various degenerative diseases such as rheumatoid arthritis, multiple sclerosis, lupus, particularly cancer, and most recently, AIDS, Naessens has been able to associate the development of the forms in the sixteen stage pathological cycle with all of these diseases. More importantly, he has been able to predict the eventual onset of such diseases long before any clinical sign of them have put in an appearance. And most importantly, he has come to demonstrate that such afflictions have a common functional principle, or basis, and must therefore not be considered as separate, unrelated phenomena as they have been for so long in allopathic medical circles.

Having established the cycle in all its fullness, Naessens was able, in a parallel series of brilliant research steps, to develop a treatment for strengthening the immune system, the resistance against diseases. The product he developed is derived from camphor, a natural substance produced by an East Asian tree of the same name. Unlike many medicinals, it is injected into the body, not intra-muscularly or intravenously, but intra-lymphatically – into the lymph system, via a lymph node, or ganglion, in the groin. The medical fraternity holds this to be impossible. Yet the fact remains that such injection is not only possible, but also simple for most people to accomplish, once they are properly instructed how to find the node. While doctors are not taught this technique in medical school, it is so easy that laymen have been taught within a few hours to inject, even to self-inject, the camphor-derived product. The product, named '714-X', when skilfully injected, has in over 75% of cases re-stabilised, strengthened, or otherwise enhanced the powers of the immune system, which results in a natural healing of the diseased tissue.

Naessens concluded that the somatid is no less than what could be termed a concretisation of energy. This particle, which has materialised in the life process, possesses energetic properties transmissible to living organisms, animal or vegetal. Underlying that conclusion is the finding that, in the absence of the normal three-stage cycle, no cellular division can take place. Why can it not? Because it is the normal cycle that produces a special growth hormone that permits such division. The hormone appears to be trephone which was discovered by the French Nobel Laureate, Alexis Carrel. The somatids, the smallest ever found living condensers of energy, are simply precursors of DNA. Now there's a new one!

Precursors of DNA means that somatids somehow are a 'missing link' in our understanding of that remarkable genetic molecule that up to now has been considered as an all but irreducible building block in the life process. If somatids are that missing link between the living and the non-living, what then would be the difference between them and the so-called viruses? We know that to continue its existence the virus needs a supportive environment in a living cellular structure like a single cell from an organism, a one-cell living organism (amoeba, bacteria), or an egg. The somatid on the other hand is able to live autonomously wherever. This difference stems from the fact that a virus is a particle of DNA, a piece of it, and the somatid is a precursor, something that leads to the creation of that DNA.

Naessens' experiments showed that, as a group, the somatids contain the hereditary characteristics of each and every individual being. Somatids, extracted from the blood of a rabbit with white fur, are then injected at a dose of one cubic centimetre per day, into the bloodstream of a rabbit with black fur, for a period of two weeks running. Within approximately one month, the fur of the black rabbit begins to turn greyish, half of the hairs of the black rabbit having turned white. This 'genetic engineering' via the transfer of somatids also now allows for skin transplants from the white rabbit to the black one without any sign of immune rejection.

Not only has Naessens proved the dictum that 'germs are a result, not the cause of the disease', but he had also shown that DNA is not the 'independent' ruler of life as it has been portrayed by the medical authorities. DNA is built from bits that come before it, and specifically those bits correspond directly to the environmental vibrational energetic state in the way they will develop living forms.

Hippocrates, and well before his time, the Hebrews and the Egyptians, already attributed the major part of morbid incidents to troubled humours. By 'humour' we mean the extra-cellular liquids of the organism. In modern science we can now demonstrate the existence of inhibitors in the cell surroundings which keep the powerful special growth hormone under control, and stops the somatid cycle at stage three (normal). The first stage of an impending illness shows itself as a diminished level of inhibitors which allows the natural evolution to move on to the appearance of diverse forms of germs grown out of the environment itself. This lack of inhibition occurs when any kind of stress is put upon the system; the more prolonged, the greater and longer lasting the effect. Illness now prevails.

Now then! Who needs more proof?

The Test of Time

Pasteur himself, hailed to be the father of the 'germ-theory', proclaimed, "the only sovereign judge must be history!" And who could argue with that? So let's see what time can teach us.

We already know the ocean of difference that separated Pasteur from Béchamp. And we read in the Memoirs of the Academy of Science how different their experimental work was, both in timing and execution. Let's remind ourselves of the principles on which the germ-theory is based and its implications for the treatment of diseases following infestation.

Each bacterial species is rigidly fixed and invariable. It exists as a stable organism and there is no likelihood of the transformation of the typhoid bacillus into the cholera vibrio. Time has already proven this to be false.

Each specific illness is caused by an invasion of a specific aerobic bacterium into the body of the animal or human. The infection occurs when the bacterium is passed from one diseased body to another body via the air, via water or via direct contact. The theory was based on the experimental proof that air, water and other materials contained 'germs'; and on the fact that the anthrax bacillus had been cultivated from the blood of infected cattle and had reproduced the disease when other animals had been injected with the cultivated anthrax bacillus. (April 30th 1878)

Dr Robert Koch, discoverer of the tuberculin bacillus, formulated a set of rules for the recognition of supposed disease-germs. These must be:

1. **Found in every case of the disease.**
2. **Never found in another disease or without the disease.**
3. **Capable of being cultured outside the body.**
4. **Capable of producing, by injection, the same disease as that undergone by the body from which they were taken.**

Here we see the basic theory of the air-borne disease-germ doctrine contradicted by the last postulate. To invoke disease, organisms are required to be taken from bodies, either directly or else intermediately through cultures, and need to be injected into healthy organisms, what evidence is to be deducted with regards to the responsibility of invaders from the atmosphere? It is noteworthy that neither Pasteur nor any of his successors have ever induced a disease by the inoculation of air-carried bacteria, but only by injection from bodily sources, heavily contaminated with rotting material. Furthermore, the verdict of time is coming down extremely hard upon the microbe rules of engagement, and even medical authorities have reluctantly acknowledged that 'Koch postulates are rarely, if ever, complied with'. Truth is that, to this day, not one single example of a properly executed scientific study has proven these postulates to actually occur in nature. No single experiment has succeeded in creating a specific disease in healthy individuals by exposing them to air-born germs or germs carried by water droplets.

Experts have been educated from the start to consider micro-organic life from the Pasteurian standpoint and to accept these theories as though they were axioms. Thus it is perhaps understandable why it is only from an unbiased vantage point that the contradictions of the germ-theory of disease are seen to make Pasteur's theory ridiculous. Its rules, the postulates of Dr Robert Koch, state, inter alia, that a causative disease-germ should be present in every case of a disease and never found apart from it. What are the facts? One of the original props of Pasteurian orthodoxy, the Klebs Loefler bacillus, arraigned as the agent of diphtheria, was, by Loefler himself, found wanting in twenty-five percent of all cases, while on the other hand, it is constantly revealed in the throats of healthy subjects.

The followers of Pasteur, however, have their method of overcoming the theoretical difficulty, namely, the carrier-theory, by which healthy people are accused of propagating certain 'germs', certain so called pathogens, which they are supposed to disseminate. This accusation has been brought against those who have never in their whole life suffered from the specific disease complaints that they are accused of distributing. This carrier-theory is also constantly invoked in connection with diphtheria. At Alperton in Middlesex 200 children were, after examination, accused of being diphtheria carriers and were put in isolation. One outstanding weakness of the theory is that we never seem to hear of the isolation of prominent bacteriologists, who obviously should set the example in undergoing microscopic and chemical tests and the subsequent quarantine. So far, apparently, this is only advocated for other people! In the same way that obstetricians are not vaccinated against rubella, but are surely a major possible source of contact infection for any pregnant woman.

Pasteur then proceeded to announce that he had found a real preventative, a vaccine, all the while dodging questions and remarks regarding the unsound testing procedure that was used to prove the validity of the vaccine-approach. At the Academy of Medicine voices were raised against the germ-theory of disease, and in particular M. Peter ridiculed the all-conquering microbe. It was easy for him to do this as in March 1882 the boasted success of the vaccine for anthrax had met with a disastrous downfall. In Italy a Commission composed of Members of the University of Turin thought it worthwhile to perform experiments such as Pasteur had described and thus test the prophylactic value of the vaccine. As a result, all the vaccinated sheep had succumbed to the inoculation. In spite of demonstrating the ineffectiveness of vaccination programmes, bacteriological institutes for experimentation upon living animals and for the production and sale of vaccines and sera came into being all over the world, modelled upon the one opened in 1888 in Paris.

Every vaccination programme that any government has rolled out over the last century and a half has been riddled with problems. So much so that many have been abandoned by national governments because it became impossible to maintain the story of 'safe and effective' to a population that visibly experienced the opposite. The questions about the safety and efficacy of vaccines do not need to be answered. Vaccines are hailed to be the way to prevent infectious diseases because it helps your immune system to fight off the pathogenic intruders. As infectious diseases are not caused by the invasion of any germ at all there simply is no need for 'protection' against such an attack. Hence, there is no need for any vaccine at all. This is scientifically definitely not the correct way 'to prevent' an infectious disease.

Quantum Physics

Quantum physics is a well-established scientific theory about the way life is structured. About one hundred years ago, scientist had to formulate a completely different theory about the structure and the function of the universe and life within it. They had to move away from the idea that life basically was a mechanical machine that operates through the physical interactions of atoms. This idea simply does not explain what scientists have been observing. Now it was time to make a big change in how we viewed the world and the way nature functions.

One of the major changes involves the way information is getting from one place to another. It is no longer acceptable to view this as a displacement of atoms or molecules. Information 'travels' by way of energy waves. For living organisms that means that their connection and interaction with their environment happens at the level of energy exchanges, of vibrational influences. It turns out that matter is nothing more than a condensation of energy and that it still is that energy that gives the matter its form and allows its function. Living organisms are condensed energy and changes that occur within any matter are an expression of changes that are happening within the energy field that has created that matter. So everything we observe within the material world is an expression of an energy field, and every change to what we observe is the result of changes that are happening within that field.

This is established non-questionable science. And yet, our education system ignores that and continues to teach material physics. Authorities are very reluctant to introduce people to this new understanding of reality and when it is done, the science behind it remains hidden and obscured. Authorities apply the science but don't share the knowledge behind the applications. Understanding that it isn't matter that directly influences other matter turns many structures and beliefs of our society upside down, including our approach to health.

If the observed changes within matter are not caused by the interference of other matter then an outside germ can never be held responsible for a disease occurring within a living organism. Surely, the cause of the malfunctioning must be looked for within the organism itself, and more specifically within the energy field that creates the organism. Then the explanation for an infectious disease would sound a bit like this. A change has occurred within the energy balance of the field of that organism, which results in a change in the way the matter of that energy expression looks and functions. Cellular changes will become clear and, at times, even different cells, such as bacteria and other 'germs', may appear out of nowhere, created as a result of the changed energy balance within the field. This means that the real disease is the imbalance within the energies of the organism and the way the matter presents itself is an expression of that imbalance, of that disease. The natural system of the organism will try and pull the energy disturbance back into its previous balance and restore its equilibrium and with that also the 'normal' state of the tissues.

The medical profession is making us believe that they totally ignore this scientific understanding of life. Everything they portray as their 'scientific' research is still focussed on molecules, proteins, hormones, electrical impulses and how these material things influence your health. They still treat the body as a mechanical machine and they still look for 'causes' of diseases in the physical world, even if they have to invent invisible and undetectable elements, from bacteria to viruses, to keep the illusion alive. No wonder we all believe that our health depends on physical factors such as food, exercises, pollution, electromagnetic fields, viruses and so on. The reality of the medical research shows a totally different picture.

As far back as the 1960's, documents were leaked from the big pharmaceutical company Merck Sharpe & Dohme, revealing that they had all the products and molecules they were working on listed by their specific frequencies. The research is not focussing on the physical characteristics of molecules and atomic structures but on the frequencies they emit. The messages that a physical structure, such as the human body, receives are influences it responds to through changes in frequencies. By changing the energetic qualities of a field one changes the function of the physical matter within that field. As an example, in order to alter the way your brain functions one simply has to send it different energetic messages, one has to put that brain in a different 'energetic environment'. Hence, the medical research is focussed on how they can alter your physical function, be it brain or reproduction or anything else, by means of unnoticed energetic influences, using the understanding and the possibilities science has discovered. But just as they have done since the introduction of allopathic medicine, using natural substances to make unnatural equivalents and convincing people that the natural substances are bad for you while the artificial ones are good, they are now using the knowledge about energies, vibrations and frequencies as if they own it and have the explicit right to use it.

Energies are everywhere and energies are being influenced by other energies. We are energy. We can influence other energy fields. This means that we do not need 'experts' to influence the way we function in life. We can do this ourselves. However, in order to do this efficiently and specifically as an individual you need to be aware of these energies and of the way nature functions. It is with that awareness that you can alter the function of your brain or of your reproductive system or of anything else about your physical life. But if you can do it yourself, you do not need a medical industry to guide you. So from the industry point of view it is best to keep quiet about this, which is not difficult if you already control the entire information distribution around the world. They didn't want people to help themselves with herbs and all kinds of healing methods. They confiscated 'healing' and they got handed exclusive ownership of anything to do with health and illness. Now they have confiscated the human energy field and make you believe it is all to do with genes. Once again, as they did with viruses, they talk about matters of life in terms and concepts that nobody understands and therefore nobody can question. The truth of life is that all physical expressions are a manifestation of energy, and that includes your genetic makeup. To the outside world it looks as if they are desperately trying to hold on to the myth of life that it is a mechanical machine, whilst hurriedly looking for a way to switch their total control over the population from a physical control to a mind control, an energetic control and influence system. Such a system is made more secure – ensuring a more reliable and direct control – by the introduction of 'message receivers' within the physical structure of the human body. That way the 'local' mast sends out the required messages from within, which is much more difficult for the cells of your body to ignore. The receivers will then be tuned to a control centre where various signals will be sent into the human energetic field, which is part of the earth's energetic field, picked up by the specific antennae they have introduced into the bodies of their subjects...

Allopathic medicine is not shifting towards genetic and epigenetic medicine. Underneath that cover it is shifting towards energy control. Remember that in order to heal, you do not need an expert to tell you how to do it. You simply need to be aware of your own energetic balance and then you can adjust it yourself by changing your attitude, your beliefs, your habits. So allopathic medicine is not about the health of the population, it is about the control of the population. The emergence of allopathic medicine and their coup d'état on the health of the population clearly demonstrates that it never has been about the health of the population.

And Then There is the Small Matter of a Conclusion

All the scientific research, and with it the people whose names are attached to it, have been brushed of the table by our establishment, by the powers that be. The information you can find about the work and the findings of these scientists is labelled 'erroneous'. These people simply had it wrong. Luckily, we have Pasteur and Koch. No scientific discussion is allowed on this subject matter. Simply trust us. We have 'examined' it for you and it is quite clear that their theories about the importance of the environment and the energy basis of life are wrong. Here is what you should believe to be right: germs cause diseases. And this is 'proven' by mountains of evidence, all of which is being produced and gathered by allopathic laboratories, setting out 'to prove' what they must maintain to be right. They are even willing to completely ignore the fact that such a work method is totally unscientific to begin with.

The world still flounders in the confusion created by Pasteur, champion go-getter of the nineteenth century. When we shall have finally uprooted the dogmas with which he enchained us, and acquired a broad, well-integrated, philosophic view of the entire matter, then we may look for progress. In the meantime, we draw some simple conclusions from the evidence before us.

Germs emerge from within diseased tissue. First the tissue becomes diseased, as a result of an energetic imbalance within the field of the individual, and then the spontaneous healing reaction of the system may involve the creation of germs. Germs are made by your body in an effort to clear up a messy environment. Once this has been achieved they will automatically disappear again. Proven several times in the last 150 years alone, and still not accepted in our world, because the experts of allopathic medicine say that it is wrong.

Don't be cynical: it has nothing whatsoever to do with vaccines and germ killing substances, and the financial lucrative businesses of making and selling them; not to mention the high regard in which all these clever brains are held and the value of the jobs they are holding onto. They are all part of a mass control structure, which was first set up as a control over the health of the individual by means of controlling natural healing substances. In our current time the focus of the control issue has shifted towards influencing the energetic field of the individual, which will give the authority control over the minds of people.

In the space of a two hundred year period allopathic medicine is showing its true face. From insisting that diseases are caused by an outside - and most importantly to the individual, invisible - enemy, which gives the authority control over how 'to combat' this enemy, we have moved through stages of chemical and mechanical interventions, of chemical and disease provoking prevention measures and of chemical genetic manipulation to arrive at an invisible controlling people method, using scientific knowledge that is kept as far away as possible from all individuals.

This is made possible by the control the profession has over the public information distribution. We are constantly told it is science and therefore too complicated for us to understand. We are too dumb, and we must be grateful that they are keeping an eye on this and telling us what is the best for us. And in order that you can understand this complicated matter, we are letting you know that we fact checked it for you. The result is presented to you in an easy to understand colour coded scheme: red means 'no go', orange means 'be careful' and green is 'safe and correct'.

The Green Agenda concerns itself, so they have us believe, with the protection of the environment. The environment of the cells of our body is the energetic field they belong to. Allowing nature to be natural would mean that we do not knowingly disturb or imbalance this field. Just as not killing all insects is allowing nature to move forward in balance, so is not killing the germs that nature has created allowing healing to take place. Making nature our enemy should never be regarded as a smart move.

THE STORY OF INFECTIOUS DISEASE

Patrick Quanten MD

To understand something we need to look at its history. Knowing where and how it started as well as seeing how it has grown over time gives us a better picture of what it truly is today. It is no different with understanding the story of how viruses have become the killing machines in today's society. This story too has a beginning, a growth phase, and no doubt it will end somewhere too.

The story of viral infections tells us how something that exists in our environment enters our bodies, disturbs its function, thereby making us ill, possibly leading to our death. This kind of story wasn't invented for viruses, it was copied. In the nineteenth century the story already existed. It started its life in the medical profession.

It became apparent that tissues could start to rot with the cellular structure disintegrating, people becoming ill, sometimes very ill, in danger of losing their life. This process was observed in wounds on the outside of the body as well as in organs and internal tissues. It was proposed that a living organism, invisible to the naked eye, was responsible for this. It was said to penetrate the outline of the body and interfere with the normal function of the cells, making them diseased with possible cell death as a result. If enough cells died then the life of the person became endangered too. In the case of infections, as this situation became known, in existing wounds it was obvious that the outer lining of the body had already been broken and it should be easy for such an invisibly small creature to settle in the debris caused by the trauma. However, this idea was extended to other parts of the body, still intact in structure, being penetrated by this organism. This unknown organism was given special powers to get passed the normal bodily defences, enter the inner world, travel to specific sites and begin the destruction of the tissues. Medical researchers called these organisms bacteria.

The medical profession decided that infectious diseases were caused by the infiltration of a foreign living organism into the human body. This was a scientific theory.

The main argument for this was the fact that bacteria could be seen underneath a microscope. Not only did these 'invisible' creatures existed but on top of that they were found in abundance within diseased tissue. Their presence in those circumstances led to the claim that they must be responsible for the ravage as they were either not found or only in very small numbers in healthy tissue. The sheer fact of their presence made them look like culprits.

Here, two important statements become fixed within the minds of the medical profession.

1. Bacteria cause infections
2. Bacteria attack the body from the outside

In the first half of the nineteenth century two very important developments took place that shaped the medical profession right up to this day.

First of all, there were the scientific experiments that dismissed the theory that the bacteria that were seen within the diseased tissues were coming from the outside. Several experiments, repeated multiple times in a number of university laboratories, proved that the occurrence of the bacteria within diseased tissue was a natural phenomenon of the disease itself. It was shown that these bacteria arose from within the diseased tissue and as a direct result of that disease and that it was not an invasion of any kind. In other words, the bacteria were present but were not the cause of the disease. The disease already existed, and in some cases gave rise to bacteria originating from within the debris caused by the disease.

Secondly, trying to establish a causal link between a possible disease factor and the disease itself the medical profession worked on finding a protocol that would determine cause and effect. Professor Koch wrote down four postulates, accepted by the scientific world, that would establish a causal link between the presence of a living organism and a specific disease. Although the postulates still stand today and are scientifically sound, even Professor Koch himself deviated from them and began minimalizing their importance as he failed to find a single causal connection. Very quickly the Koch's postulates became a footnote in the medical history books as nobody, right up to today, has ever established a causal link between any bacteria said to cause any specific disease. When you have found a solid method that separates guilt from innocence and it turns out you are unable to get even one guilty verdict you can make it a lot easier on yourself by ignoring that method and simply carrying on convicting.

Scientific evidence did not support the theory that bacteria caused an infection.

Scientific evidence showed that bacteria occurred as a result of the disease and were not responsible for causing the disease.

The scientific theory about bacteria causing infections has been exposed as being false.

At that time investors chose to ignore the scientific community and to stick with the invasion story of ill-making organisms infiltrating and destroying human tissue. They supported the theory championed by people like Louis Pasteur that in order to protect ourselves from getting ill we would need to fight these organisms in our environment. Killing them in large numbers seemed like a very good idea as well as finding a way to make a human being 'immune' against such invasions. An immunisation programme was thought off and the development of suitable vaccines against one and all known disease causing bacteria became the main quest of the medical industry. It is from this point onwards in history that the term medical science is used, a clear distinction from science, suggesting that there is another type of science that will take care of your health, one outside of science itself.

The definition of science is "the intellectual and practical activity encompassing the systematic study of the structure and behaviour of the physical and natural world through observation and experiment". There is no room for a health science separate from science. Life is part of the natural world. However, the medical world has claimed, successfully, to practise science in a different way, set out and controlled by their own authority, undeterred by what theories and truth science is living by. Medicine is the science that concerns itself with diseases and cannot be judged by science, the medical authority claims.

So they start looking for their own answers and they provide their own explanations, disconnected from science. They set out their own theories and they introduce their own methods of investigation and their own ways of 'proving' the theories, using their own standards, not related to scientific methods or codes of conduct.

One of the early problems they struggle with is the fact that in many infectious diseases they fail to demonstrate even the presence of any micro-organism to blame the observed situation on. Given the basic premise that all infections must be caused by an invading micro-organism their explanation for the fact they couldn't find it was simply that it is too small to see. It was postulated that 'a virus' was responsible for those kind of infections and that one day they would find it.

Based on a theory, already proven to be inaccurate by science, the medical authorities decided to continue the invasion story by inventing a new 'invisible' infectious agent, a virus.

And they did find it. Lots of medical research was spent on finding the elusive disease causing microbe. Lots of theories were floating about with regards to the whereabouts, the working methods and the morphology of viruses, the new predicted invisible infectious agents. It was with the coming of the electron microscope in the early thirty's that they finally 'saw'

49

the culprit. Or at least they saw some tiny blobs in and around cells, which they quickly named as the virus because it just had to be what they had been looking for for so long.

The sequence of events is that they first linked specific attributes to their elusive microbe. They then decided when and where this microbe should be present and when they saw something at the site of the delictum they were quick to name it the virus they had been looking for. Got you! Ah, that is what you look like!

Because they had long abandoned the idea of proving a causal link between a named disease agent and the disease itself nobody within the medical profession thought it odd that there was no attempt made to link the image to the observed physiology of the disease.

First the culprit was named and anything that showed up in that area under those circumstances had to be 'it'. The medical profession does not prove that what they have found is actually in line with the characteristics of what they were looking for. They used a much simpler method to establish the truth: we found something, so that must be it!

The medical profession now decides to separate the study of these extremely tiny entities from the clinical information. A specialism 'virology' is being created which doesn't concern itself with patients but with viruses that exist inside a cell and that can be found in all kinds of cellular debris. The 'specialist' is locked away from any clinical setting in a laboratory in order to immerse himself in the virtual world of the unseen.

While science, observing the natural world, is proving that the bacteria that are supposed to cause infectious diseases are almost always discovered to live inside our bodies without causing any illnesses and while science is proving that bacteria are absolutely necessary for any organism to be able to live, medical science, on the contrary, is solving this problem by proposing the theory that these bacteria under certain circumstances (which ones remain a mystery!!) turn into ruthless killing machines. It is a theory that they do not prove and they invite anybody to disprove the possibility. Because science knows that, in principle, one has to consider the possibility that anything is possible, nobody can disprove any statement that includes a 'possibility'. If you were to say that under certain circumstances it might be possible for water to run uphill, science will tell you that you might be right but that currently they are unable to prove that, which doesn't, however, exclude 'the possibility'. It then becomes a rhetorical question whether or not you would consider the possibility.

Another problem the medical profession has got is about the transmission of an infection. According to them there needs to be some sort of physical contact between an infected area, where the said infective agent is present, and the person who becomes ill afterwards. Medical science cannot always detect the source of an infection. They solve the problem by assuming that one may have 'picked up' the infective agent a long time ago and that this agent has somehow survived inside the body of the infected person without causing any problems. At a given time (circumstances and triggers are unknown!!) it comes alive and the infection manifests. They now have invented the mysterious healthy carrier. Can't prove it, but more importantly, can't disprove it!

Furthermore, they put forward the suggestion that these infective agents can be 'carried' which means that you no longer need to have direct contact. You may have picked it up through the medium of air, water or a solid surface, which could be soil or any other surface that covers your requirements. And because bacteria exist everywhere you can actually show their presence wherever you require them to be. The suggestion of transference is once again impossible to disprove as science has established that all of life on earth depends upon the existence of invisible living organisms such as bacteria, fungi and parasites. This means that, indeed, you can demonstrate their presence within the vicinity of people who are falling ill. And if you simply assume, as the medical authority does, that being present equals being guilty then you have found a solution to the question "whodunit?", a solution nobody can disprove. And since they have been ignoring the need to establish a causal link right from the beginning of them coming into power and since they have been cutting themselves loose from accepted scientific practices none of their trainees, doctors and other medical personnel can identify the mistakes made. They are unable to recognise the lack of an essential requirement when, in their experience, it was never a requirement. They are unable to recognise the conflict in the infectious agent attacking from the outside and at the same time being an essential part of the structure of all life when, in their training, they have been told that those two things are not the same, that "something has changed!".

Scientific observation and experimentation does not provide evidence for these theories but that doesn't stop the medical authorities from strictly adhering to them.

Initial information about the characteristics of viruses included that these entities are not alive.

- The structure of the virus is of such simplicity that no internal organelles are present which means that the virus has no metabolism, is incapable of doing anything. **This confirms that a virus is not a living organism.**

- The virus is only 'active' inside a living cell, has an activity inside a living cell, can only 'survive' inside a living cell. **How can a not-alive thing have an activity? How does a not-alive entity survive at all?**

- The single strand, very short, genetic code inside the virus is said to infiltrate the DNA from the cell and 'forces' the cell to produce copies of the virus. **No mention *how* it would be capable of achieving this, just that it does!**

The story goes that an infected cell is forced to produce viruses until it is completely filled with viruses (copies of the original), bursts open and spills its content in its environment where it infects the neighbouring cells, causing diseases.

As viruses are impossible to demonstrate in a clinical setting there has been no scientific evidence at all about the actual activities of a virus inside a cell, nor has there been any scientific evidence about the behaviour of a virus outside a cell. To fill these gaps the medical authorities simply borrowed the bacterial infection story they created themselves without any evidence but strengthened by the fact that people have, by now, accepted the argument that it must be true because it can't be disproven.

This attitude makes almost every conspiracy theory acceptable.

So

- if the presence of infectious agents, even invisible ones, means they are responsible for an infectious disease,

- if the infectious agents can mutate from nice and helpful ones into nasty and destructive ones,

-
  if the infectious agents can be transferred via air, water and surfaces (soil),

- if the infectious agents can be present in a dormant state within a healthy individual, who then becomes an unwitting spreader of disease,

then you have constructed the grounds on which you can manoeuver in all directions in order to 'explain' without having to prove anything at all. You stick to the theory. You expand on an unproven theory. You add exception to the expansion of the unproven theory. And you dismiss any remarks and questions with the rhetorical question. Don't you think there is a possibility that ...?

Now that they have freed themselves of the burden of having to prove the theory and that they have put the onus on the opposition to disprove the theory they feel confident enough to declare all their theories as truths until they are disproven by their own methods. They can now use any of their theories to attach further assumption to, believing the theory forms a truthful basis to work with.

Early on in the story, the medical science proposed an incubation period for every infection. This may vary from 5 days to a fortnight. It is the time period between a person 'picking up' the infection, in other words when the outside attacker infiltrates the body, and the time the destruction of the cells takes place. During this time, the attacker finds a suitable place, multiplies and uses the cell's resources to feed itself, and its comrades. This leads to cell death and the physical manifestation of this has been called 'the infection'.

Early in the story, it was said that it takes an infection to become manifest in order for it to become a new source of infection itself. In other words, you can't spread the invading force around unless your own tissues have broken down as a result of the infection. It was said that in order for another person to become infected that person needed to have had direct contact with infected material originating from another person with the infection. Simply being in their presence wasn't enough to cause you becoming infected with their disease.

Observation of sources of infection and their contacts showed very quickly that new infections could not be linked to direct contact with infected material.

Observation of possible causes of infection showed that there was no link between the presence of the infective agent and the possible disease.

Observation of the speed with which an infection spread amongst the population showed clearly that, although the idea of an incubation period is a very logic one in this story, the incubation period was not being respected by nature.

The logical, scientific, approach to the story, to the theory, would have been to conclude that there is no supporting evidence for the theory.

Instead the medical authorities decided that the infected agent 'obviously' was carried around in the air, on the floor, in water droplets and so on, by which means it was spread over larger distances, away from the source of infection. They did not have to prove this, and they never did. They left it up to others to disprove it. And luckily for them nobody bothered. By this time, science had already drawn its conclusions about the validity of the infective theory with an outside source. It was null and void and deserved no further attention as everything else based on those assumptions are, per definition, scientific nonsense.

So, they no longer have to find the source of infection, which, in any case, is impossible if you don't have an accessible way of identifying the virus, they can simply name a source and challenge others to prove they are wrong. After all, it is possible, isn't it!

So, when they keep finding deviations from their description of either the morphological features of the virus or its behaviour they claim it is such a clever creature it mutates constantly in order to avoid being detected, even though in their story it never seems to be picked up by any of the body defences anyway. Millions of viruses - everyday someone in some laboratory 'discovers' a new one! - and they are all different and we need to protect ourselves against all of them. The invisible world is said to be even violent and life threatening than the physical world we live in.

So, when you widen the infectious story you are adhering to, the one you have been actively promoting by educating your personnel into wholeheartedly believing it, you can easily sell the exact same story in relation to viruses to the world you rule.

- They attack from the environment – even though you said they can only 'survive' inside a living cell.

- They invade the body and cause diseases – even though you said they have no activity except inside their host cell.

- They are carried in air, water and on surfaces – even though you said they can only 'survive' inside a living cell.

- They can be hidden inside a healthy individual for many years – even though you know that all cells of the body have a short lifespan and will die much sooner. How does the virus survive when the host cell dies, bearing in mind it isn't producing any symptoms at all during the entire time?

- They can be spread around by people without any disease

symptoms – even though there is no way out the cell unless the cell breaks open in disease or death.

- They can cause instant symptoms – even though the incubation period may be said to be seven or even fourteen days.

- They can, for no apparent reason, change from an innocent virus to a deadly one – even though they have no activity themselves.

What is the scientific problem with adopting the original infection story to viruses?

When we talk about living creatures such as bacteria, fungi or parasites, we can demonstrate their presence by visualising the organism. We can see them in motion under a microscope and we can add a sample of the disease debris to a feeding soil and see them multiply. We can then take a sample from this culture and identify the organism that grows on the nurturing soil in plain daylight by way of its morphology. In other words, we can see the creature.

Viruses can never be identified in motion. The electron microscope is a blind snap shot of some cells. The still picture shows, sometimes, configurations that have been named viruses and certain characteristics have been given to those configurations, even behavioural characteristics although nobody has ever seen the construction called a virus do anything. So there is never a certain way to identify the virus in a certain place concerning itself with a certain activity, as you can with bacteria. The medical authorities have switched their attention to a different way of 'identifying' a virus.

They have detected DNA sequences within the blobs they have named viruses. Even though they have not identified the source of those DNA sequences they have told their personnel that when such a sequence is present it 'proves' the virus is present. So identifying a very small bit of DNA (sometimes it is only a simple protein structure instead of genetic material), which every living cell – a virus is **not a living cell** – has an enormous amount of, equals identification of the virus.

Presuming a bacterial infection must be proven by true identification of the said bacteria within the diseased tissue, a viral infection must then be confirmed by showing its presence within the diseased tissue too. The presence of some chemical structures that can relate to any possible cell cannot be accepted as proof of the presence of an infectious agent. Simply calling it a viral infection is no scientific proof.

Doctors may suspect a bacterial urinary infection and they will send a sample to the laboratory where they set out a bit of the sample on a feeding soil. If a culture grows on it, they will then under a microscope be able to identify which bacteria is present, and alive, in the sample sent to the laboratory. In contrast, when you have symptoms of a bowel infection the doctor will tell you it is viral enteritis and send you home with medication. There is no need for sample taking and testing as the virus, which he holds responsible for your symptoms, can indeed not be identified by a laboratory. You do have a viral infection because your doctor says so.

What medical science has accepted as common practice for the identification of the presence of a virus is:

1. Identification of a small DNA/RNA sequence without knowing where that small bit originates from. These bits are being replicated in a laboratory so they can be found in large quantities within the cellular debris, a mixture of leftovers from disintegrating cells. – **No quantifiable amount of the same DNA sequence can be linked to any invader, nor can it be linked to any specific activity such as, for example, causing a disease. DNA/RNA sequences are not specific to any virus. Viruses are named after specific DNA sequences!**

2. Measuring a high level of antibodies in the blood as 'proof' of an immune response from the body, which, it is assumed, must be against an unidentified invader, which

must be the virus they said is causing the specific disease. – **No scientific connection has been demonstrated between any specific antibody known and any specific 'invader' of any kind. No antibody is specific to any particular disease or to any particular infectious agent.**

3.   Measuring a high level of specific cells in the blood as 'proof' of an immune response from the body which, it is assumed, must be against an unidentified invader, which must be the virus they said is causing the specific disease. – **No specific connection has been demonstrated between the type of blood cells and the level of those blood cells on the one hand and any specific 'invader' of any kind on the other. No white blood cell level is specific to any particular disease or to any particular infectious agent.**

To the medical profession, any one of these will do as 'proof', not only for the identification and confirmation of the disease you are suffering from, but also as 'proof' for the disease causing agent! To them, it works in every direction: the virus, and only the virus, provides a positive test result and a positive test result tells you specifically which virus.

May we ask the question as to how far medical science has removed itself from science?

In the first half of the twentieth century science took a giant leap forward once it was understood that all matter is formed out of energy by compression and cooling. It means that every change one observes in the structure or the function of any material has been caused by a change within the energetic field that creates that matter. Hence, when a body begins to function differently or is struggling to function normally it means we need to look for the answer to the question why within the energetic field of that body, not within the body itself. Medical science has simply rejected this new insight of science completely and has ensured that their personnel was safely trained in looking for explanations about health and disease within the material part of life, the body and the physical environment itself.

Science says that a change in energy of the person may lead to a malfunctioning of the body, to an inflammation within the tissues or an infection. There is no infective agent being transferred from one organism to another!

Medical science is looking in a pitch black cellar for a black cat, that they know isn't there. I guess they must have a reason to keep on doing this!

It must be clear by now that what they like to refer to as 'medical science' was set aside from science about two hundred years ago when some business investors choose to go allopathic, focussing on fighting the symptoms without concerning themselves with real causes and without adhering to well established scientific practices. Since that time they have removed themselves step by step further and further away from science and they have been successful at that because they have, at the same time, managed to influence the entire world to become industrial, starting in what is referred to as the Western World. They manoeuvred themselves into the most powerful position inside governments, pushing economy as the new god. They set out governmental policies and were able to declare their newly invented medicine as 'the one and only' true medicine, turning millennia of knowledge and skills into illegal practices.

Controlling governments, media and finances has allowed medical authorities to dream about taking over the world, about putting an end to science, about ending free thinking and about determining and controlling the truth. This is their last stand. They are reaching their final station, the end of the line.

In the end, when all is said and done, it goes back to simplicity. Science begins with observation. No matter how hard you try, no matter how much manipulation influence you possess, you cannot stop everybody from observing. People that make their own observations will begin to created their own theory and that is the basis of science!

You can't stop science. You can hijack it for some time but your time in charge is limited.

In the end, an infection will be, as it always has been, an expression of a system that is struggling to continue to function in the manner it used to function. An infection is a period of cleaning up debris that diseased tissues have created. An infection is a sign of the body healing itself from a struggle.

Embrace your infection.
Encourage your infection.
Make the necessary changes to avoid your system having to do it again.
Become infection free.

VIRUSES

Patrick Quanten MD

Let's start with a medically well-known fact: **viruses aren't themselves alive.** They are a lot smaller and simpler than bacteria and by themselves they are inert and harmless. So, the immediate question then has to be: How can you 'catch' a virus if it isn't a living thing?

The answer is: You can't.

Researchers have incubated viruses for the common cold, placed them directly on the mucous lining of the nose, and found that their subjects came down with colds only 12% of the time. These odds could not be increased by exposing the subjects to cold drafts, putting their feet in ice water to give them chills, or anything else that was purely physical.

Swine flu is a known viral infection, which was considered non-dangerous and normal, but for an unknown reason during an outbreak in the spring of 1918 in the US it mutated into a severe form that killed a large number of people. The medical authorities were pressurised (by themselves!) into developing a vaccine in order to stop the spread of this now lethal disease. They conducted experiments on volunteers, which they recruited from a military prison on Deer Island in Boston harbour. The prisoners, sitting out a life sentence, were promised complete pardon if they survived a series of rigorous tests. In order to infect the volunteers with the deadly virus they were injected with infected lung tissue taken from the dead. If this failed they had their eyes, nose and mouth sprayed with infectious aerosols. After that, they had their throats swabbed with discharges taken from the sick and dying. If all else failed, they were required to sit open-mouthed while a gravely ill person was sat up slightly and made to cough into their faces. There were sixty-two chosen volunteers. Not a single one caught the flu. The only person who did was the doctor who died soon afterwards.

One of the mysteries of viral epidemics is how it can erupt suddenly in places separated by oceans, mountain ranges and other earthly impediments. Although a virus is not alive in itself, it also loses its only power, one of hijacking the genetic material of a living host cell, within a few hours of being outside the host body. The commonly heard answer that it travels in 'carriers' (people who have no symptoms but carry and distribute the virus) cannot be proven and after decades of using it as **the** explanation it remains nothing more than a shaky and desperate theory. It is made even more unlikely in the light of the fact that you cannot catch a viral infection, as apply demonstrated by medical experimentation. So even if it did travel that way, how would it 'jump' from the carrier to the victim? And even if it was still present within the cells of the carrier, it would become 'inactivated' within the water droplets he breathes out. Furthermore, how does a virus manage to lie low for several months, in the case of HIV or variant CJD we are to believe it can be up to 20 years, before erupting so explosively at more or less the same time all over? What's the trigger and why instantaneously in all those different places?

It also is a fact that some of these viral epidemics are more devastating to people in their prime than they are to infants and elderly people, who are generally considered to be more vulnerable. For some unknown reason people with a reduced resistance, a 'weaker' immune system, are seemingly more protected against viral infections. This has never been explained. This observation has simply been ignored.

Sometimes viral infections that we consider eradicated will return. There are plenty of examples of this, even in our modern times, but a well-documented story is the Russian virus known as H1N1 which caused outbreaks over wide areas in 1933. It seemed to disappear and then return with devastating effects in the 1950's and again in the 1970's. Nobody knows where it went in the meantime. In the in-between periods it was never found anywhere. These phenomena are explained by using the tale of 'dormant viruses', but nobody has ever come close to proving that this could even be a remote possibility. If you can't demonstrate the presence of the virus how do you know it is 'sleeping'? This also raises the same old two questions: *Why did it not cause any symptoms wherever it was hiding? and If it was hiding somewhere, why did it become so explosively active?*

What do we know about Viruses?

We have already mentioned that they are very very small, and they weren't detected until 1943 with the invention of the electron microscope. Many, including HIV, have ten or fewer genes, whereas the simplest bacteria require several thousand. To create a living thing you need properly organised DNA of a substantial quantity, which the virus hasn't got.

We define 'a living organism' as something that performs three tasks in succession: taking in stuff (eating, breathing), metabolising stuff (digesting, absorbing), and excreting waste. A fourth necessary task is reproduction. A virus doesn't do any of these. No virus does. Within the viral capsule there are no cellular structures that are required for a metabolic process. There is no activity at all inside the viral capsule.

Not only doesn't it look structurally as if it's alive, it also isn't alive in physiological terms.

So what is it then? As we all know, - that's what we have been told - viruses can have devastating effects on the health of plants, animals - great and small, including bacteria - and humans. How does it produce these effects, if it is not alive, can't be caught and doesn't reproduce?

Known scientific facts about viruses and the way they function are obtained from chemical analysis of cellular debris derived from diseased tissue and from looking at still pictures taken by an electron microscope. The story is pieced together, not actually observed! This means that what you are told is happening is actually a theory at best, and a fantasy story at worst.

What has actually, in simple terms, been discovered?

- Viruses contain either RNA or DNA, a small amount and mostly one or the other, but always single stranded. *Bits of genetic material of whatever kind, really, but only bits. Every living cell has a double stranded genetic structure, which is required for replication and multiplication of the cell.*

- Viruses are marked species and organ specific, and on the whole, viruses infecting plants, insects, rickettsia, bacteria and other animals are distinct from their human counterparts. This statement about viruses, lifted from the medical textbook, is very inconvenient when you want to maintain an epidemic story that starts with an animal and ends in a human being. So it gets more and more ignored. *They are specific, but now we change our tune because it is better for us.*

- Viruses may be naked with the genome only protected by a protein capsid, or they may have a lipid envelop surrounding the capsid. *Bits of genetic material in a thin simple bag, and sometimes put in a fatty bubble.*

- Viruses are seen to be 'captured' by the body cells that have specific receptors for the virus. Once inside the cell, it seems that the virus capsule is removed and the exposed bit of DNA or RNA is finding its way up into the nucleus of the cell, where it is welcomed into the genetic code of the cell. The host cell seems now to be forced to duplicate the virus genes. These bits of genetic materials are then encapsulated in a simple protein coating, and with the host cell bursting with complete viruses it will explode and the viruses are spilled into the cellular surroundings. *So, on the pictures we see a lot of genetic bits in separate bubbles within the cell. Eventually the cell burst open to release the bagged up genetic material into the extra-cellular environment. That also is a still photograph. In other words, it does not show the direction in which these bags travel.*

- Viruses in the intercellular environment are engulfed by cells from the immune system (macrophages and lymphocytes), which collect them and destroy them. *These bags that contain bits of genetic material are collected into cells from the waste management system.*

- Viruses are very difficult to demonstrate (they are extremely small) and the diagnosis of a viral infection is mostly made on clinical symptoms alone and on the assumption that it fits into a known disease pattern for which there is no causative factor known. *Virtually every time a diagnosis of viral infection is pronounced no proof is offered for this diagnosis. Rather, it is the lack of proof for any other diagnosis that makes it a viral infection.*

- Samples for the detection of the virus (not isolation of the virus!) must be obtained as early as possible during illness. It is at the very early stages of the illness that the highest levels are found and the most likely it is one can produce a positive test result. A positive test means that the replication machine has detected the specific short genetic code sequence within the cellular debris of the diseased tissue. *There are more viruses present right at the beginning of the illness than at any other stage of the disease process. If the viruses were multiplying and infecting other cells you would expect the number to rise as the disease developed.*

- Identification of viruses is done in laboratories by measuring the level of antibodies against specific viruses, not by measuring or demonstrating the virus itself. *Measuring a higher protection level, antibodies, is used as a diagnostic tool for the illness itself!*

Summarising this scientific knowledge, we can say that viral infections are not diagnosed by finding the specific virus, but by proclaiming a virus is the cause of the symptoms. In practical terms, this happens when the doctor doesn't really know what the cause is. What they 'find' at the end of complicated chemical interactions done in specific laboratories and what they then proclaim to be of viral origin is a short sequence of a genetic code and/or some proteins. It needs to be noted that these are essential parts of any cellular structure, not just the so-called virus.

With regards to the story of the viral infection itself, we now know that as soon as the symptoms start the number of viruses will very quickly dramatically reduce. There is no evidence of rapid number proliferation once the disease manifests itself. This is contrary to what is observed in case of the number of bacteria present in an infection.

Before we move on to explain the real virus story, it is worthwhile to remind ourselves of what we already know:

1. A virus is not alive.

2. You cannot catch a virus.

3. A virus disintegrates very quickly outside the host and outside of the cell.

4. A virus consists of small bits of genetic material, variable from virus to virus, surrounded by a thin coating, either protein or fat.

5. Viral materials are seen in large numbers inside the diseased host cell.

6. A full host cell breaks open and the viruses are spilled into the environment.

7. In the environment the viruses are bagged up by the cells of the waste management system (See "The Inflammation Process", available on www.activehealthcare.co.uk).

The Virus Story

If viruses are not living things they cannot multiply and they don't need a specific environment to 'survive'. They cannot appear from nowhere and they can't spread and infect other cells. They cannot be anything else but inert. Yet, on the photographs certain shapes have been named 'a virus', which begs the question, "What is that shape then?"

When a cell becomes diseased and the function of the cell begins to falter, the cell structure may start to come apart at the seams. Bits of its essential structure, the DNA and RNA, may become detached as it is falling apart. The cell will try and clean up these bits by preparing them for the rubbish bin. The small pieces of erratic genetic material, which are now floating around in the intracellular fluid, will be isolated by means of encapsulating them. As the cellular disintegration continues, more and more of these bits are seen inside the cell and more and more small 'bags' of useless genetic material will appear. Once the cell is totally dysfunctional and filled with rubbish, the cellular wall itself bursts and the contents will be spilled into the cellular outer environment. Here, the clean-up continues by packaging these small bags up even further into what has been called the lymphocytes and macrophages of the waste management system. These large vesicles now drift away into the lymphatic fluid and the blood stream, from where they will be filtered out at appropriate draining stations, like the spleen and the lymph nodes. This process continues until the whole lot has been cleared up.

This explains why the numbers of 'viruses', small rubbish bags, is the highest at the very beginning of the disease and continues to decline steadily throughout the disease process, even without treatment. This also accounts for the thousands and thousands of different 'viruses' that have been identified and for the 'mutation' of viruses. Viral behaviour is essentially totally unpredictable because the cells and the way they disintegrate is never the same. Hence, the bits of debris can vary greatly in shape and form. This variation is not due to an animal, called a virus that changes its behaviour so quickly and intelligently that nothing can keep up with it. It also does away with the idea that the 'virus' can lay dormant for an indefinite period of time and can become activated without any triggers or reasons having been identified.

How do we then explain 'viral epidemics'? Why is it then that we also get a cold the day after someone in the office starts to cough and sneeze a lot?

The medical profession has told us that viruses have incubation periods. These are said to vary from virus to virus from a few days to several years. A cold virus has an average incubation period of about a week. Now, first of all, you can't catch a virus; and secondly, if you could catch the cold virus, it would take a week before it had established itself within your body and starts to show symptoms. So the medical profession tells us. Consequently, your cold cannot have been caused by the other person's cold in the office the day before!

And then there is another small matter that seems to point in a different direction. Within the same research laboratories where people study electron microscopic pictures another story has emerged. While some people are furiously looking 'to identify' viruses others have been, unwittingly, upsetting the unified picture that the medical profession has been painting. These researchers have been looking at tiny vesicles inside cells. They are to be found in all cell material, in greater or lesser numbers, and pictures have also shown these to sometimes be attached to the cell membrane as well as being seen in the immediate cell surroundings. They named these vesicles endosomes when they are located inside the cell and exosomes when they are on the outside. The theory these researchers in medical laboratories have developed about the vesicles is that they are tiny protein bags that contain very small pieces of cellular waste. These bags are then pushed out of the cell in an effort to keep the inside of the cell clean and in perfect working order. It now turns out that these vesicles are **indistinguishable** from what others have named to be viruses.

All of this research information results in the viral story being turned inside out. It isn't the virus in the outside world that penetrates the cell membrane, dodges all cell defences, manages to break into the cell control room (the nucleus), wriggles its way into the genetic coding of the cell, forces the cell to only produce new viruses, which then make the cell die and burst open in order for those viruses to be spread in the immediate cell environment, where they can infiltrate other cells.

Wow, what a story!!

That story would now follow the same sequences but in reverse order. The cell is struggling to keep going and small bits of genetic material break off from the DNA. These 'nonsense' message could possibly get stuck in the normal cellular communication system, so the cell encapsulates these bits to prevent them disrupting and blocking the entire cell metabolism. These little bags accumulate within the cell as the rate of expulsion of the waste bags is too slow compared with the rate at which the cellular structure is disintegrating. Eventually the cell will die and burst open. All the waste bags in the outer environment are collected by the white blood cells of the organism to be carried away for recycling and disposal.

Of course, this theory must be kept in a sealed jar because not only does it directly oppose the virus theory but it also fits in with the original scientific theory of infectious diseases, which says that an infection occurs spontaneously within the tissues and is not caused by a from the outside attacking microbe. Allowing this theory, developed by their own staff, to flow into the consciousness of the population would be a large nail in the coffin of their own germ-theory.

What is seen and has been named 'a virus' starts after the cellular structure begins to disintegrate. Why does a cell start to fall apart? Because it is diseased. The disease is already there, long before any viral particles, now known as endosomes, show up in any pictures. So, then we have to ask the question why the cell has become diseased? The answer to this lies in the build-up of toxic material within the cellular structure. Waste material accumulates when the cell, the tissue, the organ, the organism is forced to burn more energy than 'normal'. When the energy field to which the cells belong becomes unbalanced, it struggles to keep functioning. This struggle requires more energy. Burning more energy leaves more waste. All of which needs to be cleaned up. As the cells and the tissues get loaded up with inappropriate material the cell will eventually be unable to cope and it will start to fall to pieces. Pieces of the genetic structure of the cell are being bagged up by the struggling, the diseased cell. It is exactly those pieces that are photographed by the electron microscope and have been named viruses, endosomes and exosomes.

Identifying a short DNA sequence in a pool of cellular debris only allows you to speculate as to its origin. There is no scientific way of proving its origin.

Photographs can show the location of something at that moment in time. It does not show the direction in which that something was travelling at that moment in time. Science has taught us that at any given moment in time one can either measure the direction of travel or the location, never both at the same time.

EPIDEMICS

Patrick Quanten MD

The word epidemic refers to the spread of a disease amongst a large number of people in a given population or group within a short period of time. Epidemics of infectious diseases are said to be caused by several factors including a change in the ecology of the host population (e.g. increased stress, increase in numbers within the species, changed living conditions), a genetic change in the pathogen that makes it more aggressive or the introduction of a new pathogen to a host population. Generally, an epidemic is said to occur when host immunity to either an established pathogen or to a newly emerging pathogen is suddenly reduced. So any epidemic is basically the result of a combination of reduced resistance within the host and an increased virulence of the pathogen or the emergence of the pathogen at a novel place. That is what we have been told so far.

What is being referred to as a pathogen or an infectious agent is a biological agent that causes disease to its hosts. These agents, microorganisms, are said to disrupt the normal physiology of a multicellular organism. So the 'knowledge' that the agent is the cause of a disease is written into the definition of an infectious agent, which means no other proof of causation is required. However, in scientific terms, one has to first prove that a said agents not only is present in the host during the illness but also, and more importantly, that it is the actual cause of that specific illness, that it is the catalytic factor in the metabolic processes of the cells. Under those conditions one can declare it to be *a pathogen.* In other words, one has *to prove* that it disrupts the normal physiology of the organism, not simply state that the normal function is disturbed and that therefore a pathogen must be the cause.

Early suggestions of a causal link between an invading organism and a specific disease resulted in the first attempts of inoculations during the 18th century. Infecting healthy persons in an attempt to build up their resistance – nowadays called immunity – turned out to be disastrous, although it did not lead to the abundance of the practice. Quite the opposite, as during the next century a coup d'état ensured that doctors were to commit fully to the idea of the invasion by a foreign pathogen as the definite cause of an infectious disease. Scientists of that time - renowned researchers, doctors and professors at numerous universities - showed that the said pathogens, seen at the site of an infection, were in fact present as a result of the infection, not as the cause.

In order to settle the argument, Robert Koch and Friedrich Loeffler formulated in 1884 the postulates designed to establish a causative relationship between a microbe and a disease. These were accepted throughout the scientific community. Refer to chapter 'A HISTORY LESSON IN GERM THEORY'.

Soon, however, Dr Koch abandoned the first of his own postulates when he had to admit that healthy people could be shown to carry bacteria that were known to cause cholera and later he noticed it was the same for typhoid fever. He also found out that the third postulate was not always happening. Not everybody got ill when a pathogen was knowingly introduced into the body. These observations, which are going against a perfectly logical approach to causation, should have led the medical world to question the theory of an invasive pathogen as the cause of infectious diseases. Instead even Professor Koch himself chose to ignore his own rules in favour of *the idea* that pathogens are responsible for the introduction of an infectious disease, in spite of his own observations to the contrary. By that time the pressure from the supporters of Louis Pasteur who advocated forcefully that infections had to be caused by an attack from the outside, was overwhelming. Investors did not want to give up the idea that humans needed to be protected against outside microorganisms as this opened up the market to *fight disease*, a market that would guarantee a fantastic return on their investment forever. It would create a dependency of an entire population on the protective measures that could only be provided by their own trained personnel. So scientific papers were destroyed, professors and researchers were threatened and alternative ideas were ridiculed and abandoned. Koch postulates were not considered worth anything as there were so many exceptions! To this day, that is what doctors, the few that even know about these postulates, accept.

It was decided that the shortcomings of the postulates were such that they are not strictly necessary to be allowed the conclusion that one infectious agent causes one specific disease. It soon, however, became evident that a single pathogen could cause several disease conditions, that a single disease condition could be caused by several different pathogens and that some so-called pathogens could not be cultured in the laboratory on traditional feeding soil (for example viruses). What more evidence does one need to seriously question the starting assumption that one invading pathogen causes one specific disease? Instead, a definite choice was made to view all these 'exceptions' as the rule and that in spite of there being more exceptions than rule the dogma was to stand firm. In doing so they abandoned the only objective evaluation scheme possible to prove a causal relationship between microorganism and disease. They could, from now on, continue, without flinching, to look for invisible infectious agents, pathogens, and name them as the cause of a disease without having to bother looking for the proof of such a statement.

In this unscientific climate the occurrence of an infectious disease within the population sets off the search for a possible organism to blame the disease on. In order to be blamed to have caused the disease the microorganism only has to be present. Nobody is interested in what it is doing there! When a similar disease occurs in a number of subjects at more or less the same time and place, one can call it an epidemic, which heightens the search for the attacker as panic spreads rapidly throughout the entire population. As it already has been decided that the disease **must be** caused by an agent either coming in from the outside or having changed its 'appearance', no other possible disease causes will be taken into account. So let's follow their lead and see what kind of agents they tell us are causing epidemics.

The World Health Organisation (WHO) states that *disease outbreaks are usually caused by an infection, transmitted through person-to-person contact, animal-to-person contact or from the environment or other media to a person. Occasionally outbreaks can follow exposure to chemicals or to radioactive materials.* When the cause is obscure it must be due to a new or modified pathogen or an undetected release of a chemical, according to the WHO. There is indeed an admission that chemicals and radioactivity can be responsible for disease outbreaks and epidemics. However bear in mind that only the WHO has the authority to declare the cause of any outbreak, which means that if there is no admission of chemical or radioactive exposure then that means that it must not be considered as a 'possible' cause.

Also bear the following in mind. However the said disease is being transmitted that does not answer the question as to where the disease came from in the first place. If humans become infected by animals it would be nice if science could then show us where the animals got the pathogen from, even if they are not being ill themselves, as very often is the case with the blamed 'origin' of the epidemic. When animals are 'carrying' the disease without there being any disease signs or symptoms then the question arises why humans aren't *always* 'catching' the disease. Where, over the centuries, have we picked up diseases that caused epidemics?

- Black death (plague) – bacteria transmitted from rodents via the bite of infected fleas
- Malaria - transmitted by mosquitoes
- Spanish flu (1918) – H1N1 virus with genes of avian origin (unknown source)
- Hong Kong flu (1968) – H3N2 virus contained genes from avian influenza

- AIDS – HIV crossed from chimps to humans in the 1920's in the Democratic Republic of Congo

- Bird flu – H5N1 and H7N9 virus coming from a dozen types of birds

- SARS – an animal virus from an unknown animal reservoir

- Ebola – an animal virus from an unknown animal reservoir

- Swine flu – H1N1 virus originating in pigs (same virus that caused Spanish flu from birds!)

- Corona flu – not identified animal reservoir (bats, pigs, cats, birds)

We started out by believing that the bacterial infectious diseases such as tuberculosis or the plague are caused by the transmission of the pathogens from an animal to a human. In both species the said bacteria can be identified under a microscope and they can be grown on culture. In other words, at least we are sure these microorganisms are present, both in the animal and in the human being. Whether the bacteria are actually causing the disease in humans or remains scientifically unproven as the postulates that would deliver such an undeniable proof are not showing the expected results. Or one could safely say that the postulates show us we are wrong in our assumptions.

Let's have a quick look at how the medical profession identifies the presence of a virus in diseased tissue. Remember that *the presence* of a virus is no proof of it being the cause of the disease! First there is the sampling of the possible virus. It says that proper sampling technique is essential to avoid potential pre-analytical errors. *Different types of samples* must be collected in appropriate tubes to maintain the integrity of the sample. It must be stored at appropriate temperatures (usually 4°C) to prevent bacterial or fungal growth within the samples. Are you sure nothing has gone wrong with the taken samples even before they reach the laboratory? You know for sure that the doctor adheres to these specific conditions for the sample taking, the storage in his surgery and the transportation to the laboratory? The information that we receive from the medical profession is that if the right conditions for the samples are not maintained all the time, unpredictable changes could happen within the sample, making the test results unreliable.

In the laboratory the virus gets 'isolated' in order for it to be used for growing on cell cultures. In order to isolate the virus the sample is *mixed with other cells,* so these can – that's the theory – become infected by the virus they suspect must be present within the sample. Cell death occurs and this debris mixture is now being used for further 'identification' testing. It is now a well-known fact that what is used for further testing cannot be proven to only contain the theoretical viral particles as there is always cellular debris mixed in with it. There is no real, no scientific, **isolation of the virus.** There is a multiplication of bits of genetic material of an unknown source. So whatever the tests identify cannot be proven to come from the theoretical virus. Scientific research has shown that when viruses from the taken samples are not mixed with other cells in the first place no virus has ever been 'isolated' or 'detected'. In other words, using the collected material in the sample directly **never** leads to finding a virus. It is an essential required for obtaining a positive test result to mix the sample material with cells, and these obviously contain genetic codes.

Further tests now detect genome parts that are being named to originate from an unknown virus, whilst it has been shown that it is impossible to prove that that specific genetic material is not a part of the normal cell genome, is not a part of the substrate the said viruses supposedly have grown on. Genetic material is inherent to all cells and when these cells break down all kinds of bits of genetic material can be found within the debris.

Other tests to detect the presence of a virus are based on the principle that a specific antibody will bind to a specific virus. In order to establish this contact the debris mixture is mixed with specific antibodies to different types of viruses. Then the tissue is exposed to a specific wavelength of light or to a chemical that allows the antibody to be visualised. Seeing the antibody should then be proof of the presence of the virus. What a shame it then is that science has established a long time ago that no antibodies are ever specific to any specific agent, whatever that 'foreign' material may be. So the laboratory may come up with lots of positive antibody tests without actually delivering any proof of the presence of a virus at all.

And then there is the electron microscopic picture. This technique is never used in routine diagnostic testing as it requires a highly specialised type of sample preparation, microscope and technical expertise. This microscope gives you blobs on a black and white badly focussed photograph whereby it is said that some of those blobs are viruses. What they do, how they got there, and whether or not these blobs are the cause of anything at all, are not questions that a still picture answers.

To be much more practical the medical profession has designed another test to allow physicians to diagnose viral infections. When a person becomes infected it is likely that the body will produce antibodies against the 'foreign invader'. This idea is part of what has been named 'the immune response' of the body. Therefore, the presence of certain antibodies in the blood stream is seen as an indication of an acute infection. So antibody testing has become the most widely used method to *identify* an infection. They screen the blood sample for a wide range of antibodies and any positive test is being translated into the presence of a specific virus, whilst no antibody is ever specific and the presence of antibodies can never be contributed to a specific infection.

The conclusion must be that there is no way of proving *beyond a shadow of a doubt the* presence of a virus in an infected person. And on top of that, as it was the case with infections related to microorganisms, *there has never been any proof of a causal link between the said presence of an agent and the disease.*

Let's return to how the medical profession proclaims a human being becomes ill as a result of an infection. From the list of epidemics as printed above we can see that the first introduction of such an invader is being blamed on contact with animals that are infected themselves or that are innocent carriers. After that we have direct transmission from human to human and a third method is via inanimate objects such as table tops, doorknobs, toothbrushes, handshakes, the list is endless. Why is that? Because none of those are proven causes of infections. It is easy to identify the presence of microorganisms in our environment because they are everywhere. When we say microorganisms we mean 'live' organisms such as bacteria, fungi, parasites. The entire living planet is based on the presence of microorganisms. However, whether their presence equals infectious diseases in human beings is a completely different matter. One that has never been proven. Even better, one that is known to be nonsense because scientists have already stated and proven that the presence of microorganisms is what keeps us all alive. They are essential to all our bodily functions and just as the sun is essential to life on earth – it is not a lethal influence! – so are microorganisms essential to life. The question of dividing them into 'good' and 'bad' ones may keep the dream alive that we need to be afraid of them and fight them, but it makes no sense whatsoever.

Viruses being identified as being present in our environment and subsequently being the cause of infectious is even more ludicrous. Viruses, so the medical textbook tells me, cannot 'survive' outside a host cell. Hence, they can't be present in dust or on doorknobs or towels. On top of that, even if they were, they too are not capable of causing any diseases whatsoever. So how are viruses then being 'identified' in our environment? Indeed, by taking samples, mixing those with other cells, causing cellular dead and 'finding' a specific genetic sequence, which we *name* as being the genome of the specific virus we were looking for. Hence you can find the corona virus in water melons, in river water, on chickens, in air – make it specific to frighten people even more: the air in the dormitory of a boarding school. You don't actually find the virus. You simple have created a positive test result by the way you have executed your search.

Ticks carry the bacterium that causes Lyme disease. Mosquitoes bring you malaria. Bats give us flu, which we might call coronavirus flu. Insects, but also other animals like badgers for bovine tuberculosis, and birds, are all possibly infecting us with germs we fall prey to. Direct contact with these animals is supposed to be the point at which the germ enters the human system. Food contamination is another blamed source, even though most of the bacteria we might pick up in decaying food are commensals, meaning they live inside our body. So no wonder you can detect them after food poisoning! And of course, direct contact with inanimate objects that possibly carry microorganisms can deliver those to our system. Germs can survive on plenty of surfaces, except viruses can't. The medical books clearly state that viruses can only survive *inside* a host cell. Water droplet, for instance, are not living cells. Viruses cannot, per definition – it is a fundamental characteristic of viruses -, survive outside of a cell. The transmission via inanimate objects as a source of infection is never scientifically proven but is always used as an argument in the frontline war against infections and the war against viral epidemics.

Contact with 'unclean' material from faeces to food to air has been blamed as a way of spreading diseases. Sometimes the presence of microorganisms can be detected but a causal link to any disease has never been established. No scientific proof is needed if nobody asks! Repeating messages of avoidance and cleanliness is enough to keep the fear alive and people maintain this kind of illusion themselves quite happily. *Better safe than sorry,* actually indicates that the statement you are adhering to doesn't have to be true, as long as you *believe* it to be safer. All attention is directed outwardly. The danger lies outside and all you need to do to prevent illness is to deal with your environment. The only mention within the medical literature of the importance of the individual in the entire infection story is that some individuals are more vulnerable to infections because of lowered immunity and weakened resistance. Sadly, the doctor informs you that there is nothing you can do about that, but he will give you cortisone and antibiotics 'to support your immune system'.

It is this part of the infective story that does not receive any attention at all. Nobody seems to be interested in why some people survive infectious diseases, epidemics, and others don't. All attention and all efforts are directed towards saving the lives of the ill and 'preventing' others from suffering the disease. Simply put, survivors are individuals who have the inner strength to overcome the impact of a disease situation, wherever the source of that disease may lie. Under these circumstances it would be beneficial to the entire population to know what it would mean to have 'high immunity' or 'great disease resistance'. How do we achieve it?

Right at the beginning it was stated that *any epidemic is basically being contributed to a combination of reduced resistance within the host and an increased virulence of the pathogen.* So the disease is the direct result of a power struggle between the inner strength of an individual and the pressures from the outside world. The medical profession efforts are all directed towards containing the environment, towards cleaning the environment, towards mastering the environment. The results of those efforts are extremely poor as we are still struggling with epidemics and pandemics in spite of their claim last century, with the emergence of the new antibiotics, that infectious diseases would soon be a thing of the past. Why have they not paid any attention to the inner resistance of an individual?

Having a high resistance against diseases surely is the most efficient and most reliable force in surviving the environment. But **inner strength** is not dependent upon an outer power. It is, per definition, something the individual can do him/herself. No expert is needed to achieve this. Inner strength, we now know, has everything to do with inner balance, with being oneself. Following instructions that are imposed upon us from the outside is not empowering inner health, whether these instructions are about what will protect us from infectious diseases or about how we have to live our lives.

Health begins with a switch from looking out to looking in.

Epidemics are not about spreading pathogens, infectious agents, from an inanimate object or an animal or a human to a human. It is much more about spreading an environment in which we as a group will feel threatened and frightened. In 2018, *Medical News Today* reported that researchers had found that chronic stress has a negative impact on memory and that it raises the risk of cardiovascular events, such as a stroke. In 2019, a study conducted by specialists from Pennsylvania State University in State College has found that negative moods may change the way in which the immune response functions, and they are associated with an increased risk of exacerbated inflammation, the precursor to infections. The results of the research — which was led by Jennifer Graham-Engeland, an associate professor at Pennsylvania State University — appear in the journal *Brain, Behaviour, and Immunity.*

Andrew Goliszek Ph.D. argues that *on-going stress makes us susceptible to illness and disease because the brain sends defence signals to the endocrine system, which then releases an array of hormones that not only gets us ready for emergency situations but severely depresses our immunity at the same time. Some experts claim that stress is responsible for as much as 90% of all illnesses and diseases, including cancer and heart disease.*

In the early 1980s, psychologist Janice Kiecolt-Glaser, PhD, and immunologist Ronald Glaser, PhD, of the Ohio State University College of Medicine, were intrigued by animal studies that linked stress and infection. From 1982 through 1992, these pioneer researchers studied medical students. Among other things, they found that the students immunity went down every year under the simple stress of the three-day exam period. Those findings opened the floodgates of research. By 2004, Suzanne Segerstrom, PhD, of the University of Kentucky, and Gregory Miller, PhD, of the University of British Columbia, had nearly 300 studies on stress and health to review. Lab studies that stressed people for a few minutes found a burst of one type of 'first responder' activity mixed with other signs of weakening. For stress of any significant duration - from a few days to a few months or years, as happens in real life - all aspects of immunity went downhill. Thus long-term or chronic stress, through too much wear and tear, can ravage the immune system. The studies also revealed that people who are older or already sick are more prone to stress-related immune changes. For example, a 2002 study by Lyanne McGuire, PhD, of John Hopkins School of Medicine with Kiecolt-Glaser and Glaser reported that even chronic, sub-clinical mild depression may suppress an older person's immune system. Participants in the study were in their early 70s and caring for someone with Alzheimer's disease. Those with chronic mild depression had weaker lymphocyte-T cell responses to two mitogens, which model how the body responds to viruses and bacteria (as believed by the medical profession conducting these studies). The immune response was down even 18 months later, and immunity declined with age. In line with the 2004 analysis, it appeared that the key immune factor was duration, not severity, of depression. And in the case of the older caregivers, their depression and age meant a double-whammy for the strength of their immunity, their resistance against disease.

These are research papers from within the medical profession and so they set up the study to look at parameters that the profession likes and appreciates. And the results are very clear about the negative impact chronic stress has on the individual's resistance to infectious diseases. And whatever may or may not be in the environment of that individual will therefore have a greater impact on his life and health.

Leaves us with the question, what is being transferred from one person to another during an epidemic? It can't be a pathogen as science has proven that one cannot introduce a specific disease by introducing the pathogen that is said to be causing the disease. It can't be a pathogen as science has proven that no pathogen has ever been found to cause any infectious disease. And yet, when one person displays an infection within a group, a separate community, others will soon display very similar symptoms. As far as normal children's infections goes, such as measles, mothers were keen to organise parties for children of similar ages in order *to catch* the disease and let nature get on with it.

Let's see what science has to say about this. Science tells us that life is a constant movement of energies and that all matter, including our physical being, is an expression of our energy field. Any changes observed within the matter, structural and/or functional, are due to changes that have happened within the energy field itself. So all interactions, those between humans and those between humans and their environment, are energetic interactions. This leads us to the possibility that what is being exchanged between people within an epidemic is energy. Different vibrations from one person may be 'picked up' by another, which is then being expressed in a very similar way. But how would that work in our everyday life?

The medical profession states that 'close contact' is, for most part, the main route for the infection to spread. So, within families, schools, military, colleagues at work the spread of the infectious disease is most pronounced. People who spend a lot of time together share the same energetic field during their time together. They are *exposed* to the same energetic messages from their environment. They all are 'having to deal with' being exposed to the same information, to the same stresses. If one person 'collapses' under the strain of this information stream and displays this collapse in a very specific way (sneezing, headache, mucus, sore throat, fever, …) then the systems of other individuals may give up their struggle against the strain and stress, give in too and collapse in a very similar fashion too. It is as if 'being ill' has become an accepted state within that group and systems all around you breathe a sigh of relief and let themselves go. When the tension is being released that way the healing process can begin.

Combine these thoughts, which are the result of quantum physics, with the information we have found in the studies done by the medical researchers concerning the immune system and a bright new epidemic picture emerges.

Chronic pressure on individuals will lower their resistance against diseases. When we have a group of people that are being put under specific chronic stress and pressure, be it at work, at school, at a community hobby centre, at a retirement home, or any other group, we will see people, for a time, not being able to cope with that pressure and becoming ill. Not only is the kind of pressure inside the group a lot similar for everybody within the group, but also the individuals within the group are very similar in crucial aspects of their life. What brings people together to form a group? A common interest or a common skill. So, the aspects of life, and therefore the bodily tissues, that are affected by the chronic pressure upon the group will be the same. Hence they will display very similar disease signs, which will lead the medical profession to declare an epidemic.

This explanation also delivers the answer to the observation that never *everybody* within an epidemic becomes ill. The exposure to the energetic pressure is the same, but the response to it is individual. As one individual, being more anxious about how they feel or having other concurrent pressures in his/her life, succumbs to the pressure and becomes ill, another is much more relaxed about life, work, etcetera, and doesn't show any signs at all. This is not about taking herbs or supplements in order to strengthen your immune system. This is simply because of a more relaxed attitude to life in general, and to the specific conditions in which the epidemic occurs in particular.

So, it would make sense, it we truly wanted to strengthen an individual's resistance against diseases, to lower the stress in his/her environment. A society that is the least invasive, the least interfering, in the personal lives of its members is the kindest and healthiest of all societies. Take note of all the pressures your life is subjected too and conclude how well your society does on this health scale, the only true health scale.

And then it is up to you to ensure you don't fall prey to pressures of the outside world. Not allowing the pressures of the outside world to penetrate your inner workings, your beliefs, ensures that you will be the one who survives the epidemic.

SOME HISTORICAL EXAMPLES

Spanish Flu 1918-1919

Also known as the Great Influenza epidemic, the Spanish Flu is possibly the main outbreak of disease in modern times that has left a huge mark on the psyche of mankind. For over a century the deaths of this period have allowed medical science, and the governments they control, to keep humanity in a state of fear waiting for the next attack. These invisible enemies, that are not even alive, seem to be able to just spring out from nowhere and go on the attack without even being seen, seemingly using tactics the famed S.A.S would be proud of. And just when we think we have gained the upper hand it mutates and we are back to square one.

As for proving the passing of this *virus* from person to person causing disease, this extract from an article by John M. Eyler, PhD, The State of Science, Microbiology, and Vaccines circa 1918, shows us how this was not just an unproven theory, but a disproven theory:

"Perhaps the most interesting epidemiological studies conducted during the 1918-1919 pandemic were the human experiments conducted by the Public Health Service and the U.S. Navy under the supervision of Milton Rosenau on Gallops Island, the quarantine station in Boston Harbor, and on Angel Island, its counterpart in San Francisco. The experiment began with 100 volunteers from the Navy who had no history of influenza. Rosenau was the first to report on the experiments conducted at Gallops Island in November and December 1918. His first volunteers received first one strain and then several strains of Pfeiffer's bacillus by spray and swab into their noses and throats and then into their eyes. When that procedure failed to produce disease, others were inoculated with mixtures of other organisms isolated from the throats and noses of influenza patients. Next, some volunteers

*received injections of blood from influenza patients. Finally,
13 of the volunteers were taken into an influenza ward and
exposed to 10 influenza patients each. Each volunteer was
to shake hands with each patient, to talk with him at close
range, and to permit him to cough directly into his face.
None of the volunteers in these experiments developed
influenza. Rosenau was clearly puzzled, and he cautioned
against drawing conclusions from negative results. He ended
his article in JAMA with a telling acknowledgement: "We
entered the outbreak with a notion that we knew the cause
of the disease, and were quite sure we knew how it was
transmitted from person to person. Perhaps, if we have
learned anything, it is that we are not quite sure what we
know about the disease." The research conducted at Angel
Island and that continued in early 1919 in Boston broadened
this research by inoculating with the Mathers streptococcus
and by including a search for filter-passing agents, but it
produced similar negative results. It seemed that what was
acknowledged to be one of the most contagious of
communicable diseases could not be transferred under
experimental conditions."*

Even one of the deadliest pandemics known to man, the Great
Spanish Flu of 1918, could not be shown to be caused by a
contagious microbe. It was based on a theory borne out of Louis
Pasteur and his germ theory and they were trying to explain an
outbreak of an illness without looking at all at all the factors that
could be involved. The belief in one 'thing' being the cause had
taken over the minds of the medical profession; a thing, though,
that they could not really see or test for. You would have thought
the medical profession and medical scientists would have come
to the conclusion that there was at least an issue with their theory,
but no. According to them the germ theory of disease was *an
established fact* that could not be challenged even when all the
evidence is against it. It seems the real powers behind medical
science could not let real science get in the way of their control
agenda.

The conditions after the First World War were of physical, environmental, emotional and psychological horror. Add to that, experimental vaccines, over-use of aspirin (Bayer), medical doctors seeming to think it best to do something rather than nothing, and with the belief in this invisible enemy putting the fear of God into people. It is hardly surprising there were mass deaths. But for that death rate to return we would need to see the return of those kinds of conditions, and remember, all of that happened without the extra means of creating, and perpetuating, the fear we have today with modern technology and social media 24/7. The mass media and government propaganda 24 hours a day is a very toxic attack indeed all by itself.

Polio

Most people think of polio as being caused by a virus. That, though, has not always been the case. Indeed it was for a long time thought of as being caused by toxic poisoning. The disease had caused paralysis and death and was not known to cause epidemics until the 1900s, when major epidemics began to occur in Europe and the US. During the 1940s and 1950s, polio would paralyze or kill over half a million people worldwide every year, mainly children, hence the new name of 'infant paralysis'.

In 1955, a polio vaccine was developed – the Salk vaccine – and put into widespread use. Polio was itself reclassified in 1954. Was this just a coincidence or a sleight of hand any magician would have been proud of? What would previously have been seen as polio could now be seen as Guillain-Barré Syndrome, transverse myelitis, coxsackie, MS, cerebral palsy. Take your pick, as long as you don't call it polio. What they still registered as 'polio' was paralytic polio, and only this form.

From The Salk 'Miracle' Myth by Marco Cáceres, published June 2, 2015:

> In 1952, a total of 52,879 people got polio. But by 1955, the numbers had already declined by 45 percent. In 1953, 35,592 contracted polio in the US. In 1954, it was 38,476. In 1955, it was 28,985.2.

So it is a fact of history that the numbers dropped precipitously before the Salk vaccine was widely distributed and it was the reclassification that a part in these statistics.

He then quotes Dr Bernard Greenberg, Head of the Department of Biostatistics of the University Of North Carolina School of Public Health on the classification of polio:

"In order to qualify for classification as paralytic poliomyelitis, the patient had to exhibit paralytic symptoms for at least 60 days after the onset of the disease. Prior to 1954, the patient had to exhibit paralytic symptoms for only 24 hours. Laboratory confirmation and the presence of residual paralysis were not required. After 1954, residual paralysis was determined 10 to 20 days"

So, it seems that polio was already in decline before the vaccine and the decline after could be a result of the reclassification alone. Ask any doctor if they are aware of this and I think the answer will be no. Control medical facts and you control medical thinking, which leads to medical treatments based on those alleged facts. Then there are the admitted cases of vaccine-induced polio which, as we will see, would not be a surprise due to the toxic nature of vaccines themselves.

In the 1940's intense debate was also happening in the US and later within the UK regarding the connection between tonsillectomy, mainly in children, and polio. With a holistic look at the body, it seems clear that inflamed tonsils would be waste/toxicity being expelled by the body via the lymphatic system doing its job. The obvious thing to do then would be to encourage that waste to be cleared out. Better out than in as they say. So, a child with reoccurring inflamed tonsils will be struggling with something in their life balance, their development and/or toxins from their environment. A tonsillectomy again is only dealing with the symptom of a problem and not the problem itself. Worse still, it is actually stopping the solution to a problem. When you eliminate the natural clean-up mechanism from a living organism, the system will need to look for another way of removing the waste products, and when it can't, or the other ways are insufficient, it will simply have 'to hide' the rubbish away into the deeper layers, away from the daily function of the system. Again this shows the total lack of holistic thinking by the allopathic medical profession who are obsessed with seeing the body as a machine that goes wrong. By naming the natural healing process, in this example the inflamed tonsils, as the actual disease and obstructing the healing process they make sure the natural system will be unable to rectify the acute problem. This turns the entire system into a chronic state of illness as the problem remains inside the tissues of the system, building a higher and higher mountain of waste.

After WWII, DDT pesticides were introduced and the polio death rate rises sharply. Although this is just showing a relationship between the two, it sure is an interesting graph showing a clear connection between polio and pesticide toxicity. Why would the medical authorities be simply ignoring data like this?

And again, a huge drop in the death rate of polio in England and Wales, BEFORE the vaccine program. Was this a reduction in pesticide use or the reclassification of polio or a combination of both? They are just factors in a complex study but for sure it was clear that at least officially polio was on the decline before the vaccine but that did not stop this medical procedure getting all the glory once again. It also shows how medical science, and governments, continue to ignore facts and data that challenge the official line of thinking.

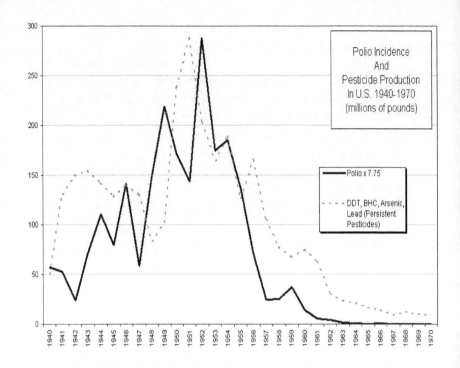

Polio Incidence
And
Pesticide Production
In U.S. 1940-1970
(millions of pounds)

Polio x 7.75

DDT, BHC, Arsenic,
Lead (Persistent
Pesticides)

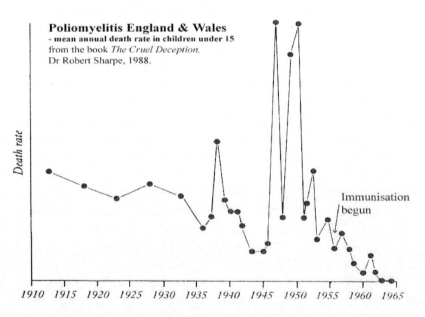

Poliomyelitis England & Wales
- mean annual death rate in children under 15
from the book *The Cruel Deception,*
Dr Robert Sharpe, 1988.

Death rate

Immunisation
begun

DDT

The previous graph shows the connection between polio and environmental toxicity. The graphs also show us that, again, it's not just about the incoming information, in this case DDT and other toxic pesticide ingredients, but how an individual responds to that information. Not everyone got polio but many people ate the food sprayed with pesticides.

In the 1940s and 1950s, DDT was heavily used as an insecticide to attack mosquitos to combat malaria and dengue fever. In 1945, DDT was made available to farmers and for domestic use in the US but fears about its safety meant that in 1972 it was banned, except for certain public health reasons. In 2004, at the Stockholm Convention on Persistent Organic Pollutant, DDT was given a global ban with the exception of vector control, mainly for use against its old foe, the mosquito. Though said to be moderately toxic, chronic exposure and accumulation can, according to Wikipedia, -

> "affect reproductive capabilities and the embryo or foetus ... Mothers with high levels of DDT circulating in their blood during pregnancy were found to be more likely to give birth to children who would go on to develop autism ... Indirect exposure of mothers through workers directly in contact with DDT is associated with an increase in spontaneous abortions and DDT is probably carcinogenic to humans."

So in the case of malaria and dengue fever we have basically just exchanged one disease for another without looking at the real cause of mosquito-borne disease? While living in the Amazon Basin in Peru for one year I asked the medical advisor, who was going into all our houses spraying them with insecticide, about the dengue fever programme. We all had to leave and they used full protection gear to go inside and spray. He told me that "the mosquito doesn't inject the dengue virus into us but rather activates it". This from a medical professional who, with a little bit more critical thinking, would be able to see a different story.

A more complete understanding of our relationship with the mosquito is available from Patrick Quanten at www.activehealthcare.co.uk article- 'The Mosquitos and I'.

So when we are seeing diseases like alleged ebola or AIDS, or more recently zika, we need to look at environmental toxins that may be affecting the human body, something the medical 'experts,' using the 'best available science,' either don't seem to understand or are willing to just ignore. The history of polio seems certainly connected to toxicity and a disease once thought of as a western disease could very well have been exported to the developing world, not as a virus but as toxic insecticides and other chemical poisoning, including the vaccine itself. Strikingly enough it wasn't just a western disease. It was also a middle class disease. Poor people who couldn't afford the 'fancy' fruit did not contract polio.

If disease is about toxicity and stress on the system, then let's face it, almost EVERYTHING about this life in this system is stressful and toxic.

HIV – Information taken out of the booklet *AIDS and The Story of Viruses* Patrcik Quanten MD 2010

In the early 1980's we were told of a highly dangerous virus that had come out of Africa and spread to the west. Again the issue was the identification of the human immune deficiency virus. The name given to the alleged, *unknown*, causal virus already includes how the virus makes the person ill. This in itself is strange. The identification, as always, was done via a PCR test that we know is not a diagnostic tool. In Africa they began diagnosing people who would otherwise have been diagnosed with other illnesses, like pneumonia, where now, because of a test result, were being diagnosed as HIV infected and they were dying of an immune deficiency disease, called AIDS. There was also huge political influence connected to this alleged disease and poor African countries were flooded with millions of dollars to go with again 'the best medical science'.

In the West we were told that this virus was affecting mostly homosexuals and drug addicts. But while the vast majority of the medical establishment went with the official narrative, of a HIV virus wreaking havoc, there were some more clear thinking doctors who had recognised the lifestyle and health condition of those who were allegedly being affected by this virus. Drug abuse, exposure to blood products, people who already had underlying health issues were now being diagnosed as HIV positive.

Then we have the anti-viral treatments themselves, the most famous being AZT, produced by the Wellcome organisation owned by the Rockefellers. AZT was developed as an anti-cancer drug to be used in chemotherapy, but it was found to be too toxic even for that! AZT's effect in the 'treatment' of cancer was to kill the cells – simple as that – not just to kill cancer cells, but to kill cells, cancerous and healthy. This is the drug of choice to treat HIV. When your immune system is compromised then the medical establishment recommends to kill off as many cells as they possibly can in order to bring you back to health. Do you find the logic in this?

The effects of the recommended treatment includes causing cancer, hepatitis, dementia, seizures, anxiety, impotence, leukopenia, severe nausea, ataxia, amongst others, and the termination of DNA synthesis. Effectively, I don't think there is another way to describe this but as AIDS/death by prescription. It destroys the immune system so causing AIDS. People were dying from the treatment, not from the virus, called HIV. AIDS is simply the breakdown of the immune system, for which there are endless causes, none of them passed on through sex. All of them relating to the way one lives life.

So it was not only people with symptoms of illness being diagnosed with HIV but also worried and afraid healthy people getting a *positive test* result via PCR and believing they had been given a death sentence. The fear then pushed them onto to anti-viral drugs which had a huge potential to make them ill.

My own experience – Rob Ryder- with HIV was in Peru when I got married over there in 2000. To get married I had to have an HIV test. At that time I had no understanding of the medical science and had a week's wait to find out if I too had a death sentence. Though I was not a drug addict, homosexual or promiscuous I still spent the whole week on edge waiting to see if I was *infected* or not. After a week with a chronic headache, stress, the test came back negative, meaningless I now know, but at the time it felt like I had been given my life back. I am not sure what would have happened if it had come back positive, and maybe it's better not to think about that. I would have probably been another victim of medical 'treatment' and I certainly would not have got married. How many lives, healthy lives, have been destroyed by this meaningless test as we will see in the next chapter, *Testing in the Medical World*.

Anti-viral Treatments

What we are told about antivirals is that they reduce the ability of viruses to multiply. Seen through the eyes of germ/viral theory, it would make sense to reduce the ability of these attackers to replicate. But by seeing these particles as our own cellular waste then that would only be storing up waste and toxicity in the cells. Even though acute symptoms may appear to go, the cells, and hence the body, will be functioning at a reduced level. This would be a classic example of suppression of an acute illness, or even suppressing the cleansing and rebalancing system in healthy people, leading to a more chronic illness, what is called 'post-viral syndrome' or as is happening now, 'long COVID'.

Antivirals may have zero benefit for human health but for well-connected people in the political and medical scientific stage they seem to produce many benefits. This is just one example of many where politicians have made enormous profit from policies passed by politicians and yet they continue to get away with it to this day.

*"Donald Rumsfeld has made a killing out of bird flu. The US
"Defence Secretary has made more than $5m (£2.9m) in capital
gains from selling shares in the biotechnology firm that
discovered and developed Tamiflu, the drug being bought in
massive amounts by Governments to treat a possible human
pandemic of the disease."*

– Independent, Sunday 12th March, 2006

TESTING IN THE MEDICAL WORLD

By Patrick Quanten

Our time is marked by an almost obsessive urge for testing and measuring in an effort to be accepted as 'scientific'. This results in statistics and conclusions that are then used as a proven tool to separate good from bad, right from wrong. Because we now believe we have got scientific proof, by way of measurement, about what is right and what is wrong, we can implement rules and laws to express that knowledge, and 'to prevent' anything from going wrong. We force everybody to accept our conclusions and we ensure that there is no room left for doubt. *Beyond reasonable doubt* is our standard for justice, so it has become our standard for life itself. We pretend.

The key to this sequence is the belief that once something has been measured, has been tested, it becomes an undeniable truth, which allows us to draw definite dividing lines between good and bad. The speed by which I drive my car denotes me as 'a good and responsible citizen' on one side of the dividing line, but when I overstep the agreed and *measured* line by even one mile per hour I become 'a danger to my fellow humans' and consequently I need to be punished. No amount of pleading, arguing or giving explanatory reasons will alter the conclusion that I have behaved in an inappropriate and dangerous manner. Once measured it becomes an established knowledge and rules flow forth from that knowledge, rules that then need to be obeyed under all circumstances.

From this point onwards the citizen has lost the freedom of choice. In the interest of the entire community the individual must obey the rule, which has been set as a result of the test done. All this in the name of science.
Humanity in its developing wisdom has always used tests to 'prove' things. Even Jesus on the cross was told that *if He truly was the Son of God* He could prove it by removing Himself from

the cross. Failing the test inevitably means that the proposition one is testing is wrong. In order to prove heresy, people were dropped in boiling fat. Failing to survive this test meant one was not protected by God and therefore deserved the punishment. Being unable to remove oneself from the stake was proof of witchcraft, a danger to the community. In today's, so much more wise and tolerant society, failure to prove one's innocence in the matter of Shaken Baby Syndrome makes one guilty, and therefore in need of punishment. Although our judiciary system states **not guilty until proven**, this mantra changes from the moment an expert is called upon for his opinion. This expert will observe and measure until he reaches a conclusion which then becomes the undeniable truth, followed by necessary punishment to all of those who contravene this 'truth'. The individual has lost its freedom and power as society has deemed what is right and what is wrong in a *measured* and therefore *scientific way.*

Strangely enough, that particular 'scientific' way has been superseded a century ago when scientists realised that nothing could be measured or observed and translated into an *objective* conclusion. In quantum mechanics, the observer and the system being observed became mysteriously linked so that the results of any observation seemed to be determined, at least in part, by actual choices made by the observer.

When a quantum observer is watching quantum mechanics it is said that particles can also behave as waves. When behaving as waves, they can simultaneously pass through several openings in a barrier and then meet again at the other side of the barrier. This meeting is known as *interference.* Strange as it may sound, interference can only occur *when no one is watching.* Once an observer begins to watch the particles going through the openings the picture changes dramatically. If a particle can be seen going through one opening, then it's clear it didn't go through another. In other words, simply because they are being watched electrons are 'forced' to behave like particles and not like waves. *Thus the mere act of observation affects the experimental findings.* This is so because we, as human beings, can only 'watch' in a very specific and limited way.

To demonstrate this, Weizmann Institute researchers built a tiny device measuring less than one micron in size, which had a barrier with two openings. They then sent a current of electrons towards the barrier. The 'observer' in this experiment wasn't human, but it was designed 'to look' in a specific way. Institute scientists used for this purpose a tiny but sophisticated electronic detector that can spot passing electrons. The quantum observer's capacity to detect electrons could be altered by changing its electrical conductivity, or the strength of the current passing through it. Apart from observing, or detecting, the electrons, the detector had no effect on the current itself. Yet the scientists found that the very presence of the detector/observer near one of the openings caused changes in the interference pattern of the electron waves passing through the openings of the barrier. In fact, this effect was dependent on the 'amount', on the intensity, of the observation. When the observer's capacity to detect electrons increased, the interference (the wave pattern) weakened. In contrast, when its capacity to detect electrons was reduced, the interference increased. Thus, by controlling the properties of the quantum observer the scientists managed to control the extent of its influence on the electrons' behaviour.

Hence, the manner in which a test is set up influences the observed results of the test. The way a laboratory 'measures' a certain substance in the blood gives a result that relates to the chemical way the test is being performed. This result, which obviously cannot be seen as *objective*, will then be interpreted by someone who *believes* it to have a particular significance. If he didn't he wouldn't do the test! This interpretation then leads to a conclusion about right or wrong, which in turn results in an action. Let's give an example.

Test: amount of immunoglobulins in the blood

Belief: level is an indication of high or low immunity

Result: low level of immunoglobulins

Action: vaccination

Belief: creates protection against infection

Result: higher level of immunoglobulins

Belief: vaccination results in a high level of protection against infection

Let's look at this briefly from a scientific point of view. Testing the level of blood immunoglobulins is no indication of the status of your immune system. Why not? Because immunity cannot be measured. We have individuals with a low blood level count and a high immunity and the other way around. Nothing can be *objectively* tested or measured! The action of vaccination in order to raise the protection level is scientific nonsense as infection occurs spontaneously from the inside and does not relate to an invasive process. Linking the observed change in the blood level to the action taken is also scientific nonsense as vaccination is not the only thing that has changed between the first and second blood test. Millions of things have changed, from the outside temperature, to my personal tiredness or stress level, to what I have been eating, thinking, feeling, hearing, reading, to the person who takes the blood and the circumstances in which the blood is taken, and so on and on and on. Which of these can you 'prove' has no influence on the test result? If you can't prove it to have a neutral influence you shouldn't scientifically dismiss it either. Everything changes constantly anyway, even if we do not vaccinate!

The conclusion has to be that testing only hands us a specific frozen picture in time, which was taken in a specific way with the purpose of showing something in a specific light. Indeed, a test result can be seen as a still photograph, a snapshot in time. What it looked like moments before the picture was taken or a few precious moments later remains a mystery. What it would have looked like if we had frozen the moment in a different way, looked at it from a different angle, nobody will ever know. In other words, what happened when you took out the camera? How did that change what was actually going on? What we might have seen if we had been looking with a different purpose, is lost in time forever. We do not have that specific picture to hand, and it can never be created as the moment is gone.

And yet, we test, we interpret, we conclude, we judge, and we act upon the judgment as if all these were steps into a true reality, although science, the very umbrella used in the cover-up, has clearly demonstrated a century ago that the reality we observe depends on the way we look at it.

Let's take a look at some of the basic tests and measuring the medical profession relies on in order to conclude what is healthy and what is diseased.

- Measuring your blood pressure. – *The real pressure inside a tube can only be measured by a probe inside the tube. Taking a measurement on the outside of one elbow does not tell you anything about the pressure in the arteries in your abdomen, heart, brain, or anywhere else in the circulation system. Taking a measurement now does not tell you what the pressure will be in two minutes time, tomorrow, next week.*

- Hearing tests and eye tests. – *A snapshot in time. Sensory effectiveness varies with changing circumstances in the outer world and with changing inner circumstances such as the level of focus, of interest, of willingness and eagerness to cooperate.*

- Taking pictures (X-Rays, scans, ultrasound). – *A snapshot in time. It doesn't tell you anything about the function of the body part you are taking pictures off. Slight angle changes will show different results. Different machine calibrations and qualities will change the resulting picture.*

- Measuring blood levels of specific molecules (hormones, vitamins, nutrients, enzymes, toxins, etc.). – *A snapshot in time. Different chemical techniques result in different measured levels. Different machine calibrations and qualities result in different measured levels. Different skills of the staff will result in different measured levels.*

- Measuring blood cells and proteins with supposedly very specific functions such as antibodies. – *A snapshot in time. Different skills, different machines, different calibrations, all influence the measured result.*

And these are just some of the commonly used physical measurements the medical profession relies on. You can imagine how many more influencing factors one can find when one is measuring your psychological state, your intelligence or your emotional state!

So the way measurements are taken and the fact that one proceeds to measure something helps to shape the result one obtains from the measurement. Surely that is a problem if we are trying to define what is good and what is bad for us. But here is some more scientific information about *what* one is proposing to measure.

- Blood pressure. – *Determining that a persons' blood pressure is too high or too low is a statement made on comparison of the measured blood pressure with the belief of what a 'good' blood pressure should be. It does not take into account what the 'normal' blood pressure for that individual is. It does not take into account that a normal blood pressure needs to respond quickly, and sometimes violently, to quickly changing circumstances. So the blood pressure of the individual adapts spontaneously every moment to the circumstances, which means that the blood pressure of the individual is ALWAYS the correct one, taking into account ALL influencing factors.*

- Sensory function. – *The sensory organs are the windows to the outside world. The 'sensing' of the outside world is a brain function. Finding 'abnormalities' in the eye does not tell you the person can and can't see properly. It is the way the brain interprets the incoming information that determines what the person sees and under what circumstances he does see it.*

- Anatomical correctness. – *Every individual is supposed to have the same anatomy and the measurements are compared to that accepted standard. In fact, each individual is an individual balance of all aspects and all functions of life. The balance of individuals created is always different, one from another. In order to know what is an anatomical 'abnormality' for an individual one needs to understand what the balance is of all aspects of his life and how he can maintain that balance. A picture is not going to tell you that because it doesn't contain any information about all the person's aspects of life.*

- Hormone levels. – *Blood hormone levels are being measured in venous blood taken from the elbow of an individual. Venous blood returns oxygen depleted blood, filled with cellular waste products, to the detoxifying organs in the abdomen and to the lungs. In this blood sample the medical profession measures the function of your kidney, of your thyroid, of your sexual hormones, of your liver, of your pancreas, of your heart, and so on. The blood sample is taken from a blood vessel that returns blood from fingers, hand, wrist and forearm. How can it contain these hormones that are produced by organs elsewhere in the body and that are used up by the cells? These can only be present in this sample if every cell of the body produces these hormones and then discards them as waste into the blood stream.*

- Levels of toxicity or nutrition. – *The blood sample is taken from a vein in the elbow. It is a sample of cellular sewage in which the profession is going to measure your nutritional status. The toxicity, however, that one can measure in such a sample is more realistic but one has to bear in mind that one is talking about toxic material that is being discarded by the cells, not something one has eaten or breathed in.*

- Antibodies. – *The blood sample is taken from a vein in the elbow. No antibodies are known to be specific. Antibodies 'against' certain pathogens or against specific toxins do not exist. Not only is there an overlap and a 'sharing' of the same antibodies for different purposes, but the level of measured antibodies can also not be related to a higher or lower resistance to disease. Nobody knows the true value of antibody levels in the venous blood.*

Scientifically speaking, no test result can be used to formulate conclusions with regards to health and disease. Scientifically speaking, nobody should ever have proposed such an idea as science itself has proven that one cannot use testing and measuring for that purpose. Scientifically speaking, testing and measuring is done to *disprove* a proposed theory. Let me give you a few examples.

- When not everybody with a high cholesterol blood level dies of heart failure then the theory that *a high cholesterol level causes heart disease* is proven to be false.

- When not everybody with a high antibody blood level is free of the infectious disease then the theory that *a high antibody level protects you from catching the infection* is proven to be false.

- When not everybody with a low red blood cell count has symptoms of anaemia then the theory that *a low red blood cell count is causing anaemia* is proven to be false.

- When not everybody with serious joint pains is shown to have arthritic changes in the joint then the theory that *joint pain is caused by arthritis* is proven to be false.

- When not everybody shows a positive test result for disease markers such as rheumatoid arthritis and cancer then the theory *that these markers are a sign of the disease* is proven to be false.

- When not everybody who has a positive test result for a specific disease, such as a viral infection, is actually ill then the theory *that the specific test indicates that specific disease* is proven to be false.

Science uses testing and measuring as a way to disprove theories. Science knows that one cannot prove the truth, one can only disprove a 'believed' truth, and even that takes up a lot of time. It takes time to observe, collect data, test data, share data and compare notes with other researchers.

Let me give you one example of how it is not done. This is how the medical profession 'handles' science and alters it to fit their requirements. This is one example but it is general practice within the profession since the emergence of allopathic medicine.

Let's have a look at how PCR testing became the standard test to 'identify' a corona virus within a sample taken from the nasal passage from a person. Here is a short version of the story, to which I added some comments in italics.

Dr. Kary Mullis received the Nobel Prize for chemistry in 1993 for inventing the Polymerase Chain Reaction (PCR) technology. It is a manufacturing technique to replicate DNA sequences millions and trillions of times. It has nothing to do with 'identifying' viruses. It is a method for replication of short sequences of genetic coding.

In December 1998 John Lauritsen, a market research executive and analyst, wrote in connection with HIV: "PCR is intended to identify substances qualitatively, but by its very nature is unsuited for estimating numbers. Although there is a common misimpression that the viral load tests actually count the number of viruses, these tests cannot detect free, infectious viruses at all. They can only detect proteins that are believed, in some cases wrongly, to be unique to HIV. The tests can detect genetic sequences of viruses, but not viruses themselves."

In early 2020, CDC (Centres for Disease Control and Prevention) developed its first laboratory test kit for use in testing patient specimens for SARS-CoV-2. The test kit is called the CDC 2019 Novel Coronavirus (2019-nCoV) Real-Time Reverse Transcriptase (RT)–PCR Diagnostic Panel.

On February 3, 2020, CDC submitted an EUA package (Emergency Use Authorisation) to expedite FDA-permitted use of the CDC diagnostic panel in the United States. FDA (Food and Drug Administration) issued the EUA the next day, and CDC sent the test kits to state and local public health laboratories.

"Under section 564 of the Federal Food, Drug, and Cosmetic Act (FD&C Act), the FDA Commissioner may allow unapproved medical products or unapproved uses of approved medical products to be used in an emergency to diagnose, treat, or prevent serious or life-threatening diseases or conditions caused by CBRN (chemical - biological - radiological - nuclear) threat agents when there are no adequate, approved, and available alternatives."

Before laboratories use a new test on samples from patients, they must verify the test performance (make sure it works as expected) using 'positive' and 'negative' control materials. The positive control should always test positive, and the negative control should always test negative. During validation of the CDC SARS-CoV-2 test, some laboratories discovered a problem with one of the test's three reagents — chemicals required to run a test. The reagent produced a positive result with the negative control, so laboratories could not verify the test performance.

To resolve the issue, CDC laboratories determined that this reagent could be left out without affecting test accuracy. The redundant design saved time by allowing the kits to be used without the reagent. FDA authorised this modification, and new test kits with the two necessary reagents were manufactured and distributed. These kits are still in use.

When it turns out the test is useless, you simply remove the factor that is in your way and you pretend the test works perfectly well without it! Or, put differently, you fiddle with the procedure until you get the result you want.

High demand for the reagents needed with this test has resulted in global shortages. Some public health laboratories have been unable to get testing reagents to support their testing volumes, resulting in testing delays. Therefore, CDC laboratories validated alternatives for processing the test:

- Four additional extraction reagents that can be used in the existing extraction methods
- An additional extraction instrument and associated reagents
- A new process that can be used in place of the extraction method when materials for the current method are limited

FDA approved these changes on June 12, 2020, in an amendment to the test's EUA to allow state public health laboratories and others to use these alternatives. Additionally, FDA approved an amendment on July 13, 2020, to add the Promega Maxwell® RSC 48 as an authorized extraction instrument for use with the CDC 2019-nCoV rRT-PCR Diagnostic Panel.

If you don't have the ingredients to do the test in the way we have pre-tested it then you are allowed to change all kind of things (chemicals, instruments, operational method) and we will pretend it is still the same test!

Lots of people started questioning the validity of the test in the context it was being used. Official reaction from the authority was vague and evasive but when pressed they had to admit that it wasn't quite what they said it was. In 2020 a spokesperson for Public Health England told Reuters: "It is important to note that detecting viral material by PCR does not indicate that the virus is fully intact and infectious, i.e. able to cause infection in other people."

> *You can't tell how much virus was present in your original sample and you can't tell if it is capable of infecting people.*

We need to know where the RNA for which the PCR tests are calibrated comes from.

As textbooks as well as leading virus researchers such as Luc Montagnier or Dominic Dwyer state, particle purification — i.e. the separation of an object from everything else that is not that object — is an essential pre-requisite for proving the existence of a virus, and thus to prove that the RNA from the particle in question comes from a new virus. The reason for this is that PCR is extremely sensitive, which means it can detect even the smallest pieces of DNA or RNA — but it cannot determine *where these particles came from*. That has to be determined beforehand. And because the PCR tests are calibrated for gene sequences (in this case RNA sequences because SARS-CoV-2 is believed to be a RNA virus), we have to know that these gene snippets are part of the looked-for virus. And to know that, correct isolation and purification of the presumed virus has to be executed.

None of the studies with regard to the existence of SARS-CoV-2, or any other virus for that matter, have been able to confirm that the viruses they worked on had been purified. Most studies clearly stated the virus had not been purified.

> *In scientific terms, in reality, no virus has ever been isolated. Every paper claiming otherwise has been shown to make false assumptions with regards to the definition of 'isolation' and 'purification'. It is for this reason that the medical world and the health industry has switched to using the term 'identification'. However, if one has never isolated a virus, never seen the virus in its entirety, never been able to identify every part of an intact virus, one cannot identify any virus by one of its parts.*

Finding genetic material in any sample taken from anywhere can easily be done when one mixes the sample with cells, allows those cells to disintegrate and die and then pcr-test the mixture for a specific genetic coding. If you look long enough, if you repeat the test cycle often enough, you will find whatever genetic coding you are looking for. And when you find it you claim this to be the genetic material that was inside a virus. Claim, not prove. Then you claim that this virus causes the disease the sample giver is suffering from. Claim, not prove. And when it turns out that he is not ill at all, you claim he is still a danger to the rest of the population because he spreads the virus and the disease. Claim, not prove. Then you isolate him from other human beings and you claim this will protect others from catching the disease. Claim, not prove.

Seriously! This is so far removed from scientific methodology, scientific practice and scientific thinking that it is impossible to judge how far down the dark tunnel of manipulation and deceit the medical profession has already travelled. I am convinced that they can never find their way out of the tunnel anymore.

Truthful science-based-medicine would apologize to the people it cares for and it would scrap it, test-based-medicine, immediately. Science is observation and, hence, science-based-medicine would in the first place observe and not interfere. It would observe the individual, as a whole. It would observe the pathway of health within the individual, his balance in health, as time passes by. It would observe the individual requirements for supporting the system to maintain its balance. Its actions would remain limited to simple, individual and moment based changes in behaviour. It would mean the end of 'the war': war against cancer, war against dementia, war against super-bugs, war against obesity, and so on. It would mean the end of the war industry that provides huge profits for owners and investors. When health is no longer a war, is no longer a fight one has to fight in order to survive, there is no more money to be made in healthcare.

Please follow these simple rules if you want to base your healthcare on science.

- Gather data by observing the natural trail from illness back to health.

- When formulating a theory about possible causes of a disease incorporate accepted scientific energy theories.

- When testing the theory understand that testing can only disprove the theory and that a positive test result does not prove that the theory is absolutely right.

- When a theory is proven to be wrong then discard it and share this information with everybody.

MEASLES GOES TO COURT

The previous article leads nicely in to how medical testing has been used to push a perception within the medical profession and the general public.

On November 24th, 2011 Dr Stephan Lanka offered a prize of €100,000 for a scientific publication in which the alleged 'measles virus' could be proven to exist. *"The reward will be paid, if a scientific publication is presented, in which the existence of the measles virus is not only asserted, but also proven and in which, among other things, the diameter of the measles virus is determined."*

On January 2012, Dr. David Bardens took Dr. Lanka up on his challenge and put forward six papers to show in his opinion the existence of the alleged measles virus.

Here is s short summary from researcher Tracy Northern, (a link at the end of the book to her many years of research) who translated Dr Lanka's article from German to English. It is important to know the difference between putting data forward, six papers, to propose the existence of a measles virus and actually isolating the alleged virus itself, measuring it and showing via Koch Postulates it can cause disease. If a measles virus actually does exist then the obvious first thing to do would be to isolate it from everything else and say, look guy's here it is! Initially at The court of judgement, the regional court (LG) Ravensburg, Dr Lanka describes the presiding judge Matthias Schneider as coming under pressure and panicking.

"By overstretching law and statute and ignoring all the facts presented in writing, Judge Schneider came in on March 12, 2015, in the first part of the oral hearing, before the expert's approval and before the further steps of civil proceedings, prescribed a so-called 'chair judgment'. Chair judgments are judgments given without the otherwise specified necessary time

for reflection by the court and the parties. In civil law, chair judgments may only be made in cases of very simple and unambiguous facts".

"By this ruling, the Ravensburg Regional Court prevented me from being able to refute the statements of the court-appointed expert after their legally regulated submission of evidence at the oral hearing by means of the prepared documentation, which the court had been informed of by my lawyers. The rebuttal came therefore later at a heavy cost using the appeal procedure before the Stuttgart Higher Regional Court. If I hadn't raised and deposited a huge sum of money (over €150,000) necessary for an appeal within a very short time, it would not have come to the appeal proceedings and to the Court of Justice. It is difficult to get justice in Germany without lots of money"

"With the ambush-style "chair judgment" being given the LG Ravensburg prevented any possibility of: "The parties negotiating contentiously over the evidence" as it is wrongly written in the minutes of the hearing, without proper hearing of evidence having been carried out and concluded and without the plaintiff's subsidiary action having been negotiated. The plaintiff claimed I should pay him € 492.54 plus interest, without the alleged charge being judicially established or heard. With the rushed, inadmissible chair judgment (the assessor and clerk of the court asked decisive questions that refuted the expert during the expert testimony) Judge Schneider prevented me from submitting my prepared refutations to the expert's testimony"

*"**As** a precaution, at the beginning of the hearing, the presiding judge Matthias Schneider forbade me to ask the expert questions myself. The judge knew that I had scientifically published expertise in the field of virology to be presented and that the judicial reviewer who was not a specialist in the field had no knowledge of any scientifically published expertise in the field of virology. The judge sentenced me to pay the prize money of €100,000 plus a high rate of interest, all expenses and*

high appraisal costs. The judge also ruled that the plaintiff could claim these sums even if I appeal. The plaintiff did this immediately and with maximum possible effort. He even applied for an arrest warrant for me and publicly, untruthfully claimed that it had become effective. The plaintiff himself did not provide the security required by law to demand a provisionally enforceable judgment. This "gross misjudgement" by the Ravensburg Regional Court was overturned on February 16, 2016 due to my successful appeal at the Stuttgart Higher Regional Court. To date (February 28, 2017: as of going to press), the plaintiff has not released the €121,000 I paid and has not paid the legal, court or expert fees, even though the judgment of the Higher Regional Court Stuttgart of February 16, 2016 became final with the decision of BGH on December 1st, 2016"

The Bundesgerichtshof lets the belief in viruses perish.

"In the five-year measles virus trial, the Federal Court of Justice in Karlsruhe confirmed the sensational judgment of the Stuttgart Higher Regional Court of February 16, 2016 on December 1, 2016. As of December 1, 2016, the highest court ruling in Germany stipulates that all claims regarding the infection called measles, measles vaccinations and the measles virus have no scientific basis."

The legally appointed expert Professor Podbielski in court stated, "Thus, at this point, a publication about the existence of the measles virus that stands the test of good science has yet to be delivered."

The trial showed clearly that the symptoms we call measles are in fact a process and not a *thing* caused by a disease causing agent called a virus. Did this change anything in the real world of medical science? Well clearly not. If they, the medical cabal, can't disprove your evidence then they think it best to simply ignore it.

Measles Testing

The case clearly showed the lack of proof of an actual measles virus. So it seems that all along the idea of an infectious agent called a virus was at best a poor untested theory. When actually put to the test, even with modern technology, the isolation of an actual disease causing measles virus could not be demonstrated. Even with €100,000 at stake it could not be shown in a single paper that the said virus had been isolated and measured. Yet at the same time the testing for a measles virus, one that had never been found, was regularly done to prove a child was 'infected' or not.

Measles notifications (confirmed cases) England and Wales 1995-2013 by quarter. The table below shows only the cases confirmed by oral fluid IgM antibody tests and/or PCR in each quarter compared to the number of notified cases.

Year	Quarter	Uncorrected Notified Cases	Tested Number	%	Confirmed Number	%
2013*1	4th	535#	620	116.0%	17	2.7%
2013*1	3rd	872	770	88.3%	83	10.8%
2013*1	2nd	3167	2654	83.8%	402	15.1%
2013*	1st	2222	1369	61.6%	383	28.0%
2012*	4th	1664	944	56.7%	309	32.7%
2012	3rd	1307	873	66.8%	241	27.6%
2012	2nd	1192#	1454	121.9%	419	28.8%

2012	1st	982#	1277	130 %	168	13.2%
2011	4th	451#	627	139.0%	138	22.0%
2011	3rd	477#	610	127.8%	154	25.2%
2011	2nd	862#	1208	140.1%	346	28.6%
2011	1st	538#	722	134.2%	151	20.9%
2010	4th	370#	458	123.8%	31	6.8%
2010	3rd	579#	646	111.6%	134	20.7%
2010	2nd	736	641	87.1%	71	11.1%
2010	1st	543	452	83.2%	13	2.9%
2009	4th	519	398	76.7%	4	1.0%
200 9	3rd	830	558	62.2%	86	11.1%
2009	2nd	2113	1811	84.9%	482	26.6%
2009	1st	1781	1704	95.7%	304	17.8%

1 England only data

• Provisional

Oral fluid specimens were submitted early from suspected cases and may not have been subsequently notified, thus the proportion tested is artificially high in this quarter.

My notes: - Over a four-year period doctors notifications of measles which ended in a positive test with antibody or PCR method ranged from 1% to 32.7% with an average positive result of 17.68%. With antibody tests non-specific and PCR tests not able to detect a complete virus even if it existed, which has been clearly shown it does not, then it is easy to state that these test results are totally meaningless. But again, look at it from the medical point of view, believing these tests provide you with an objective diagnostic result, the only conclusion they could come to is that either doctors are mainly wrong in their guess or the test is very inaccurate. Either way, considering that these are the tests that are deciding if a child has a measles infection or not. If, by any chance, they determine a cluster of positive tests, which the medical profession can turn into an outbreak, they can then push out fear propaganda and pressure parents, who have chosen not to vaccinate, to change their minds to protect their child and others around them.

Another thing to mention is that the sensitivity of the tests can be prepared beforehand. This means that you could have an 'outbreak' of many positive tests, 'cases', depending on how the tests were calibrated. So if the sensitivity of the tests can be altered then that would leave it wide open to be used for political purposes if people were inclined to do so. Basically 'outbreaks' could be created at will. This is something well known by the medical profession themselves. With an almost infinite number of genetic sequences that could be used as primers in PCR tests the 'new variant' game being played out could go on as long as ignorance and fear control the population.

BBC NEWS 6 SEPT 2020

"Coronavirus: Tests 'could be picking up dead virus'

The main test used to diagnose coronavirus is so sensitive it could be picking up fragments of dead virus from old infections, scientists say.

Most people are infectious only for about a week, but could test positive weeks afterwards. Researchers say this could be leading to an over-estimate of the current scale of the pandemic. But some experts say it is uncertain how a reliable test can be produced that doesn't risk missing cases.

Prof Carl Heneghan, one of the study's authors, said instead of giving a "yes/no" result based on whether any virus is detected, tests should have a cut-off point so that very small amounts of virus do not trigger a positive result. He believes the detection of traces of old virus could partly explain why the number of cases is rising while hospital admissions remain stable.

Prof Peter Openshaw at Imperial College London said PCR was a highly sensitive "method of detecting residual viral genetic material".

Yes, even during 'The Pandemic' it was well known that adjusting the sensitivity of the test would result in more positive cases, whether people were ill or not. Yes, the only time in history when you were critically ill without showing any symptoms at all! It would then also be possible to make the test less sensitive to show a drop in cases with which this data could then be used to show any government measures to control the virus were working.

A 2019 Caixin Global article, *'Why Aren't People in China Dying of the Flu?'* may provide a clue:

In 2016 and 2017, China reported only 56 and 41 deaths respectively, according to NHC data. Meanwhile, the U.S. — which counts deaths by flu season, rather than year — saw an estimated 51,000 deaths in the 2016-2017 flu season, according to the country's Centers for Disease Control and Prevention (CDC).

One possible reason for China's unusually low flu death numbers is that health officials in the country depend on reports of deaths for their data, rather than the statistical modelling used by authorities elsewhere in the world.

The number of deaths provided by Chinese authorities this week is "likely to be reported deaths in patients with influenza, which will massively underestimate influenza deaths, because most patients in hospitals in China are not tested for influenza," Ben Cowling, a professor at the Hong Kong University School of Public Health, told Caixin. Additionally, not all cases may be reported to the authorities.

"I would predict that more than 100,000 people in China have died from influenza or the complications following influenza virus infection this winter," Cowling said, citing previous studies on flu mortality.

Additionally, doctors in China tend to attribute flu-related deaths to the underlying conditions or complications that make patients more vulnerable to the influenza virus, Rath Li Dongzeng, deputy director of the infectious disease center at Beijing You'an Hospital, told Caixin after the 2017 flu season that he believed it was inaccurate to attribute the deaths of patients to the flu if there were other factors at play, like pneumonia or heart disease, which occur commonly in high-risk groups.er than the flu itself.

Medical professionals have argued that not attributing deaths to influenza isn't just a question of statistics and may have a harmful real-world impact.

"The general perception that seasonal influenza does not cause substantial mortality in China may contribute to the underutilization of influenza vaccines in the country," according to a 2012 World Health Organization (WHO) bulletin authored by a team of Chinese and U.S. researchers.

The World Health Organization considers flu vaccines the most effective protection against severe bouts of the flu, and recommends annual vaccination by people at risk, including older and pregnant people, as well as young children.

But a relatively small percentage of the Chinese population gets vaccinated against the flu each year — only 2% in 2018, according to the state-run People's Daily. In contrast, around 44% of people in the U.S. were vaccinated against the flu by mid-November 2018, according to the CDC.

So here we can see a theme that is present throughout the

book: how can we define an illness? Can we define an illness by the microorganism or an alleged viral particle present even if it is found in healthy people? This is the biggest question the medical profession and medical science choose not to look at. As you can see, defining an illness will bring statistics to life.

Does China really have low influenza rates? If so, why? Does the western world really have high influenza rates and if so, why? With high uptake on influenza vaccines why does the West still have high rates of mortality? With low influenza vaccine rates why does China have low mortality? Why does China take into account underlying conditions more so than the West? Who is right and who is wrong? It is well documented that the main factors in pneumonia are poverty, air pollution, malnutrition, poor sanitation and that the gap between rich and poor countries is great. Surprisingly, China comes out low in the countries with mortality from pneumonia and especially influenza.

Data from an article from the *BMJ, PETER DOSHI, DEC 10 2005:*

USA 2001 62,034 DEATHS FROM COMBINED PNEUMONIA AND FLU

61,777-PNEUMONIA

257-FLU

ONLY 18 OF WHICH WERE CLINICALLY TESTED AS POSITIVE FOR INFLUENZA VIRUS

USA 1979-2001 AVERAGE OF 1,348 FLU ONLY DEATHS (257-3006)

So, again, we have all the mass hysteria about getting your annual flu jab, yet hardly anyone seems to be dying of it. It being the alleged influenza viral particles they claim are in circulation and causing the symptoms seen, named as flu. Similar to the measles data you would think the medical profession would look at the test results and come to the conclusion flu is not really an issue in the US. If in the US the death rate from influenza is low then why in other papers is it said to be high and everyone needs the jab to protect themselves. And why is it that the rates in China are low yet it is really high, but they don't really know either way. Confusion seems to be the accepted norm by the scientific community and they don't seem to be questioning the obvious: what are the environmental and social circumstances surrounding an outbreak of flu like illness. The issue of testing is covered by Patrick Quanten in the chapter *'Testing in the Medical World'*. Here though this is just an example of how tests can mean many things, all things, contradicting each other and meaning nothing all at. It all depends on how you look at the tests and what you are testing for. All this at a time when we are constantly told that our glorious leaders are using the 'best available science'.

Just to repeat words from Patrick Quanten to remind us

- PCR test.

- *PCR test does not identify viruses*

- *PCR test has not been standardised and results are therefore not comparable.*

- *The origin of the detected genetic material has not been established.*

When it was clear Koch's Postulates could not be used for viruses new criteria were put in place.

Here are Koch's Postulates for the 21st century as suggested by Fredricks and Relman:

Fredericks DN,& Relman DA (1996). Sequence-based identification of microbial pathogens: a reconsideration of Koch's Postulates.

- *A nucleic acid sequence belonging to a putative pathogen should be present in most cases of an infectious disease. Microbial nucleic acids should be found preferentially in those organs or gross anatomic sites known to be diseased, and not in those organs that lack pathology.*

- *Fewer, or no, copy numbers of pathogen-associated nucleic acid sequences should occur in hosts or tissues without disease.*

- *With resolution of disease, the copy number of pathogen-associated nucleic acid sequences should decrease or become undetectable. With clinical relapse, the opposite should occur.*

- *When sequence detection predates disease, or sequence copy number correlates with severity of disease or pathology, the sequence-disease association is more likely to be a causal relationship.*

- *The nature of the microorganism inferred from the available sequence should be consistent with the known biological characteristics of that group of organisms.*

- *Tissue-sequence correlates should be sought at the cellular level: efforts should be made to demonstrate specific in situ hybridization of microbial sequence to areas of tissue pathology and to visible microorganisms or to areas where microorganisms are presumed to be located.*

- *These sequence-based forms of evidence for microbial causation should be reproducible.*

With that criteria and the knowledge that many microbes and cell debris containing genetic sequences are found in healthy people, it would certainly be easy to come to any desired conclusion. The original criteria, Koch's Postulates, were very precise and clear. As they were aimed at demonstrating the presence of an organism, accused of causing diseases, which could be seen under a microscope, in a life form, it quickly became apparent whether or not the scientifically sound postulates confirmed or rebutted the accusation. When one makes the same scientifically sound rules for 'organisms' that cannot be demonstrated in any scientific way, then it becomes easy to create an illusion of 'demonstration'. The only task for the ruling authority would then be to convince their public, mesmerize them, with the brilliance of their magic show. Make the illusion seem real, and one has total power over the minds of the audience. They see what you want them to see. They believe what you want them to believe. Then there is no further need for truth investigation, as 'the truth' is known by *everybody*.

"If the 'germ theory of disease' were correct, there'd be no one living to believe it."

– Bartlett, Joshua Palmer, 1882-1961, father of chiropractic

VACCINATION ON TRIAL

Is it safe and is it effective?

"Vaccination is a barbarous practice and one of the most fatal of all the delusions current in our time. Conscientious objectors to vaccination should stand alone, if need be, against the whole world, in defence of their conviction."

– Mahatma Ghandi

"When people ask me what are the great threats to civilisation, it's true that very unlikely things like asteroid impacts, there are those threats out there in the universe, but really I think the biggest threat to our civilisation at the moment is the disconnect in democratic societies between facts or data and the understanding of our electorates." Cox said the anti-vaccination movement *"baffled"* him. *"In terms of vaccination, one of the great human achievements was the eradication of smallpox through a worldwide co-ordinated vaccination programme. It's probably one of the greatest achievements of modern civilisation. It killed hundreds of thousands, even millions of people throughout Europe and beyond, and it went gone. But it's clear that these childhood diseases that we've largely controlled or eradicated are going to begin rise back again if we, as a society, don't properly vaccinate our children. It's a huge risk."*

– Professor Brian Cox

Two very different views on vaccination.

I would be very interested in knowing if Brian Cox, the glamour boy of modern science, has ever seen the data that follows. If he did, would he change his mind? He is a scientist after all, and it is the data that decides the truth, allegedly.

We are told:

Vaccination simulates disease

Stimulates the immune system

Creates antibodies that protect us

Saved us from infectious disease

Wiped out smallpox

Are safe and the benefits outweigh the small risk

Unvaccinated = no protection and herd immunity protects the weak

Reality

Vaccination in no way simulates disease as it has never been proven that invading microbes are the cause of infectious disease. Germ Theory is still just that, a theory. In fact as we now know it's a disproven theory. We know disease is a process that can be triggered by many factors and is not the same for every individual, and that it is a process initiated by the body to cleanse itself from a build-up of waste, toxaemia. *Disease is a process and not a thing.* Rather than stimulate the immune system, (cleansing and rebalancing system) vaccination actually bypasses over 80% of that system, the digestive tract, gut flora and internal membranes, and poisons the rest with access to the internal organs, blood and brain.

Antibodies are no indication of protection; they are not specific to a particular pathogen or toxin, therefore tests can be inaccurate at best. It is not clear whether the test means you are *infected* or *protected* using their own science but in reality we now know it means neither. Indeed Dr Clements of the World Health Organisation and Expanded Programme on Immunisation, in a reply to Trevor Gunn on behalf of The Informed Parent in 1995, agreed, *"there is not a precise relationship between seroresponse* (antibody production) *and protection"*. He was replying to the fact that Trevor pointed out that people with high levels of antibodies could be seen to be ill and yet people with low or no traceable antibodies could remain healthy. Also a blood antibody response could be the sign of a poor functioning system as it could mean the body, and especially the digestive tract, is not dealing with waste and toxicity well and it is leaking deeper into the system. So by promoting the production of antibodies, it seems we are promoting the body to function in a way known to be of someone who has poor natural immune functioning.

External antibodies like those produced to protect people allergic to pollen, are not the body going wrong or an overactive immune system, surely it is the body saying that for some reason, "I don't like this, it's getting inside me and affecting me, hence I'm going to stop (mark it) it on arrival." So, blood antibodies, it seems, are produced by the body when toxicity becomes internalised. Surely it would be better to ask why that is happening. Why, though, is not a question allopathic thinking allows.

When they say a vaccine is 95% effective what they mean is in tests, mainly in the lab, a certain vaccine produced an *immune response*, an antibody reaction, 95% of the time, and as antibodies are not specific, how can you be sure as to which ingredient in the vaccine the body is reacting to? Remember, adjuvants are used in vaccines to actually get the immune system to respond, and again, as above, we know antibodies do not equate to *protection*. This statistic cannot be used to promote effectiveness in a real disease situation, it is completely irrelevant. Yes, the whole basis of their vaccination programme, *antibodies protect us*, is flawed and they know it, yet they continue with this regardless.

The graphs and letters at the end of this chapter show us vaccination never saved us from infectious disease; things like clean water and sanitation and better living conditions should take all the glory, and not Big Pharma, again supporting Soil Theory.

The smallpox death rate increased dramatically, with compulsory vaccination in the mid-1800s, then dropped off again with all infectious disease worldwide. Indeed, as Trevor Gunn mentions, symptoms of smallpox are still found in the world today under other names like monkey pox. I even remember a couple of years ago a mainstream newspaper stating a case of monkey pox in England and it being "like smallpox". Also in 1885, the people of Leicester in England came out protesting the compulsory smallpox vaccine they believed was causing damage and killing people. An estimated 100,000 people from the city and the surrounding areas went out in the streets and successfully over turned the strict compulsory vaccine law. The city introduced strict public hygiene measures and isolation of the sick, not the healthy.

With the massive fall in vaccination and the introduction of these new measures the whole world sat back and waited for a disaster to unfold. It didn't happen and in fact when other areas were still having large outbreaks and deaths with almost total vaccination rates, Leicester saw their death rate drop dramatically. Strange coincidence that Leicester was the first city in England on a regional lockdown. I think some people have long memories.This information has been kept alive in the book, *Dissolving Illusions: Disease, Vaccines, and The Forgotten History*. Suzanne Humphries MD and Roman Bystrianyk.

Here is the data deemed correct by the Dept of Health in the UK:

> *"In England free smallpox vaccines were introduced in 1840 and made compulsory in 1853. Between 1857 and 1859 there were 14,244 deaths from smallpox. Between 1863 and 1865 after a population rise of 7% the death rate rose by 40.8% to 20,059. In 1867 evaders of vaccination were prosecuted. Those left unvaccinated were very few. Between 1870 and 1872 after a population rise of 9% the death rate rose by 123% to 44,840."*

Did vaccines save us from smallpox? Make up your own mind.

In the 1868 book *Essay on Vaccination* by Dr Charles T. Pearce, you will see another version of the history surrounding the smallpox vaccine and its alleged success.
https://www.informedparent.co.uk/wp-content/uploads/2017/11/1868-The-Vaccination-An-Essay-Dr-Pearce.pdf

> *"Yet the Report of the Committee of the House of Commons on Jenner's discovery—on which report the money grant was made to Jenner—stated, upon the evidence given,*
>
> *1st. That vaccination effectually secured the patient from small-pox.*
>
> *2nd. That it never was followed by eruptions.*
>
> *3rd. That it had never been known to be fatal.*
>
> *Every one of these assertions has been falsified. It is evident that conclusions were too hastily drawn. So fatal had been the epidemic, that a panic had seized the Parliament and the people, and then upon insufficient evidence a medical theory was established and bought most dearly by Parliament. The highest medical authorities of that day, either denounced the theory and practice of vaccination, or declined to give their assent."*

Sounds familiar when you look at government policies today and the lack of science backing them up.

Since the start of the Vaccine Damage Fund on 22nd March 1979, until 30th April 2017, the scheme in the UK has paid out **£74,130,000**. In the US the sum amounts to billions of dollars and worldwide we can only guess at a lot more. You have to be at least 60% disabled and a child/baby has to be two years or older for the parent to apply, hence any damage done at a younger age when you would think the baby's system would be more fragile and less able to deal with the toxins, does not count or at least will be very difficult to prove way after the fact. A one-off £120,000 is awarded, a pittance for a destroyed life, and this award can even affect any other benefits you may have.

With ingredients like formaldehyde, antibiotics, aluminium which is well-known to be neurotoxic, mercury-based thimerosal, animal products, human foetal cells and more, it does not take a genius to see that this can't end well. It has been well stated that the number of children actually damaged or killed by vaccines is massively underestimated due to lack of studies and nobody knows the true figure; it could be the tip of a very big iceberg.

The book, 'Vaccination - 100 years of Orthodox Research Shows that Vaccines Represent a Medical Assault on the Immune System' by Viera Scheibner Ph.D. is now hard to find even on Amazon books. She showed many studies demonstrating a direct connection between vaccines and Shaken Baby Syndrome. The original link to her website is now being used by another business and her work is hard to find. What exactly is being hid?

To say vaccines are safe is simply not true. Vaccine damage payments clearly show things do go wrong and as it is the governments themselves who pay out the damages, and that itself comes from taxpayer money so we end up paying ourselves as a society for the damage done by vaccine companies. Not a bad earner if you can get it. All the profits with none of the liabilities and this policy is also going to protect the new coronavirus vaccine makers from any damages caused even though they are being pushed to rush out a vaccine in record time.

The Sunday Times, 24/10/10: "40 deaths linked to child vaccines over seven years."

Express, 30/12/12: "ten deaths linked to having flu jab." For 2011.

Even when proven to have been damaged, some people still don't get the payment.

> *"Imagine taking your healthy previously unvaccinated toddler for the MMR to see her suffer fits and never recover. Jodie is now 25 and is 80% disabled; her brain damage means that she is non-verbal and her epilepsy has caused daily fits. Years after the injury the medical records revealed that actually 8 vaccines were given, 5 without consent or knowledge. The complexity, legal aid issues and the mix up with the Vaccine damage payment unit means that the family have never been compensated."*

-Justice for Jodie Appeal via arnica.co.uk

If vaccines are safe why does the WHO have a vaccine safety summit?

As for the benefits, well, this letter from the WHO should explain a lot.

Trevor Gunn, a self-employed homeopath working free for *'The Informed Parent'*, a non-profit subscription magazine, asked for evidence of successful vaccine campaigns regarding measles. He was sent half a dozen studies or so from the developing world, not the developed world interestingly enough, and after *'diligence'* in his examination, exposing all the flaws in the reports, this was his reply.

For a full history of this letter and another great book for vaccines read *'Vaccines - This Book Could Remove Your Fear of Childhood Illness '*– Trevor Gunn

10 February 1998

Dear Mr Gunn

Thank you for your long letter dated 16 January. May I compliment you on your careful and expansive response to my earlier letter. I very much respect your diligence at looking at

the literature and carefully considering the issues.

You ask many questions in the text of your letter which would entail a considerable amount of work on my part to answer. While of great interest to you and me, I am not sure that really benefits lay audiences. The point is that the Expanded Programme on Immunisation continues to believe in the value of child immunisations as being of overwhelming value to the human race. Until the unlikely moment we have developed perfect vaccines administered by perfect vaccinators there will remain problems from time to time. But these problems in no way mitigate against the widespread use of the vaccines. Nonetheless, national policy makers must make wise (and often difficult) decisions on what vaccines to include in the national schedule.

I do not feel that it is the right medium to embark on a scientific point-by-point defence of vaccines. My concession to this is to add that Vitamin A administration with immunisation is part of EPI's policy.

Yours sincerely

Dr C J Clements

Medical Officer, Expanded Programme on Immunisation

So the man at the head of the WHO immunisation programme and with unlimited resources didn't have the time to answer the questions raised. He said the issues raised would not *'really benefit lay audiences'*, meaning the fact that he can't stand up to the challenge of showing vaccines prevent measles is not something you and me need to know about.

He states the WHO *'continues to believe in the value of child immunisations as being of overwhelming value to the human race'*. This confirms that vaccination benefiting mankind is a belief system and not a scientifically proven fact.

As Trevor highlighted Vitamin A deficiency as a factor in the severity of measles, they agree to *'add that Vitamin A administration with immunisation is part of EPI's policy.'* So knowing this, how, when a measles vaccination campaign is underway, would you know if any benefit was due to the supplement or the vaccine? What do you think will take the credit?

It turns out that despite its claims and when challenged medical science cannot show one single successful vaccine campaign EVER, or simply they don't have the time and we should just take their word for it. This is where people will have to do deep study, look at their own lives and the way they function and make up their own minds about wanting to prevent a disease or stop a disease process. How much of their thinking is driven by fear, lack of knowledge or laziness, or a combination of all, and how much of that they are projecting onto other people? How much of a benefit is it to try and *prevent* an illness if in doing so it builds up more problems for the future? How much of a benefit is it to kill the mosquito to avoid malaria if the consequences are other diseases like polio? How much of a benefit is it to your own growth if you are always giving your decision making to 'experts' in white coats?

As for unvaccinated meaning 'unprotected', again, we have to go back to germ theory and ask ourselves, protected from what? Look up the story of the 'Hopewood Children' in Australia who were raised in a purely natural way without drugs or vaccines. The drop in disease due to clean water and sanitation shows clearly that 'protection' is not needed and in fact just a focus on health is all that is needed to promote health in individuals and communities.

As for 'herd immunity', well, that is a relatively new term and based on germ theory which we now know is wrong It is based on killing the microbe or alleged virus and then not giving it space to survive and reproduce so that it just dies out and therefore can never come back. They say 95% herd immunity is needed for this to happen but as Patrick Quanten has pointed out, does the enemy suddenly give up with only 5% space left to live in? Of course not, and as we know viruses are not alive anyway. Life always tries to continue and to survive. Their scientific theories do not even make sense with their own germ theory of disease.

And we know that even full 'herd immunity' (if it existed) doesn't even seem to work.

"Whooping cough outbreak closes Texas school despite 100-percent vaccination rate: officials."

– 19th December, 2019, Fox News

If we need vaccine-induced herd immunity to protect us, how on earth are the human race and all the domestic animals now being vaccinated, still alive? Remember, modern vaccines are a relatively new invention. So if, again, the origin of germs and viruses is within our own tissues, then the idea of wiping a disease out so there is not one trace of it or even one microbe left is nonsense. As it is the conditions we live in that create disease and diseased tissues create germs from within them to clear up the waste, and viruses are just part of that waste. The idea of fighting disease is a war that can never be won, does not need to be fought and will not end well.

In an interview I did with Dr Patrick Quanten on the history of vaccination and infections (YouTube Dr Patrick Quanten UK Column Interview live) we talk about immunity in connection to childhood illness. Meaning, if childhood illness is about development, then going through that process and allowing it to happen, not suppressing it, and allowing the changes to be made, the child will then become *'immune'*. Not immune from a microbial or viral attack but simply immune in the sense of not needing to go through that development process again. The body really does know what it is doing.

Herd immunity in the end is unscientific emotional blackmail and an easy way to turn people who are pro-vaccination against those who choose not to. It is claimed those who don't vaccinate put those who can't, and in some cases even those who do, at risk. Basically they are throwing their fears onto other people, a bit like the mask wearers and social distance people of today.

If vaccines protect and you are vaccinated then why attack those who don't? If vaccines are so safe then why are certain people with health issues not allowed to vaccinate?

Boosters

As Patrick points out, a vaccine is a toxic injection into the body; the body then has to prioritise the clearing-out of the toxins so any development stage (childhood illness) that the child is ready for, has to be delayed until the toxins are cleared. For allopathic doctors this means a period of 'vaccine protection'. When the toxins are cleared out the body now has enough energy and can look to go through a development stage (childhood illness). He/she is now 'susceptible' in the eyes of medical doctors but in the eyes of a holistic practitioner he/she is now ready for the next development stage. So the medical profession gives a booster, toxic injection, which then the body has to prioritise so the development stage is again put on hold. Again, in the eyes of the doctor this means a period of 'protection' due to the vaccine's success in protecting from a virus/bacteria, simply because no illness is recorded, when in fact, according to Patrick Quanten and others, the development stage is again delayed to clear out the toxins. Then when a child is older and has had all the boosters, he/she may then get an illness he/she should have had when they were five or six, and as we know, these illness seem to be more severe in older children or young adults.

Nits and worms have also been known for a long time to be connected to cleaning up the system after some kind of development which has left behind waste. The waste being pushed through the scalp would provide food for the nits and in turn they help clean up the waste.

The same could be said for worms. Where did they come from? What are they feeding on? Where and why do they seem to just go on their own? Again, why does this seem to be only in young children?

Pick your own truth. Vaccines protect from childhood illness or vaccines delay illness? Vaccines give immunity or vaccines delay immunity? Immunity is protection from a pathogen or prevention of the proliferation of certain microbes due to the terrain? The benefits are worth the risk? The choice is an individual one and not one to be chosen by society as a whole? I'm a victim or I'm in control?

Possible scenario

With the information that has been put forward now about the nature of disease and symptoms, imagine a young child having some vaccines. We know it is an injection that delivers toxins internally into the system of that child. The child then has to deal with those toxins and excrete them from the body. Maybe a day later, a week later, a month or longer the child develops a fever. The mother panics as the child seems unwell and is afraid of the high fever. In panic she gives the child Calpol which is an over-the-counter drug. The fever drops and all seems well again.

What has actually just happened? Even mainstream medicine is now accepting the benefits of fever in cleansing out the system.

The NICE guidelines state: *"Do not use antipyretic agents with the sole aim of reducing body temperature in children with fever."* And to put to rest the dreaded fear of febrile convulsions: *"Antipyretic agents do not prevent febrile convulsions and should not be used specifically for this purpose."*

The truth is, no one would know why a child has a fever, but if the child has had a vaccine it would be perfectly logical that in the near future a fever could be used to cleanse out the toxins. The problem is allopathic thinking sees this as a side effect whereas holistic thinking sees this as an intelligent reaction. But again, using critical thinking, if the body was cleansing itself of the toxins but that cleansing was suppressed, what could be the possible consequences?

Dr Jane Donegan, in her articles in *The Informed Parent*, has written about many patients with meningitis who have had previous fever suppressions. http://www.jayne-donegan.co.uk/

Does it seem possible to you that by stopping the process of fever, the toxins are just pushed further internally and the outcome may be meningitis? And the big question. Are our decisions driven by fear or logic?

Data not widely published

The following are graphs, Dept. of Health's own graphs, I copied out of the booklet 'Comparing Natural Immunity with Vaccination' by Trevor Gunn and sent to the Dept. of Health through my MP. Knowing the protocol is they have to reply if it comes through your MP, I decided it was the best way to get confirmation that the graphs were known to be correct. Obviously Trevor Gunn knew they were correct but I had to be sure myself and wanted proof that they knew too.

Here are copies of the graphs; sorry for the quality but it is the data that is important, and the three replies I got from the Dept. of Health. I say data not widely published but I can tell you I have not spoken to any medical professional yet, apart from Patrick Quanten, who is aware of the following data.
Decide for yourself whether it is 'relevant' or not.

Unclear dates on graphs

Diphtheria Notifications: 0-1200, Date: 1950-1988, Death Rate: 0-1000, Date: 1866-1969

Whooping Cough Notifications: 0-200,000, Date: 1950-1985

Scarlet Fever Death Rate: 0-2500, Date: 1866-1969

135

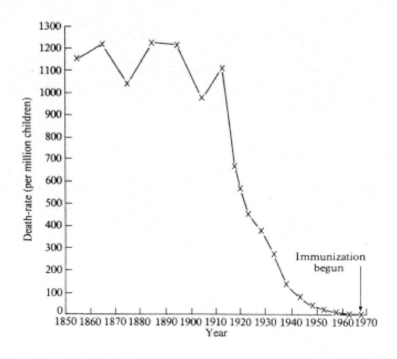

Measles

This is an example of a graph that doctors will **not** get in their 'Green Book'. It is a very powerful graph showing a very clear story. How could you imagine that this graph would not be considered "relevant" by the authorities? How has it even been possible to keep this graph away from public view and even doctors themselves? The fact that it has, really does show how controlled information is in this world. This graph, if released, could end the fear of measles and the risk of not vaccinating in one day. Do you think anybody would actually risk their child's health with a vaccine based on this alleged risk? Do you believe the same authorities who are hiding this information will be telling you the truth about 'The Pandemic'?

It is not for me to tell anyone what conclusions to come to or who to trust but it should be very clear that we are not being told the whole truth.

136

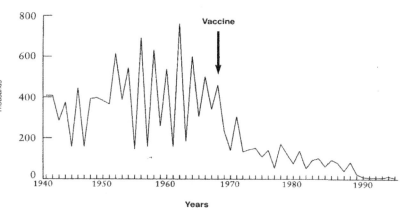

Notifications of Measles to ONS
England and Wales (1940-1995)

Notice the difference between when the death rate figures start and the notifications. Strange that most graphs they make public, the notifications start just before the time of the vaccine programmes. They claim they didn't have good information of notifications before that date but they did, though, have good data on deaths. Remember, as Patrick Quanten mentions in the interviews, notifications are really just a guess and even alleged confirmed cases are still not really an accurate figure. People dying, though, with certain symptoms, gives us a clearer picture of the health of the population in dealing with certain illnesses/disease processes. Getting an illness or 'testing positive' is one thing and doesn't really mean anything too worrying is going on, people dying on the other hand, would be a worry and require more investigation.

Imagine yourself as a doctor at medical school and looking at those graphs of notifications; it would surely give you the impression that vaccination is a valuable tool in preventing disease. But when you then look at the deaths the picture certainly changes and would clearly give the impression that something other than vaccines caused a massive drop in disease BEFORE vaccine programmes. Look at scarlet fever, once the biggest child killer fell to ZERO with no vaccine programme at all.

137

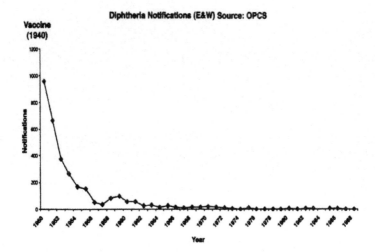

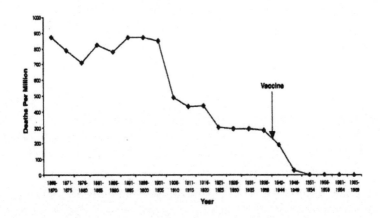

Diphtheria

Top – notifications; bottom – deaths

138

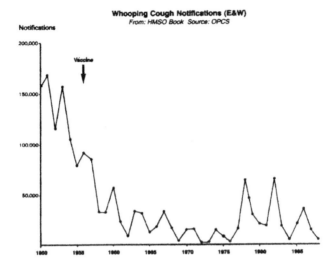

Whooping Cough Notifications (E&W)
From: HMSO Book Source: OPCS

Notifications

200,000

Vaccine

150,000

100,000

50,000

1850   1855   1860   1865   1870   1875   1980   1985

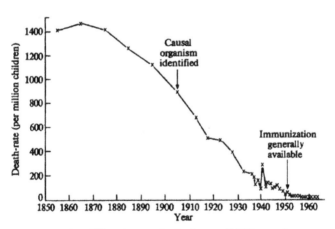

FIGURE 8.12. Whooping cough: death rates of children under 15: England and Wales.

Whooping cough

Top – notifications; bottom – deaths

139

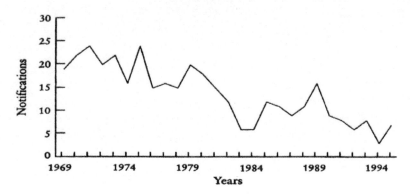

Tetanus notification to ONS
England and Wales (1969-1995)

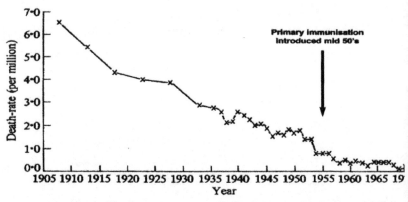

FIGURE 8.11. Tetanus: mean annual death rates: England and Wales

Tetanus:

Top – notifications; bottom – deaths

140

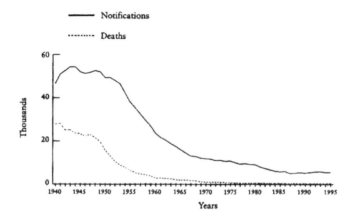

Notifications of tuberculosis and deaths to ONS
England and Wales (1940-1995)

——— Notifications

········ Deaths

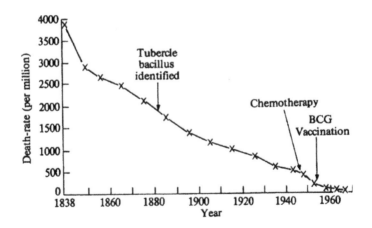

Respiratory tuberculosis: mean annual death-rates E&W.

Tuberculosis

141

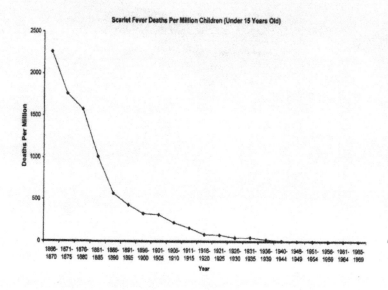

Above is the graph for scarlet fever, once the biggest child killer, falling to zero with no vaccine programme at all.

Fraud

> "A false representation of a matter of facts whether by words or conduct, by false or misleading allegations, or by concealment of what should have been disclosed-that deceives and is intended to deceive another so that the individual will act upon it to her or his legal injury."

Below are the two letters I received from Jane Ellison MP, the Parliamentary Undersecretary of State for Public Health at the time, regarding my questions about vaccines and cancer. Apologies for the quality, but I wanted to use the original copies.

Department
of Health

From Jane ENson MP
Parliamentary Under Secretary of State for Public Health

Your Ref: 14/18.1/ag/ew

PO00000841071

Richmond House
79 Whitehall
London
SW1A 2NS

Tel: 020 7210 4850

Andrew George MP
Trewolla
18 Mennaye Road
Penzance TR18 4NG

0 6 MAR 2014

Dear Andrew

Thank you for your letter of 6 February on behalf of your constituent about the publication *Comparing Natural Immunity with Vaccination* by Trevor Gunn.

Public Health England (PHE), the national organisation for the improvement of public health outcomes, has provided the following information.

As Mr Ryder may be aware, the Government is advised on all immunisation matters by the Joint Committee on Vaccination and Immunisation (JCVI), which is an independent Departmental Expert Committee and a statutory body. In providing advice and making recommendations, it considers all currently available relevant evidence, including both published and unpublished information from a variety of sources. These sources include, but are not limited to, publications by scientists in peer-reviewed journals, opinion of experts in the field and information provided by vaccine manufacturers. Data from the Office for National Statistics, some of which are unpublished, may also be reviewed. The recommendations of the JCVI are translated into guidelines for best practice which are published in the 'Green Book' *Immunisation against infectious disease*, a PHE publication.

Comparing Natural Immunity with Vaccination is the opinion of one individual and is not a peer-reviewed publication. It would not be considered as a reliable source of information for consideration by the JCVI. The JCVI takes into account reliable data on disease and death as a result of vaccine-preventable infectious diseases. These data are provided by surveillance schemes such as those run by PHE. More information on these surveillance schemes and links to reports and data can be found on the website www.hpa.org.uk by selecting 'topics A-Z' and then 'vaccinations'.

Such data are considered when JCVI decisions are made and used to develop information which appears in the Green Book.

Mr Gunn criticises a solely orthodox medical approach to health and illness and suggests that there are other ways in which serious disease can be avoided. Unfortunately, the data in the publication, which   included in his letter, only show death rates in England and Wales. By failing to consider the effects of vaccination on the impact of serious disease (as well as death), these graphs do not give an accurate picture of the impact of immunisation on public health.

The very large decreases in death rates in England and Wales that are shown in the figures since the late 1800s may be due to a variety of factors, including improved sanitation and a better understanding of the ways in which transmission of infectious diseases can be prevented. There is no evidence to suggest that the transient increase in death rates due to smallpox in the 1870s was causally related to the introduction of the vaccine. The introduction of the smallpox vaccine had a dramatic effect on the incidence of disease and death worldwide and resulted in the World Health Organization announcing in 1980 that smallpox had officially been eradicated.

With regard to issues of consent, immunisation in the United Kingdom is based on informed consent. Consent must be obtained before starting any treatment or physical investigation or before providing personal care for a patient. This includes the administration of all vaccines.

The NHS Choices website states that *for consent to be valid, it must be voluntary and informed, and the person consenting must have the capacity to make the decision"* and that *the person must be given full information about what the treatment involves, including the benefits and risks, whether there are reasonable alternative treatments, and what will happen if treatment does not go ahead.*

PHE provides a range of leaflets, newsletters and other sources of information which are freely available and which enable people to make informed decisions about accepting medical treatment, including vaccination. In addition, healthcare workers discuss the possible implications of treatment (both positive and negative) with individuals prior to that treatment being given.

Finally, the JCVI, PHE and the Department of Health only consider issues which affect human, not animal, health and so I am unable to comment on any possible relationship between immunisation programmes in people and vaccination of badgers as a means of controlling bovine TB. This issue is one for the Department for Environment, Food and Rural Affairs.   may therefore wish to contact that Department for more information. The contact details are:

Department
of Health

Department for Environment, Food and Rural Affairs
Nobel House
17 Smith Square
London SW1P 3JR

I hope this reply is helpful.

Kind regards
Jane

JANE ELLISON

Notes on letter

The government is advised by the JCVI in *"providing advice and making recommendations"* and *"considers all currently available relevant evidence"*, which is "translated into guidelines for best practice which are published in the Green Book immunisation against infectious disease".

So to be clear, the JCVI does not think it is *"relevant"* to publish to doctors the massive fall in death rate from infectious disease, total fall in case of scarlet fever, happening BEFORE vaccine programmes. They say that the book which I used to quote the data, *Comparing Natural Immunity with Vaccination* by Trevor Gunn, would *"not be considered a reliable source of information for consideration by the JCVI"*. But the source of the information is the ONS, a government organisation which takes data from the medical profession. So are they saying their own data is not reliable?

They also claim the JCVI would not consider it a reliable source of information. So the question is, have the JCVI even seen this data? Is it being deliberately withheld? Have they seen it but decided themselves it is not *"relevant"*? The source of the data is the Dept. of Health put together by the ONS.

Jane Ellison admits the *"very large decreases in death rate"* were due to *"a variety of factors including improved sanitation"*. And on seeing the smallpox data shown earlier with the rise with compulsory vaccines, she admitted there was a *"transient increase in death rate due to smallpox"* but it was not *"causally related to the introduction of the vaccine"*. So without any investigation it was just a coincidence. She stated, *"the introduction of the smallpox vaccine had a dramatic effect on the incidence of the disease and death worldwide"*. In this she is right but the dramatic effect was the dramatic rise in the death rate.

I have only used the England and Wales figures as those are the ones I can confirm with our own Dept. of Health but by reading the book '*Dissolving Illusions: Disease, Vaccines, and The Forgotten History*'. Suzanne Humphries MD and Roman Bystrianyk, you will be able to see other world figures showing the same story with a rise in death from smallpox with the vaccine.

Reading the book *Nature Cure* by Henry Lindllar you will see another version of the smallpox history and view of the 'famous freemason' hero Edward Jenner, and that it wasn't true that those milk maids who had cowpox were immune to smallpox; in fact it is another story similar to that other hero Louis Pasteur, in that a particular viewpoint was taken on board as truth despite having very little scientific basis and many scientists in their time not agreeing with their conclusions.

Surely to use the term 'vaccine preventable infectious disease' you would need to show they actually prevent it in the first place. The 'law of consent' is mentioned so she must be fully aware of what it entails.

Law of Consent

Consent from a patient is needed regardless of the procedure, whether it's a physical examination, organ donation or something else.

Defining consent

For consent to be valid, it must be voluntary and informed, and the person consenting must have the capacity to make the decision.

Voluntary – the decision to either consent or not to consent to treatment must be made by the person, and must not be influenced by pressure from medical staff, friends or family.

Informed – the person must be given all of the information about what the treatment involves, including the benefits and risks, whether there are reasonable alternative treatments, and what will happen if treatment does not go ahead.

Capacity – the person must be capable of giving consent, which means they understand the information given to them and can use it to make an informed decision.

Consent is not needed (in their opinion) when someone *"is a risk to public health as a result of rabies, cholera or T.B."* (Seems COVID-19 has just been added to that list.)

In your opinion are we being 'informed'? I personally don't think so, and after years of research I am actually shocked at how little doctors know about vaccines and their history.

Department of Health

Your Ref: 14/18.1/ag/cw

PO00000865738

Andrew George MP
Trewella
18 Mennaye Road
Penzance TR18 4NG

- 7 JUL 2014

From Jane Ellison MP
Parliamentary Under Secretary of State for Public Health

Richmond House
79 Whitehall
London
SW1A 2NS

Tel: 020 7210 4850

0 3 JUL 2014

Dear Andrew

Thank you for your letter of 4 June on behalf of your constituent Mr Robert Ryder of ▓▓▓▓▓▓▓▓▓▓▓▓▓▓▓▓▓ about immunisation.

Research from around the world shows that immunisation is the safest way to protect a child's health. The vaccinations included in the NHS routine childhood immunisation schedule have been recommended by experts, after consideration of a wide range of evidence, including evidence about efficacy and adverse reactions. The vaccines have undergone rigorous testing with large numbers of people before being licensed and their safety is continuously monitored to discover and assess any rare side effects. These recommended vaccines are among the safest medicines.

Immunisation protects children against diseases which, even today in developed countries, can cause serious long-term ill-health, including mental and/or physical disability, and even kill. The childhood immunisation programme in the UK has resulted in the incidence of childhood diseases being at very low levels.

In the UK, these diseases are kept at bay by high immunisation rates. Around the world, more than 15 million people a year die from infectious diseases. More than half of these are children under the age of five. Most of these deaths could be prevented by immunisation. As more people travel abroad and more people come to visit this country, there is a risk that they will bring these diseases into the UK. The diseases may spread to people who have not been immunised.

As set out in my previous reply (our ref: PO00000841071), the Government is advised on all immunisation matters by the Joint Committee on Vaccination and Immunisation (JCVI), and Mr Ryder, or you on his behalf, may therefore wish to contact it directly.

149

With regard to Mr Ryder's concerns about cancer, the Department of Health is fully committed to clinical and applied research into treatment and cures for cancer. The Department's National Institute for Health Research (NIHR) welcomes funding applications for research into any aspect of human health, including cancer. These applications are subject to peer review and judged in open competition, with awards being made on the basis of the scientific quality of the proposals made. The NIHR spends around £100million annually on cancer research.

In August 2011, the Department of Health announced the UK's largest ever investment, £800million, in 'early stage' health research that will fund advances in diagnosis, prevention and treatment, benefiting patients with diseases including cancer, diabetes and heart disease. Of the £800million, £61.5million is for the NIHR biomedical research unit in cancer, a partnership between the Royal Marsden Hospital and the Institute of Cancer Research.

I hope this reply is helpful.

Kind regards
Jane

JANE ELLISON

After just repeating the theme about vaccines, in the final letter Jane Ellison also addresses my concerns over cancer. It seems, as usual, the same reply of just totally ignoring any possible investments into natural therapies and as on other NHS pages, they just attack 'alternative' therapies or say there is no evidence. Well, if you don't look, you won't find. The truth is, cancer is a multi-billion-pound business and there are too many invested interests to risk anyone finding a cure, especially if that cure lay within the body of the individual. Like all diseases, cancer is a process and not a thing and by understanding how it advances we may come to understand how to reverse it. To do that, though, would take holistic thinking and a desire to give health and not make profit.

One thing for sure from looking at the data and seeing the letters, is that we are not being told the truth and in that case, how can the *law of consent* be applied?

Looking at *'the Coronavirus Act 2020'* you can see a clear attack on the law of consent. Even for a physical examination consent is needed but it seems the Coronavirus Act has taken that protection away completely, as we will see further on.

So where do we now stand exactly? Is a law that has been passed by a process and put in place to protect our natural rights under common law now not valid because of an alleged state of emergency? It does seem now that the word of one man, Boris Johnson, can overpower the laws of a nation; this is clearly a dictator's actions. So looking at the law, please now examine your experience when being asked to vaccinate or for that matter take any medical treatment or drug. Clearly by not giving us, or even doctors in their Green Book, all the evidence, then it is impossible for doctors to give out full information on the benefits of vaccines if they are given such a one-sided view. I would also surely doubt they are aware of the massive vaccine damage pay-outs and I have never known them to give alternatives.

Dr Jane Donegan was charged with serious professional misconduct after being accused by senior judge of using 'junk science' after she wrote two reports for a case heard in 2002 in the family division of the High Court, relating to two families who were unconnected but whose cases became linked in the courts. Although the courts lodged no complaint, the GMC began an investigation and announced that Dr Donegan would face a charge of serious professional misconduct. In 2007 after a three-week hearing in Manchester, the GMC panel concluded that all of the substantive charges against Dr Donegan were unproved except for the charge of quoting selectively from research. The panel declared, however, that *"it is normal practice in the preparation of reports to quote selectively from references, which indeed you did."*

Sheila Hewitt, who chaired the panel, told Dr Donegan: *"The panel were sure that at no stage did you allow any views that you held to overrule your duty to the court and the litigants. You demonstrated to the panel that your report did not derive from your deeply held views, and your evidence supported this."*

What was Dr Donegan's crime?

She backed the mothers' stance in opposing the MMR and other childhood immunisations.

In July 2023 the medical authorities finally won their war of terror against Dr Jane Donegan for allegedly giving one-sided views regarding vaccination to parents at her public lectures. A brave and defiant former Doctor Jane Donegan on being struck off declared it was a *"small price to pay for taking a lawful ethical stand for the safety of British children"* and claimed her tribunal hearing a *"politically motivated show trial"*.

Jane, along with Patrick Quanten, writes for 'The Informed Parent'.

The Informed Parent was founded by Magda Taylor who has done nearly 31 years of amazing research into the history of vaccines and infectious disease.

The Informed Parent was originally set up in September 1992 to counter frustration and isolation experienced by parents in their efforts to seek information about immunisation, following uncertainty about its safety and effectiveness.

'The Informed Parent' is one of few organisations I support and I can recommend subscribing and helping Magda in her incredible work.

I will now pass you on to Patrick for a deeper understanding of vaccine science and especially the recent 'new technology'. In the book 'Brave New World' I always noted the only physical genetic engineering took place at the creation of the first cell. After that first cell it was total social engineering so I did not fit right with me that this 'new technology' vaccine was direct 'gene therapy'. We have to understand that in the system we are subject to there are games within games. And they are all mind games.

VACCINE SCIENCE

Patrick Quanten MD

So much information is pushed into the public domain about the results of laboratory work surrounding viruses and vaccines that I sometimes wonder what the purpose is. Who understands all that stuff? Who had, until very recently, heard of mRNA? Of nanoparticles? Of spike proteins? What is all that? What does it mean, if anything at all? Maybe it is time to calm down, to sit down with a relaxing drink and to take a look at some of the reality and the meaning of such information.

They tell us that vaccines work by *imitating* an infection so that the body's natural defences are being engaged. This reaction should then build up an alertness and a readiness towards a specific disease *before* the actual disease arrives, *before* one comes in contact with the actual disease, as direct contact with the disease causing agent is the pathway they advocate for 'catching' the disease. For the natural defences to become engaged, one requires an 'active' ingredient, the stuff the body is going to react to. They say that the active ingredient in all vaccines is an antigen, which is the name for any substance that causes the immune system to begin producing antibodies.

No scientific proof has ever been produced that shows that the presence of antibodies provides protection against a specific disease.

Scientific research has shown that there does not exist any antibody that is specific against any particular disease.

In a vaccine, an antigen can be:

* weakened or killed bacteria or viruses – *Viruses are shown not to be alive and can therefore, by definition, not be weakened or killed.*

* bits of their exterior surface or genetic material (RNA) – *As viruses have never been isolated nobody can actually prove*

that any protein, any genetic material or any other structural component belongs to a virus.

- bacterial toxin treated to make it non-toxic – *Here the immune response is triggered by a toxin said to have been produced by a specific bacteria, not the bacteria itself. How would the alerted immune system then recognize the bacteria if it hasn't been given any information about the bacteria itself? How can a toxin imitate an infection? A toxin can have multiple origins and cannot be solely linked to one specific bacteria.*

Newer vaccines contain the blueprint for producing antigens rather than the antigen itself. What they mean by that is that the vaccine contains instructions on how to produce the antigen and they propose that these antigens are then made by the cells of the vaccinated body itself.

Without providing any scientific proof for this theory, they propose that the cells are induced by the vaccine, containing the blueprint, to manufacture the antigen. It can't be a 'weakened or killed bacteria or viruses'. So it must be 'bits of the exterior surface or genetic material of those bacteria or viruses', in other words a protein. This protein should then convey the message to the organism that it is being attacked. In response to that 'feeling' of being attacked the organism is then going to produce the appropriate antibodies. Why do you want to make the protein inside the cells of the organism when you could simply isolate it from the virus and introduce it directly into the system of the organism?

No virus has ever been isolated. This means that no single part of the said construction of a virus, be it a genetic sequence or a piece of the protein mantle, can be scientifically proven to originate from that virus.

Besides the active ingredient the vaccines all contain other elements. The old vaccines all contain at least one element from the following categories:

- Stabilizers - to protect the integrity of the active ingredients during manufacture, storage and transport

  o Sugars: lactose (danger: allergic reactions), sucrose, sorbitol (both artificial sweeteners linked to several cancers)

  o Amino acids: glycine, monosodium glutamate (MSG – controversial food additive)

  o Proteins: human or bovine serum albumin

  o Gelatin (bovine or porcupine): dangers include anaphylactic shock

- Adjuvants – creates a stronger immune response

  o Aluminium – side-effects include bone and brain diseases

  o Cervarix – side-effects include headache, myalgia (muscle pain), fatigue (tiredness), and reactions at the site of injection including pain, redness and swelling

  o ASo3 – side-effects include both injection site (pain mainly) and general symptoms (such as irritability and drowsiness in young children; myalgia, headache and fatigue in older children and adults)

  o MF59 – releases ATP from muscles (is a sign of injured or inflamed muscles) – side-effects include local swelling, myalgia, atopic dermatitis, narcolepsy

  o CpG 1018 – side-effects include pain/soreness/redness/swelling at the injection site, fever, headache, tiredness, sore throat, nausea, diarrhoea, loss of appetite, and dizziness

  o ASo1B – side-effects include headache, muscle pain, tiredness, fever

- Residual cell culture materials – leftovers from the culture the active ingredient has been grown on in the laboratory. These can be human cell lines, HEK 293 cell lines, animal cell lines, genetically modified organisms, recombinant DNA technology (using enzymes and various laboratory techniques to manipulate and isolate DNA segments), bovine products.

- Residual antibiotics – causes allergic reactions as well as antibiotic resistance

- Preservatives

  o Thimerosal – side-effects are neurotoxicity (nervous system) and nephrotoxicity (kidneys)

  o Formaldehyde – side-effects include irritation of the eyes, nose, and throat, even at low levels for short periods. Longer exposure or higher doses can cause coughing or choking. Severe exposure can cause death from throat swelling or from chemical burns to the lungs. It is listed as a carcinogenic.

  Scientific research has shown that vaccines without adjuvants do not create any immune response at all. Adjuvants and preservatives are in fact the 'active ingredients' of any vaccine. The key characteristic is the toxic effect these products have on the cells and on the entire organism.

  We can now understand why the so-called bacterial toxin, one of the possible antigens, creates an immune response, because what they measure and call 'an immune response' is basically the reaction of the organism to any toxin, whatever its origin.

One type of vaccine that contains the so-called blueprint for the production of an antigen is a new type called mRNA vaccine. This allows your body to trigger an immune response without using the actual germ to train your immune system. Instead, it trains your immune response using a piece of the virus so your system will protect you from getting infected if and when you encounter the said virus. Here is a list of the generalized ingredients of the mRNA vaccines.

- There is only one active ingredient in these vaccines, nucleoside-modified messenger ribonucleic acid (mRNA). mRNA are genetic instructions that train your body how to make the viral proteins (spike proteins in the case of SARS-CoV-2) that are present on the virus. Since this is a foreign protein, your body responds by building an immune response in the form of antibodies that will later recognize the same spike protein on the live virus.

- There are four main categories for the inactive ingredients: lipids, salts, acids/acid stabilizers, and sugars. These make up the rest of the vaccine or 99.7-99.8%!

  o Lipids are molecules that are insoluble in water like oils. They are used in this vaccine to protect and deliver the mRNA to the cell. Examples of some of these lipids in the COVID-19 vaccines include:

    - Cholesterol, a common lipid that is found in many foods and in your body

    - ((4-hydroxybutyl)azanediyl)bis(hexane-6,1-diyl)bis(2-hexyldecanoate), a specialized lipid designed for these vaccines specifically - made in a laboratory, unnatural, toxic to the system

  o Salts are molecules soluble in water that balance the acidity and maintain the pH in your body after receiving the vaccine. Examples of some of these salts in the COVID-19 vaccines include:

    - Potassium chloride, found in many frozen foods, sports drinks, and baby formula – side-effects include severe throat irritation, nausea, vomiting, diarrhoea, gas, bloating, stomach pains – signs of high potassium level: nausea, weakness, tingly feeling, chest pain, irregular heartbeats, loss of movement; or signs of stomach bleeding: bloody or tarry stools, coughing up blood or vomit that looks like coffee grounds.

    - Sodium chloride – side-effects include fast heartbeat, fever, hives, itching, or rash, hoarseness, irritation, joint pain, stiffness, or swelling of the joint, redness of the skin, shortness of breath, swelling of the eyelids, face, lips, hands or feet, tightness in the chest, troubled breathing or swallowing o Acids/acid stabilizers are hydrogen-containing molecules with a pH less than 7. These are similar to the salts in that they help maintain the pH to that of your body, but these also help stabilize the vaccine to last longer and at lower temperatures for ease in transportation. Here are a few examples of acids/acid stabilizers in the COVID-19 vaccines:

- acetic acid, the main ingredient in vinegar – side-effects include hives, difficulty breathing, swelling of your face, lips, tongue, or throat, and severe burning or irritation in the ears (ear drops)

- tromethamine, currently used as a blood/urine acid reducer by doctors in a hospital or clinic setting and often used after heart bypass surgery or cardiac arrest – side-effects include allergic reactions, wheezing; tightness in the chest or throat, troubled swallowing or talking, unusual hoarseness, swelling of the mouth, face, lips, tongue, or throat, fever - signs of low blood sugar like dizziness, headache, feeling sleepy, feeling weak, shaking, a fast heartbeat, confusion, hunger, or sweating - signs of high potassium levels like an abnormal heartbeat, confusion general weakness, light-headedness or dizziness, numbness or tingling

o Lastly, sugars are the sweet-tasting, water-soluble molecules that specifically contain carbon, hydrogen, and oxygen. These help the other molecules such as mRNA to maintain their shapes while frozen/during freezing, allowing the vaccines to last longer. Here is an example of sugars in the COVID-19 vaccines:

-Sucrose (artificial sweetener) – side-effects include digestive issues, increased blood sugar levels, a higher risk of cancer, increased blood pressure and adverse effects on those with pre-existing mood disorders

Once again it is explained that all the extra ingredients are needed to elicit a 'proper' immune response with the active ingredient.

The active ingredient in the new mRNA vaccines is one of the possible active ingredients used in the older type vaccines. It is simply a very short RNA sequence, from whatever origin. Hence, if the active ingredient of the new vaccines is not new, what makes the vaccines 'new' then?

It may be obvious when you look at the additional ingredients in both vaccine types. These are completely different. The important factor they have in common is that they both contain seriously toxic ingredients. In the newer vaccines we specifically note an artificial lipid and tromethamine.

This could explain the said measurement of an immune response in both types of vaccines. But then the question remains: why is there an urgent need to change to a new format? One reason could be that it became increasingly more difficult to wave away concerns regarding the toxic elements in the older vaccines, such as aluminium, thimerosal, mercury, formaldehyde. But maybe there is more to it.

The information about the new type of vaccines seems to focus entirely on viruses. No mention anywhere of the need for a new approach towards bacterial infections and the corresponding vaccination programme.

The main difference between the old style vaccines and the new ones is not the active ingredient. It is the use of lipids. Also note that no 'spike protein' is present in the vaccine. The claim is that the mRNA is the blueprint that will 'force' the cell to produce the protein itself. Once the cell has done this it is then supposed to come up with an immune response directed towards its own manufactured product. The first obstacle to possibly achieving this is to get the genetic code into the cell. The cell membrane consists of a lipid bilayer. Cell membranes serve as barriers and gatekeepers. They are semi-permeable, which means that some molecules can diffuse across the lipid bilayer but others cannot. Small hydrophobic molecules and gases like oxygen and carbon dioxide cross membranes rapidly. Small polar molecules, such as water and ethanol, can also pass through membranes, but they do so more slowly. On the other hand, cell membranes restrict diffusion of highly charged molecules, such as ions, and large molecules, such as sugars and amino acids (the base elements of the genetic coding). The passage of these molecules relies on specific transport proteins embedded in the membrane. Other transmembrane proteins have communication-related jobs.

> *The cell has no mechanism to take up genetic material from their environment. It barely allows the building blocks for the genetic structure to pass through. There is no structured genetic material in the outer environment, no matter how small, and if there was, by accident, the cell has no interest in it.*

Various lipids have been tried and researched to be used as an effective delivery vehicle for the nucleic acids. One key consideration in the design of lipids for nucleic acids delivery systems is how to overcome the innate cellular membrane defences. You need to get passed 'the border control' unseen.

However, nanoparticles' efficient and controlled entry/trafficking into cells, the method of choice, remains a major challenge. Before the nanoparticles reach the exterior membranes of the target cells, they must interact with the microenvironment around the target cells. Furthermore, that microenvironment, including fibrosis, extracellular matrix, various micro-environmental factors, pH and so on, can also change the properties of nanoparticles themselves and affect their interactions with the cell membrane. So what you expose the cell membrane to might not be the same thing you manufactured to do the job. The area of nanoparticle-cell interactions can also be affected by the interplay of various micro-environmental factors, such as bradykinin, vascular endothelial growth factor, prostaglandins, and matrix metalloproteinases. Moreover, characteristics of the microenvironment such as pH can affect the nanoparticle-cell interactions and the entry of nanoparticles. When the nanoparticles reach the exterior membrane of a cell, they can interact with components of the plasma membrane or extracellular matrix and enter the cell, mainly through endocytosis. That is what they say.

The lipids in the vaccine are needed to disrupt the lipid bilayer of the cell membrane in order to break through the barrier and move the content of the lipid vesicles inside the cell. We know that natural and synthetic fatty acids may modify the structure of the lipid membrane, altering its micro-domain organization and other physical properties, and provoking changes in cell signalling. Therefore, by modulating fatty acids it is possible 'to regulate' the structure of the membrane. It may, in theory, be possible but achieving it is still a different matter.

Lipid nucleic acid nanoparticles (LNP) have emerged as the most promising delivery systems for clinical applications among the various non-viral delivery systems. Various lipids have been reported for intracellular delivery of nucleic acids in the past decades. The lipid structures play the most important role for safe and efficient intracellular delivery of nucleic acids. One key consideration in the design of lipids for nucleic acids delivery is to overcome endosomal barriers for efficient intracellular delivery. The pH-sensitive protonatable or ionizable lipids have emerged as the most promising class of lipids for efficient intracellular nucleic acid delivery. While the role of nanoparticle properties in inducing membrane damage has received significant attention, the role of the lipid chemical structure in regulating such interactions is less explored.

All these findings suggest that mRNA transfection mediated by lipid nanoparticles is an overly complex process, strongly influenced by several factors, such as uptake mechanism, endosomal maturation, endosomal recycling, and may vary widely between different cell types. Inefficient endosomal escape efficacy and precise tissue/cell targeting efficiency remain the major challenges for mRNA delivery by lipid-based nano-platforms. For example, while cationic lipids offer great promise as carriers for the delivery of fragile compounds such as nucleic acids, some cationic lipids cause cytotoxicity. In some cases, cationic lipids reduce mitosis in cells, form vacuoles in the cytoplasm of the cells, and cause detrimental effects on key cellular proteins such as protein kinase C. So they tell us.

Under laboratory conditions, in vitro experiments are struggling to deliver RNA inside any cell. In vivo, the challenges are even greater and the scientific literature indicates that they are still a long way from understanding how it works and achieving it in an efficient manner.

The normal function of the cell membrane is seriously disturbed by the nanoparticles, to the extent that the cell begins to leak fluid and on many occasions simply breaks open and dies. The nanoparticles have done what they are supposed to do, to disrupt the cell membrane function in order to allow foreign material to cross the barrier. However, in the process the entire cell has died.

Apart from using this method in the new vaccines, a great deal of attention has been focused on nanoparticles for cancer therapy, with the promise of tumour-selective delivery. However, despite intense work in the field over many years, the biggest obstacle to this vision remains extremely low delivery efficiency of nanoparticles into tumours. Due to the cost, time, and impact on the animals for *in vivo* studies, the nanoparticle field predominantly uses cellular uptake assays (laboratory cell experiments) as a proxy to predict *in vivo* outcomes.

Effective delivery of therapeutic and diagnostic nanoparticles is dependent on their ability to accumulate in diseased tissues. However, most nanoparticles end up in liver macrophages regardless of nanoparticle design after administration. Liver macrophages have significant advantages in interacting with circulating nanoparticles over most target cells and tissues in the body because the natural task of macrophages is 'to swallow' unwanted material. Nanoparticles undergo opsonization and subsequent uptake by resident macrophages. This results in high accumulation of nanoparticles in organs, such as the spleen and the liver, contributing to nonspecific distribution of nanotherapeutics to healthy organs. Indeed, healthy organs, mainly the detoxifying organs of the body, accumulate the nanoparticles, not the cancer cells.

In vivo, in real life, virtually all nanoparticles end up in detoxifying organs where macrophages, cells that remove all kinds of debris and potentially dangerous material from the system, clean up the rubbish. The liver and spleen will then break down this debris and recycle the useful elements.

So it turns out that, outside a viral laboratory, there is no evidence of any significant 'uptake' of genetic material brought to the cells of the organism.

Remember that delivering the RNA, the blueprint for the spike protein that identifies the virus to the body, is only the first step in the process. Once inside the cell, this mRNA then has to make its way through the cytoplasm, avoiding the internal defence mechanisms of the cell, crossing the membrane into the cell nucleus. The critical function of the nuclear membranes (an inner and an outer membrane) is to act as a barrier that separates the contents of the nucleus from the cytoplasm. Like other cell membranes, the nuclear membranes are phospholipid bilayers, which are permeable only to small nonpolar molecules. Other molecules are unable to diffuse through the phospholipid bilayer. The inner and outer nuclear membranes are joined at nuclear pore complexes, the sole channels through which small polar molecules and macromolecules are able to travel through the nuclear envelope. The nuclear pore complex is a complicated structure that is responsible for the selective traffic of proteins and RNAs from the nucleus to the cytoplasm, not in the opposite direction.

Indeed, nobody has explained how the mRNA, if it all gets to the gates of the cell nucleus, can possibly enter the nucleus. The mRNA has been disrobed at crossing the cell membrane, leaving its lipid nanoparticles behind. On top of that, the cell has a perfect mechanism to release mRNA, the normal way in which the cellular genetic material organizes messages and dispatches these into the cytoplasm. It doesn't allow any genetic code to come back to the chromosomes, the genetic storage room and command centre. There is no reason why a genetic code should be allowed back into the nucleus. It is meant to be a one way system. Instructions are written down inside the nucleus and dispatched to the cell factory. And that is it!

In spite of all this scientific evidence and knowledge they claim that the 'viral' mRNA enters the nucleus of the cell, attaches itself to the 'appropriate' spot on the cell's DNA and instructs the cell to produce the spike protein, for which the blueprint is contained within the genetic code that was brought to the cell's DNA. This process they call *reverse transcription*.

DNA transcription is the process by which the genetic information contained within DNA is re-written into messenger RNA (mRNA) by RNA polymerase. This mRNA then exits the nucleus, where it acts as the basis for the translation of DNA. By controlling the production of mRNA within the nucleus, the cell regulates the rate of gene expression. Research has shown that the instructions stored within DNA are 'read' in two steps: transcription and translation. In transcription, a portion of the double-stranded DNA template gives rise to a single-stranded RNA molecule. In some cases, the RNA molecule itself is a 'finished product' that serves some important function within the cell. Often, however, transcription of an RNA molecule is followed by a translation step, which ultimately results in the production of a protein molecule.

Reverse transcriptase (RT), also known as RNA-dependent DNA polymerase, is a DNA polymerase enzyme that transcribes single-stranded RNA into DNA. So now RNA can be transformed into DNA. This mechanism, so they tell us, is how the viral information, the blueprint for the manufacturing of the spike protein that identifies the specific virus, gets incorporated into the cell's DNA. Once the RNA, the messenger, has been turned into a DNA code (reverse transcription), the cell will, so they tell us, begin to copy this information into mRNA (transcription), thereby instructing the cell factory to keep producing this protein (translation). It is then, according to their expert sources, that the immune system of the body recognizes this 'foreign' protein and the same cells then begin to produce antibodies against this protein. Because the protein, so they tell us, is part of the outer casing of a specific virus these antibodies will recognize the protein, therefore the virus, and instruct the body to destroy the viral invader. This entire 'process' begins with *reverse transcription*.

The DNA that is produced by the process of reverse transcription is called cDNA (short for copy DNA; also called complementary DNA). This is synthetic DNA that has been transcribed from a specific mRNA through a reaction using the enzyme reverse transcriptase. While DNA is composed of both coding and non-coding sequences, cDNA contains only coding sequences. Scientists often synthesize and use cDNA as a tool in gene cloning and other research experiments.

Reverse transcription is done in a laboratory. As an example, AMV Reverse Transcriptase synthesizes single-stranded cDNA from total or poly(A)+ isolated RNA. The Reverse Transcription System provides lot-tested reagents to efficiently reverse transcribe poly(A)+ mRNA or total RNA in 15 minutes. cDNA synthesized with the Reverse Transcription System can be used directly in PCR.

> *Reverse transcription only exists within a laboratory setting. It is a technique used to artificially make short DNA sequences to be used in further genetic laboratory experiments.*

> *Cells don't do reverse transcription. They have no need for it. It doesn't exist in real life.*

Where does that leave us with regards to the newly developed so-called vaccines?

The change in 'inactive ingredients' we encounter in the new vaccines is the most significant part of the story. These no longer, compared to the old vaccines, create a toxic effect within the organism, but they break open the cells of the organism. All this cellular debris needs to be cleaned up by the organism. Hence, one notices a massive reaction of the entire organism to stop the onslaught. As mainly the macrophages of the liver and the spleen seem to be involved, the major overload on the system will manifest in the overall toxicity of the system and within the circulation system. This means on the one hand that heart and blood vessel cells will have less capacity, less energy available, to do the normal repairs and to maintain a normal function, and on the other hand that the general level of toxicity within the cells and their environment increases massively. The latter will show itself mostly where the individual already was seriously stressed before he got vaccinated, be it the nervous system, the breathing, or the mobility system.

When an individual has enough 'spare' energy he is able to perform a good clean-up and has no ill health effects from the injection. It will cost him a lot of energy though, which of course can then not be used for any other essential work. When one keeps repeating this process more and more people will fall ill as a result of repeated injections. However, if the authority manages to blame the symptoms on a disease rather than on their intervention nobody will be any the wiser.

Maybe it is time to give you some bullet points to remember.

- Germs, pathogens, microorganisms do not cause diseases. So there is no need for any protection against them.
- The old vaccines create a response, which is said to be an immune response, because of the toxicity of the injection.
- An increase in antibodies and/or lymphatic cells, the so-called immune response, does not provide protection against any disease.
- The so-called 'active ingredient' of the new vaccine does not differ from that of the old vaccines. The genetic material is not 'the' active ingredient.
- All information about the new vaccines is obtained from cell experiments under laboratory conditions.
- The new vaccines create a so-called immune response as a result of their impact on the cell membranes. It penetrates the membrane which results in leaks and cell death.
- In real life, the 'introduced' genetic code (mRNA) is found in organ cells responsible for the clean-up of the organism, not in ordinary cells. It is their clean-up cells that capture the nanoparticles that contain the genetic code.
- In real life, there is no penetration of the membrane of the nucleus. The 'introduced' genetic code does not get

167

anywhere near the genetic code of the cells.

- In real life, there is no reverse transcription. This is only a laboratory technique.

- In real life, the 'introduction' of a messenger RNA does not trigger the production of a protein.

In real life, the danger of the vaccination programme lies in the story it tells us. It is the message that does the damage to our health. It is message of helplessness, of vulnerability, of weakness. It is message of fear, fear for our life, fear to inadvertedly kill someone, even a loved one. It is fear that weakens our resistance against all diseases. It is fear that drains our life energy. And it is fear that makes us pray for the saving grace, for the guardian angel, for the knowledge and skills that will save us. It is fear that allows an industry to rule our lives, to do whatever they please with us.

Because we begged them for it!

THE HISTORY OF MODERN MEDICINE

"To find health should be the object of the doctor. Anyone can find disease."

– Andrew Taylor Still, 1828-1917. Father of osteopathy.

Modern medicine, allopathic medicine, means to oppose what the body is doing, to work against it. This is the only accepted scientific method, thinking and truth but it wasn't always like this. In fact, as Patrick Quanten points out it is actually modern medicine which is the alternative. Traditional means what is longstanding and as far as history is concerned modern medicine is a newcomer.

Around the time of modern medicine getting started and changing the way we see,and therefore treat disease, a peasant farmer, in Gräfenberg, Austria, lay the foundations of what became known as Nature Cure. Vincenz Priessnitz, 1799-1851. Born into a farmer's family he grew up observing nature and especially what animals did when ill or suffering wounds. Copying their methods, he became very well versed in what would become to be known as hydrotherapy, using water to heal, with the addition of other natural therapies such as vegetarian food, air, sunlight, exercise, rest, water, fasting and traditional medicine (remember, traditional means longstanding). His reputation grew and in 1822 he extended his father's home to build a healing spa for the incoming patients.

His therapies, which did not use modern drugs or even herbal remedies, were focused on removing waste and foreign matter from the body, this build-up of waste became known as 'toxaemia'. Waste is a matter of life; we take in food, air and liquids and in the modern world toxins in the diet and environment. The idea is the body removes the waste so it remains at a balanced level which does not disturb the functioning of the body. Many things like poor diet, overeating, lack of exercise, a toxic environment and poor organ function that may be due to stress, can build up waste.

In recent times, through ' *German New Medicine'* and other practices, we now know how the emotions can affect the body, certain emotions affecting certain parts of the body and therefore how it functions. When waste builds up and goes beyond your balance point then an extra effort is needed by the body to remove the excess waste and restore balance; this was the principle behind his healing and something only the body itself could do. We could help it by removing stresses and partaking in certain natural therapies but the healing was up to the body.

The success of his natural nontoxic methods saw him even treating royalty and in 1846, Priessnitz was awarded a medal by the Emperor. The world though, would soon forget the peasant farmer from Austria and was given a path instead that would see modern medicine not just creating a near monopoly on health and disease but even attacking the more traditional practitioners as 'Quacks'.

In 1914 Hendry Lindlahr MD published his book *'Nature Cure'*. Along with *'The Science of Health' and Healing* and *'The Biology of Belief'* it is another great addition for someone wanting to study natural health. Lindlahr exposes germ theory, allopathic thinking and modern medicine as unscientific and shows his own natural techniques, which mainly consisted of rest, sunlight, clean air, breathing, fasting and simple foods, were enough to cure even the most severe illnesses. He tells the story of a fellow doctor who travelled the world and came back stating he saw no chronic illness in native tribes living simple lives. They went through the acute illness stage and because they had no access to modern suppressive drugs it did not progress to the chronic. Also they ate local natural foods, had no access to processed foods and the stresses of modern life in the 'civilized' world.

Toxic Takeover

The American Medical Association (AMA) was founded in 1847 and incorporated in 1897, is the largest association of physicians – both MDs and DOs – and medical students in the United States. Their mission was to *"to promote the art and science of medicine and the betterment of public health."* Its founder, Nathan Smith Davis, also founded the Journal of the American Medical Association in 1883 and was behind pushing laws for compulsory smallpox vaccines in 1889.

In 1904 the AMA created the Council on Medical Education (CME) with the aim of restructuring the American medical education. In 1908 the CME contacted the 'Carnegie Foundation for the Advancement of Teaching' to survey the American medical education. Abraham Flexner was chosen to conduct the survey although he was neither a physician, scientist nor medical educator. After visiting 155 of the medical schools in America, all very diverse in their thinking, he came back using the John Hopkins School of Medicine as his ideal in 1910 and with these recommendations:

Reduce the number of medical schools (from 155 to 31) and poorly trained physicians.

Increase the prerequisites to enter medical training.

Train physicians to practice in a scientific manner and engage medical faculty in research.

Give medical schools control of clinical instruction in hospitals.

Strengthen state regulation of medical licensure.

This report was then pushed through the colleges and hospitals with an initial donation of $100 from John D. Rockefeller; many hundreds of millions followed. The report basically regulated all of medical thinking and training with oversight given to the AMA and made allopathic thinking and germ theory unchallenged as the only acceptable scientific way to deal with illness and disease. From this day on disease became a massive business, one that the Rockefeller Foundation invested in – yes, invested in, and not donated. We then saw an onslaught against any other health practices such as homeopathy, chiropractic, osteopathy, naturopathy and more and also an attack on anyone against the use of vaccines to prevent disease; the term 'quackery' had been invented.

I find it also interesting that a similar attack on marijuana happened in the US around the same time. A plant well known for its many uses and medicinal qualities. After years of attacks in regulating it, the 1937 Marijuana Tax Act was the beginning of the end for this highly useful bit of nature. It was then classified as a narcotic drug in the US, bringing an end to the easy access of this wonder of nature. Strangely, again, this plant was a huge competitor to the now-Rockefeller-backed big pharma and even his oil business. Maybe the competition was just pushed out of the way?

The later establishment of the WHO was, again, centred on allopathic thinking and germ theory, came with mass promotion of vaccines and claims they wiped out smallpox with vaccines. But to understand the Flexner Report is to understand the position we find ourselves in today and how the WHO and the Rockefeller-backed science took hold of the world. The same family who were well known to use homeopathy themselves.

This is the same Rockefeller Foundation that in 1939 formed an alliance with the German chemical company I.G. Farben. I.G. Farben was once the largest chemical and pharmaceutical company in the world and owned the Monowitz concentration camp, which was a subcamp of the main Auschwitz concentration camp, and used to produce chemicals for I.G. Farben with the slave labour provided by the Nazis from the main concentration camp at a cheap rate. Employees of the Bayer group at I.G. Farben conducted medical experiments on concentration camp inmates and the company was a massive powerful ally and funder of the Nazis.

After the war I.G. Farben was broken up into its original companies and one of them, Bayer, in 2016 bought the infamous Monsanto Company for $66 billion and took control of GMO seeds. Bayer was also the creators of aspirin before they merged into I.G. Farben, an interesting fact we went into when looking at treatments of the great Spanish Flu.

At the Nuremberg trials directors of I.G. Farben were put on trial for war crimes and thirteen were found guilty. Also research 'Operation Paperclip' for information on how Nazi scientists were brought to the West after the war ended.

There is a massive story surrounding the Nazis and private companies that could entail a book by itself but the point I want to make is that the people who run and control medical thinking, allegedly to help human suffering, took part in some of the worst atrocities against human beings.

This modern way of looking at things goes against the well-established sciences going back thousands of years from Ayurveda and later Chinese medicine. These sciences took into account the whole human being and not just the physical symptom; life was about energy and an expression of energy, something we knew from before the time of Einstein, yet have continued to ignore in medical science to this day and to the detriment of human health. Until the true nature of what we are, energetic and emotional, is incorporated into health and our understanding of disease, I'm afraid human health will only deteriorate as big pharma profits rise.

In the UK: The Cancer Act 1939

"No person shall take part in the publication of any advertisement

A: containing an offer to treat any person for cancer or to prescribe any remedy therefor, or to give any advice in connection with the treatment thereof."

Here, we now see medical science and big pharma using government to take total control of the treatment of disease, even criminalising anyone claiming to treat or cure cancer without the' correct' method. Only a medical doctor can now treat cancer and the main three methods they have used for decades is chemotherapy, radiotherapy and surgery, and yet cases rise and the cost of treating continues to go into the billions. Welcome to the cancer business.

As for alternatives, well look at what happened to the Gerson Institute in the US. Banned. Despite having many documented cases of curing cancer with natural detoxification therapies using natural juices and supplements. They were kicked out and moved into Mexico for their 'crimes'. This attack continues today in the UK with David Noakes being imprisoned for four charges relating to the manufacture, sale and supply of an unlicensed medicine, GcMAF. Though GcMAF is not a pharmaceutical drug and derived from a naturally occurring human protein, the medical establishment, the government and the courts all waged war against this man who, similar to the Gerson Therapy, had many testimonials to the effectiveness of treating cancer without the awful and sometimes deadly side effects of modern medical treatments. The evidence seemed clear, it was safe and could actually be a major breakthrough in treating cancer, but that did not matter, he wasn't a doctor and he didn't follow protocol, therefore he is a criminal. Not that he had actually harmed anyone, in fact the opposite, but in the eyes of the establishment he was a danger to society. Rick Simpson and his hemp oil is also another example of someone taking a natural treatment, having success and then being shut down. His documentary 'Run from the Cure' can still be found on YouTube. I am not personally stating here I believe these are cures for cancer. I am saying they have acquired huge amounts of data to show they actually help people with no side effects and instead of being investigated to find out if there is some truth in this that could benefit mankind they are investigated as criminals. Their crimes though are not against humanity, but against the rulers of the medical profession who fear losing their money, power and control.

Patrick Quanten has been asked many times at seminars I have arranged *"what is the cure for cancer?"* His answer was always the same *"pack your bags up and leave!"*

For Patrick, and myself, cancer is a symptom of a life that has been a long time out of balance. When the life you are living is slowly killing you then a huge change in life is needed and packing up and leaving for new shores is the most radical way to change your life as you have to change. Of course not everyone can do that, but it is a simple statement that tells people very clearly that whatever they are doing is killing them so they need to change. Even if it's not clear what exactly needs changing, change is for sure needed.

Toxic Psychiatry

There is a stunning book, *'Toxic Psychiatry'*.Peter R Breggin MD. I recommend reading it to get an insight into the massive damage modern medical thinking, doctors and drug companies have done to humanity over the last century. Psychiatry is really just an extension of this system concentrating on what is known as 'mental illness'. Psychiatrists are in fact medical doctors so we see straight away how they are trained in medical school, this time seeing mental illness or psychiatric problems as things going wrong and again, based on materialism. A look into the history and the same names come up again.

Ernest Rudin, 1874-1922, worked under Emil Kraepelin who was known as the founder of modern scientific psychiatry, psychopharmacology and psychiatric genetics. Rudin was a Swiss-born German psychiatrist, geneticist, eugenicist and Nazi. He has been credited as a pioneer of psychiatric inheritance studies and in 1932 he became President of the International Federation of Eugenics Organizations. Rüdin joined the Nazi Party in 1937 and in 1939, he was awarded a 'Goethe medal for art and science' handed to him personally by Hitler, who honoured him as the 'pioneer of the racial-hygienic measures of the Third Reich'. In 1944 he received a bronze Nazi eagle medal, with Hitler calling him the 'pathfinder in the field of hereditary hygiene'. He also held the post of professor of psychiatry at the Kaiser Wilhelm Institute in Munich which later inspired and conducted Eugenics experiments in the Third Reich, the same institute that when having financial problems in the early 1930s, was bailed out by that family again, the Rockefeller Foundation. He was also a visitor in America with the support of that other great family; yes, you guessed it, the Carnegie Foundation. As Breggin states in his book *"it was Rudin who influenced Hitler, not Hitler who influenced Rudin"*.

During the late 1920s, the Rockefeller Foundation created the 'Medical Sciences Division' which was known for making large contributions to research across several fields of psychiatry. The horrific legacy of this is well-documented in *'Toxic Psychiatry'*. It was an era with the Rockefeller Foundation giving massive donations to the fields of psychiatry, social sciences and genetics and they continued funding Nazi racial studies even after it was clear that this research was being used to rationalise the demonising of Jews and other groups. They continued to fund Nazi racial science studies at the Kaiser Wilhelm Institute of Anthropology, Human Heredity, and Eugenics up until 1939, four years after the 1935 Nuremberg Laws which were a racist assault on all non-Germans by the Nazi Party.

If we think of what is happening to our children in schools today with all the 'safety' rules to follow, all the consequences for 'wrong' behaviour, or even just questioning the self-proclaimed authority, then think of what Peter Breggin said in chapter 12 of his book, entitled: *'abandoning responsibility for our children'*.

"Nothing measures the quality of a society better then how it treats its children. Nothing predicts the future of a society better then how it nurtures and educates its children."

And on how psychiatry moved in on children he states:

"In blaming the child-victim, psychiatry takes the pressure of the parents, the family, the schools, and society. By diagnosing, drugging and hospitalizing children, psychiatry enforces the worst attitudes towards children in our culture today and exonerates those adult institutions that need reform. Psychiatry has been joined by factions within behavioural educational psychology in exonerating the schools and blaming the children. The question asked by John Holt, "Why can't Jonny read?" Has been answered. Because he has a learning disability."

How are we treating our children at the moment? What kind of future are we nurturing? Why do we look at the children and judge how they are behaving without asking why?

The education system worldwide now, and especially in the West, has been infiltrated by trained 'experts' who seem to have a similar view of how children should behave and if they don't fit into the mould they will need to be guided.

From Aldous Huxley's *Brave New World,* chapter 3:

"From a neighbouring shrubbery emerged a nurse, leading by the hand a small boy, who howled as he went. An anxious looking little girl trotted at her heels. "What's the matter?" asked the Director. The nurse shrugged her shoulders. "Nothing much," she answered. "It's just that this little boy seems rather reluctant to join in the ordinary erotic play. I'd noticed it once or twice before. And now again today. He started yelling just now..."

"Honestly," put in the anxious-looking little girl, "I didn't mean to hurt him or anything. Honestly." "Of course you didn't, dear," said the nurse reassuringly. "And so," she went on, turning back to the Director, "I'm taking him in to see the Assistant Superintendent of Psychology. Just to see if anything's at all abnormal."

Tyranny Funded by Philanthropy

Other Rockefeller Foundation donations and funding went to:

American Red Cross

International Health Commission

World's first school of Hygiene and Public Health, at Johns Hopkins University

China Medical Board

Department of Industrial Relations

Social Science Research Council

Eugenics Record Office, with the Carnegie Foundation

Supporters of Henry Kissinger

Council on Foreign Relations

Royal Institute of International Affairs in London

Carnegie Endowment for International Peace

Brookings Institution

World Bank

Harvard, Yale, Princeton and Columbia Universities

University of the Philippines, Los Baños

McGill University

Montreal Neurological Institute

University of Lyon, France

Library of Congress

Bodleian Library at Oxford University

Population Council of New York

Social Science Research Council

National Institute of Public Health of Japan

Group of Thirty

National Bureau of Economic Research

London School of Economics

Trinidad Regional Virus Laboratory

Agriculture and The Green Revolution

The Bellagio Center

Rockefeller Foundation Communication for Social Change Network which supports grassroots/community-based and international non-governmental organisations, (This sounds very much to me like the 'Common Purpose' charity in the UK which we will come to later.)

The 100 Resilient Cities initiative

Cultural Innovation Fund

And of course the United Nations.

An estimated $14 billion over the years gets a lot of fingers in many pies and with others like the Carnegie Foundation and the new king of giving, Bill Gates, it seems a lot of the things that run societies are actually being funded by very few individuals trying to put life into their own personal 'visions'.

A quote from the Rockefeller Foundation Bellagio Center:

"Since 1959 The Rockefeller Foundation Bellagio Center has hosted thousands of artists, policymakers, scholars, authors, practitioners, and scientists from all over the world enabling them time and space to work, to learn from each other, and to turn ideas into actions that change the world."

These Rockefeller funded organisations show how much influence this one family has on the development of society world-wide. Now we shall look at another elite family.

Bill & Melinda Gates Foundation

Launched in 2000 and is reported to be the largest private foundation in the world, holding $46.8 billion in assets globally, and whose main goals are to 'enhance healthcare and reduce extreme poverty', and, in the US, to 'expand educational opportunities and access to information technology'.

So, again, similar to the Rockefeller Foundation and Carnegie Foundation, this is a very rich family whose goals are to help needy people, especially in healthcare. By expanding educational opportunities it seems clear to me they want again to tell people what to think and therefore how to behave and using technology. Search patent '060606' to see what visions' they may have.

> *"This is a large part of the reason that Melinda and I got into philanthropy. One of our first big investments was to an organization called Gavi, the Vaccine Alliance. Since 2000, Gavi and partners have immunized more than 760 million children, saving over 13 million lives. And now, Gavi has a new effort underway to purchase COVID-19 vaccines for lower-income countries as soon as they are available."*

So from the off his main project was to vaccinate the whole world, already claiming to have saved 13 million lives. How that claim can be proven nobody knows but he said it so I guess it must be true.

> *"Our resources alone are not enough, so we work to change public policies, attitudes, and behaviors to improve lives."*

Again, we see some wanting to change public behaviour, which means changing beliefs.

> *"We partner with governments and the public and private sectors, and foster greater public awareness of urgent global issues."*

So they work with all areas of society to tell us what we need to be afraid of, therefore what actions we need to take to avoid these disasters. Remember, we have seen interviews of Bill Gates on TV telling us all we need to know about 'the pandemic' and how and when we will be out of lockdown. Yes, this private business man was holding the world in a lockdown (prison term) until his vaccine comes along to free us all. Bill speaks and all the world's politicians listen, what a guy.

In 2018/19 the WHO top four donors were the USA – $851.6 million, UK – $463.4 million, Bill and Melinda Gates Foundation – $455.3 million and GAVI – $388.7 million.

With Gates behind his Foundation and GAVI, this is basically one man funding, and therefore controlling, the WHO, and remember the WHO was founded on allopathic thinking and germ theory, which was funded into existence by the Carnegie and Rockefeller Foundations through the Flexner Report. It must be clear now that 'EVENT 201', which remember was funded by the Gates Foundation, the World Economic Forum and the WHO, who had for years been priming us with the inevitable *viral outbreak* threatening mankind, could easily have the wealth and power to utilise the elite-controlled mainstream media. It is estimated that just five companies own over 90% of the world's media, the 2008 financial crash has already shown us very clearly that world governments represent big banks and corporations and not people. Bailing out banks and not people clearly shows what their priorities are.

Tony Blair, who, evidence shows, lied about 'weapons of mass destruction', was never put on trial and was even rewarded by the rich organisations for his actions that resulted in hundreds of thousands of innocent people being murdered by western military action in Iraq, destroying a country for regime change, which resulted in western companies going in to take control of the resources and even getting contracts to rebuild the country that had just been destroyed. This war criminal is still doing the rounds and still has a political voice.

So it is clear that a mass media campaign and controlling the government narrative would be easy work and also using those same outlets for promoting the philanthropy of Gates, to paint him as some kind as saviour. If you do some simple research you will see he is a very astute business man and doesn't invest (donate) in things if he is not going to get some kind of return.

According to Wikipedia these are the top organisations that received recorded funding in millions of $ between 2009 and 2015 by the Gates Foundation:

GAVI Alliance	3,152.8
World Health Organization	1,535.1
The Global Fund to Fight AIDS, Tuberculosis and Malaria	777.6
PATH	635.2
United States Fund for UNICEF	461.1
The Rotary Foundation of Rotary International	400.1
International Bank for Reconstruction and Development	340.0
Global Alliance for TB Drug Development	338.4
Medicines for Malaria Venture	334.1
PATH Vaccine Solutions	333.4
UNICEF Headquarters	277.6
Johns Hopkins University	265.4
Aeras	227.6
Clinton Health Access Initiative Inc	199.5
International Development Association	174.7
CARE	166.2
World Health Organization Nigeria Country Office	166.1
Agence Française de Développement	165.0
Centro Internacional de Mejoramiento de Maíz y Trigo	153.1
Cornell University	146.7
Alliance for a Green Revolution in Africa	146.4
United Nations Foundation	143.0

University of Washington Foundation	138.2
Foundation for the National Institutes of Health	136.2
Emory University	123.2
University of California San Francisco	123.1
Population Services International	122.5
University of Oxford	117.8
International Food Policy Research Institute	110.7
International Institute of Tropical Agriculture	104.8

From Microsoft they also have investments in companies like FedEx, United Parcel Service, Walmart, Televisa and many more and when looking at these 'philanthropists' it is important to ask, are they donating or are they investing?

Other noted funding is to Imperial College London, to the department 'Imperial Network for Vaccine Research'. Also in May 2009, Bill and Melinda Gates visited Imperial College London after which the Foundation *"awarded grants to several Imperial research programmes, including major projects tackling neglected tropical diseases and HIV"*. Yes, the same institution that gave us Neil Ferguson, who has also benefited from their funding, has over the years been given tens of millions of pounds by the Gates Foundation and GAVI. The British Government themselves are the largest funder of GAVI and this year during 'the pandemic' GAVI were promised £330 million per year over the next five years by Boris Johnson. On the 5th June 2020 at the Global Vaccine Summit 2020, hosted by UK Prime Minister Boris Johnson, world leaders pledged US$ 8.8 billion for GAVI, the Vaccine Alliance, far exceeding the target of US$ 7.4 billion.

So let's get things clear, a private business man is working with world governments and is funding mass vaccination programmes around the world which will clearly lead to massive profits for vaccine makers. As you will see later, especially in line with any SARS-coV-2 vaccine, there will be no liability if things go wrong. Now this may seem to you a good man who has done well financially and wants to give back to the world. Why not indeed? But as we have seen, the agenda to vaccinate the world for the health benefits of mankind has not got science behind it and in fact has a legacy of death and suffering and zero evidence of improving health. And also who does Mr Johnson think he is giving this man our money without even asking us? It seems he doesn't think he needs our permission for anything.

The Gates Foundation also donates massive amounts of money to 'Planned Parenthood' over the globe, promoting contraception, abortion and emergency contraception as well as other areas of sexual health. In fact Bill Gates Senior, another rich philanthropist, has spent time on the board of Planned Parenthood. Its history goes back to Brooklyn, New York, when in 1916 Margaret Sanger, who had close connections to the American Eugenics Society, opened the first birth control clinic in the US. Later, in 1921 she founded the American Birth Control League which evolved into Planned Parenthood in 1942.

Planned Parenthood's push to reform abortion law is normally pushed as a positive move; for example if it is clear there is a seriously deformed child who simply will not survive and is putting the life of the mother at risk, or maybe when a woman is raped and early intervention, especially before about ten weeks before the human form is created, could save her from massive emotional and psychological pain. These examples are where maybe you could see abortion being used to the benefit of individual women but as always, this is the starting point and the finishing point is very far from the starting line.

When looking at the history of Planned Parenthood and Eugenics and the connections to today's 'Reproductive Health' programmes sponsored by Planned Parenthood and the Gates Foundation, there is a feeling that all is not as it seems. After the fall of the Nazis, Eugenics certainly had a bad name; it had an elitist ideology and a belief in an elite race to rule humanity, and that humanity should be culled of the weak and undesirable. Basically through breeding, their vision of how humanity should be structured could be made manifest. Putting themselves above God and Nature is an underestimation to say the least. There is clearly no compassion, or what we call humanity, in this ideology and it gives the impression they see themselves as farmers of human beings to be used as slaves. Just as cattle farmers want to breed the best stock for their own gains, these people see us as cattle to be bred or culled to fit their own needs and visions.

What people like Bruce Lipton showed, though, was that genes are the way cells hold onto the information of the history and present of that person but they do not control life. Life works through the genes but is not controlled by genes; that control comes down to the perception, and as he showed, the belief of the individual. So instead of wanting to improve the human race they are actually deliberately holding us back through controlled education and control of perception through instilling beliefs from a young age. The great thing about this truth, though, is we don't need technology or elite help to positively evolve ourselves, we just need to become aware of how life works and focus on opening our own minds and hearts. Yes, there are clearly massive problems within different cultures who maintain unhealthy beliefs but we have to ask ourselves how many of those beliefs were put in place by a level of people above us all, and whose desire is to control us all.

Eugenics never went away, it was just rebranded and its true agenda is one of population control, control in numbers and control in perfecting the perfect slave, and when Mr Gates and Elon Musk get us all chipped and connect us to AI then they have an opportunity to create and control humanity as desired, the perfection of the slave race through Trans-humanism.

It is worth noting that they talk about birth control as if nature doesn't provide a way, well it does, and it's been known for centuries or more by primitive people, it is commonly known as the Billings Method. It's safe, effective and teaches young girls, and men, discipline, control, respect and how nature works. By showing a young woman how her body works and the difference between different vaginal discharges she can learn when it is possible to conceive or not. There is a certain discharge a sperm needs to survive in the womb; without this, pregnancy cannot occur as the environment is too hostile for the sperm. Mass education in this fact could change the world for young women and men all over the world without using any body-changing toxic drugs and at the same time teaching us how amazing nature is. This knowledge though gives humanity independence and freedom to control our own lives and that doesn't go down well if you have a master plan to control the world.

The Legacy of Modern Medicine

Barbara Starfield MD, MDH, 26 JULY 2000, published in American Medical Association:

12 000 deaths/year from unnecessary surgery

7000 deaths/year from medication errors in hospitals

20 000 deaths/year from other errors in hospitals

80 000 deaths/year from nosocomial infections in hospitals

106 000 deaths/year from none error, adverse effects of medications

These total 225,000 deaths per year from iatrogenic causes. This conservative study shows modern allopathic doctors as the third biggest killers behind heart disease and cancer in the US. With our new understanding of how chronic illness takes hold in the body the question regarding those figures is, how many of those deaths from heart disease and cancer are caused by modern medicine and allopathic thinking?

Research conducted by university academics in Manchester, Sheffield and York in England published in Feb 2018 shown

"712 deaths in England every year result from avoidable adverse drug reactions"

An article in the Independent Feb 23 2018 stated from the report

"We estimate that 61.4 million and 4.8 million errors occur in England per annum that have potential to cause moderate or severe harm, respectively." The report also stated *"prescribing errors and mix-ups which contribute to as many as 22,300 deaths a year."*

In his speech at the *'World Patient Safety, Science and Technology Summit'* in London on 23 February, 2018, Secretary of state for health and social care, Jeremy Hunt, said that while NHS England

"does well in international comparisons, this new study shows medication error in the NHS and globally is a far bigger problem than generally recognised, causing appalling levels of harm and death that are totally preventable".

Translated into simple English he is admitting modern medicine is killing and damaging a lot of people in England but by world standards we are doing ok. It is totally accepted now that modern medicine and its practices kills people, something that cannot be said for resting, sleeping, sunlight and drinking clean water. But then again that actually works and is free.

That is the legacy of this 'scientific method' used by 'experts'. Where is the outrage against modern medicine? Where is the precautionary measure towards modern medicine? Where is the propaganda warning of this killer? How would the world be today using methods of a peasant farmer from Austria? What is the true legacy of modern medical thinking and its practices on our bodies and on our minds? Not really a good reason to be going outside and clapping and hitting pots and pans, now, is it!

And last but certainly not least, never forget Thalidomide!

"Medical science has made such tremendous progress that there is hardly a healthy human left"

- Aldous Huxley

MEDICAL DOCTORS

The UK General Medical Council, direct from their website:

Our role

We are an independent organisation that helps to protect patients and improve medical education and practice across the UK.

We decide which doctors are qualified to work here and we oversee UK medical education and training.

We set the standards that doctors need to follow, and make sure that they continue to meet these standards throughout their careers.

We take action to prevent a doctor from putting the safety of patients, or the public's confidence in doctors, at risk.

Every patient should receive a high standard of care. Our role is to help achieve that by working closely with doctors, their employers and patients, to make sure that the trust patients have in their doctors is fully justified.

Duties of a doctor

The duties of a doctor registered with the General Medical Council

Patients must be able to trust doctors with their lives and health. To justify that trust you must show respect for human life and make sure your practice meets the standards expected of you in four domains.

Knowledge, skills and performance

- *Make the care of your patient your first concern.*
- *Provide a good standard of practice and care.*

- *Keep your professional knowledge and skills up to date.*
- *Recognise and work within the limits of your competence.*

Safety and quality

- *Take prompt action if you think that patient safety, dignity or comfort is being compromised.*
- *Protect and promote the health of patients and the public.*

Communication, partnership and teamwork

- *Treat patients as individuals and respect their dignity.*
- *Treat patients politely and considerately.*
- *Respect patients' right to confidentiality.*
- *Work in partnership with patients.*
- *Listen to, and respond to, their concerns and preferences.*
- *Give patients the information they want or need in a way they can understand.*
- *Respect patients' right to reach decisions with you about their treatment and care.*
- *Support patients in caring for themselves to improve and maintain their health.*
- *Work with colleagues in the ways that best serve patients' interests.*

Maintaining trust

- *Be honest and open and act with integrity.*
- *Never discriminate unfairly against patients or colleagues.*
- *Never abuse your patients' trust in you or the public's trust in the profession.*

You are personally accountable for your professional practice and must always be prepared to justify your decisions and actions.

PLEASE REMEMBER ALL THESE DUTIES OF A DOCTOR THE NEXT TIME YOU ARE ASKED FOR YOUR CONSENT TO VACCINATE, BE TESTED OR ARE OFFERED OTHER TREATMENTS AND DRUGS, OR IF YOU WANT TO ASK ABOUT ALTERNATIVE NATURAL THERAPIES.

Extracts from the Hippocratic oath

> "I will use those dietary regimens which will benefit my patients according to my greatest ability and judgment, and I will do no harm or injustice to them. Neither will I administer a poison to anybody when asked to do so, nor will I suggest such a course."

> "Into whatsoever houses I enter, I will enter to help the sick, and I will abstain from all intentional wrong-doing and harm, especially from abusing the bodies of man or woman, bond or free."

I think maybe a return to the Hippocratic oath would put us in a better position to stay safe and healthy than the 'Coronavirus Act 2020' which will do harm, injustice and potentially administer poison. And with its powers to enter our homes I think we could do with that protection and boundaries at this moment in time.

THE GLOBAL PANDEMIC
– WHAT JUST HAPPENED?

We have tried our best to give you as much information as we can, but in a condensed way, to take us through the next chapters on recent events here in the UK and worldwide. We have tried to show that away from the mainstream media and science there is another way to think of disease. We have also tried to show you that there are many invested interests of very rich people in maintaining a belief that drugs are needed for human health and to fight disease and vaccination programmes to prevent disease. We will now try and take you through the events of 'the pandemic' and how it started, and try and show you where humanity may end up if we keep following the men who claim to be 'experts' and also claim they can tell us what to believe and how to behave and when.

The main thing is to try and start with a blank piece of paper and just go with the data and the information shown and also do your own research. See if things add up and if they don't, stop, think, question and research some more. Make up your own mind and don't be swayed by the popular opinion, our opinion or especially the 'experts'. Find your own truth and come to your own conclusions. The aim of this book is to open up people's minds and not just ingrain our own personal belief so you exchange one lot of nonsense for another.

So the story begins of the greatest threat to mankind. A story that doesn't begin in China, but in New York.

EVENT 201 – YOUTUBE 'Event 201 Pandemic Exercise'

"Event 201" is a pandemic table top exercise hosted by The Johns Hopkins Center for Health Security in partnership with the World Economic Forum and the Bill and Melinda Gates Foundation on October 18, 2019, in New York, NY. The exercise illustrated the

pandemic preparedness efforts needed to diminish the large-scale economic and societal consequences of a severe pandemic. Drawing from actual events, Event 201 identifies important policy issues and preparedness challenges that could be solved with sufficient political will and attention. These issues were designed in a narrative to engage and educate the participants and the audience."

– Dr Michael Ryan, Executive Director WHO Health Emergencies Programme

This is the beginning of his introduction:

"The issues we will be dealing with over the next hours may be table top exercises today but they address real and critical threats which we at WHO take very seriously. Without a question epidemic risk has become a Global Strategic Concern. I don't think we've ever been in a situation where we have had to respond to so many health emergencies at once. This is the NEW NORMAL. I don't expect the frequency of these epidemics to reduce and in fact vulnerabilities all over the world in developed and developing countries have increased not decreased, driven by many factors mainly through human behaviour, economic development, population densities and many others. The scenario you will be presented with this morning could easily become one shared reality one day. I fully expect that we will be confronted by a fast moving and highly lethal pandemic of a respiratory pathogen."

What was the scenario they were presented with? An outbreak of coronavirus.

Extract from "epilogue chapter 4":

"The outcome of the CAPS (Coronavirus Associated Pulmonary Syndrome) pandemic in Event 201 was catastrophic. 65 million people dead in the first 18 months. The outbreak was small at first and initially seemed controllable but then it started spreading in densely crowded and impoverished neighbourhoods of mega cities. From that point on the spread of the disease was explosive.

Within 6 months cases were occurring in nearly every country."

Pandemic preparedness exercises in themselves are not unusual. In the UK in 2016 we had *Exercise Cygnus*. *'Exercise Cygnus was a Tier 1(national level) exercise which took place from Oct 18-20 2016'.*

> *"Pandemic influenza is one of the most severe natural phenomena to affect the UK and the most severe civil emergency risk. As such pandemic influenza remains at the top of the UK Government National Risk Register. During the exercise, participants considered their capacity and capability to operate at the peak of a pandemic affecting up to 50% of the UK population and which could cause between 200-400,000 excess deaths in the UK."*

https://assets.publishing.service.gov.uk/government/uploads/system/uploads/attac hment_data/file/927770/exercise-cygnus-report.pdf

So to be clear, the UK Government have completed exercises to deal with possible influenza pandemic that could cause 200-400,000 deaths. I am not here promoting the science of 'viral pandemics' at all. I am showing here how the minds of the people who would be dealing with an alleged attack would be primed, and psychologically prepared, to perceive a said attack a certain way and follow certain protocols in the belief that they were saving lives.

Wuhan, China

From WHO website:

WHO Statement regarding cluster of pneumonia cases in Wuhan, China 9 January 2020

Statement

China

Chinese authorities have made a preliminary determination of a novel (or new) coronavirus, identified in a hospitalized person with pneumonia in Wuhan. Chinese investigators conducted gene

sequencing of the virus, using an isolate from one positive patient sample. Preliminary identification of a novel virus in a short period of time is a notable achievement and demonstrates China's increased capacity to manage new outbreaks.

Initial information about the cases of pneumonia in Wuhan provided by Chinese authorities last week – including the occupation, location and symptom profile of the people affected – pointed to a coronavirus (CoV) as a possible pathogen causing this cluster. Chinese authorities subsequently reported that laboratory tests ruled out SARS-CoV, MERS-CoV, influenza, avian influenza, adenovirus and other common respiratory pathogens.

Coronaviruses are a large family of viruses with some causing less-severe disease, such as the common cold, and others more severe disease such as MERS and SARS. Some transmit easily from person to person, while others do not. According to Chinese authorities, the virus in question can cause severe illness in some patients and does not transmit readily between people.

Globally, novel coronaviruses emerge periodically in different areas, including SARS in 2002 and MERS in 2012. Several known coronaviruses are circulating in animals that have not yet infected humans. As surveillance improves more coronaviruses are likely to be identified.

China has strong public health capacities and resources to respond and manage respiratory disease outbreaks. In addition to treating the patients in care and isolating new cases as they may be identified, public health officials remain focused on continued contact tracing, conducting environmental assessments at the seafood market, and investigations to identify the pathogen causing the outbreak.

In the coming weeks, more comprehensive information is required to understand the current status and epidemiology of the outbreak, and the clinical picture. Further investigations are also required to determine the source, modes of transmission, extent of infection and countermeasures implemented. WHO continues to monitor the situation closely and, together with its partners, is ready to provide technical support to China to investigate and respond to this outbreak.

The preliminary determination of a novel virus will assist authorities in other countries to conduct disease detection and response. Over the past week, people with symptoms of pneumonia and reported travel history to Wuhan have been identified at international airports.

WHO does not recommend any specific measures for travellers. WHO advises against the application of any travel or trade restrictions on China based on the information currently available.

So, initially, we have someone ill in hospital with pneumonia and the alleged isolation of a 'novel virus' and sequences of the genetic code. No other usual suspects virus-wise seemed to be present indicating this to be the cause. This new virus was said to cause severe illness in some but did not easily spread between people.

This extract is from an article by James Griffiths, July 11th 2019, for CNN:

China has made major progress on air pollution. Wuhan protests show there's still a long way to go. At 146 globally on the AirVisual list, Wuhan, in northeastern China, is not among China's most polluted cities, but residents aren't taking any chances. Recent weeks have seen major protests there – in themselves a rarity in China – over plans for a new garbage incineration plant.

Holding banners with slogans such as "we don't want to be poisoned, we just need a breath of fresh air," thousands of people took to the city's streets over two weeks in June and July calling for the suspension of plans to build the plant.

"We are fearful that the plant is too close to residence area," one protester in the city of 10 million people told state media. Others expressed concern that emissions could worsen air

pollution and harm residents' health.

Local officials were apparently surprised by the scale and size of the protests, which came after several similar waste plants were reportedly found to be giving off dangerous emissions. Photos and videos shared on social media showed large crowds marching in the streets near where the plant was to be built, and police arresting numerous protesters.

The government has since suspended building of the plant, which locals said had halted protests, but a heavy police presence remains in the city where the situation is tense.

So it is clear that the residents in Wuhan were worried about pollution and toxicity in the environment. Wuhan is the largest city in central China with a population of over 11 million. Well known for its steel industry and now 5 car manufacturers, and is an industrial centre in China. The article also shows China along with India, having the worst deaths attributable to air pollution in 2017. So does it surprise you that people living in a heavily polluted country, and in fact in one of the industrial centres, already protesting about pollution and the environment and in the presence of what history has shown to be a ruthless Communist government (remember tank man.), may come down with an illness with breathing difficulties as a main symptom?

Why the obsession with finding a 'new novel virus' as the cause of illness? Why is there zero holistic thinking into the issues of illness and disease coming from the medical authorities, the self-proclaimed 'experts'? We all saw the pictures coming out of China, the mayhem, the ruthless control, the madness of people in laboratory protection gear disinfecting whole streets, and people. Is this sheer stupidity, a total lack of awareness or something more sinister? It may be a mixture of all of the above.

A New Novel Virus

Let's now have a look into the scientific method used which brought them to the conclusion that it was a virus that was passing from person to person and killing people.

First, it was noted that a number of people were coming down with a severe flu-like issue that manifested in severe breathing difficulties in a wet market. The 'experts' took samples, then out of the samples looked for the culprit, assuming it had to be a virus. They do that a lot. How many times have you been to the doctors feeling under the weather and been told "*it must be a bug/virus going around*"? Hardly a deep investigation and not an ounce of proof needed. They don't really know so it must therefore be a virus.

So they took the samples and found the enemy. They managed to filter out and claimed to isolate a virus previously unknown to them. So now, without any more tests they have found the enemy; they presume it is new and presume it wasn't there before so in that case it **must** be the cause.

Science, though, tells us we must look at all information and all factors when doing our best to come to some sort of conclusion. So the obvious information left out is, what about the physical, energetic and emotional environment of the patients and what else was found in the samples of tissue taken from the patients? Obvious things to look for would be toxins in the environment and if the same toxins are found in the samples. Also the other influences in the environment and what other toxins and waste, whether from the outer world or inner cellular waste, were in the samples? This, you would think would be a proper scientific method to at least have a good idea of what is going on and what the influences are on the patient to make them ill or die. This is what we would call holistic thinking, something that has no room in the world of modern medicine.

Science is just an observation and then asking the questions – why and how did that happen? It doesn't have to take place in a lab and you don't need a white coat and a degree in anything to be scientific. Anyone can be scientific; in fact most of us do make scientific observations every day. We all have the right to observe and think and come to our own conclusions. Don't think you should leave it to the 'experts'"to tell you what to think and let them tell you their version of events is more accurate than yours because they have letters after their name and use words that most of us don't understand. Look at all observations around an event and bring in all factors and then maybe, just maybe, you may be able to come up with a reasonable idea of why and how.

Medical science and science are not the same thing. Medical science wants to promote predetermined 'truths' whereas real science observes to try and find real objective truths.

The Paper that Locked Down the World

A Novel Coronavirus from Patients with Pneumonia in China, 2019

https://scholar.harvard.edu/files/kleelerner/files/20200124_nejm_-_a_novel_coronavirus_from_patients_with_pneumonia_in_china_2019_01.pdf

Feb 20 2020

Summary

In December 2019, a cluster of patients with pneumonia of unknown cause was linked to a seafood wholesale market in Wuhan, China. A previously unknown betacoronavirus was discovered through the use of unbiased sequencing in samples from patients with pneumonia. Human airway epithelial cells were used to isolate a novel coronavirus, named 2019-nCoV, which formed a clade within the subgenus sarbecovirus, Orthocoronavirinae subfamily. Different from both MERS-CoV and SARS-CoV, 2019-nCoV is the seventh member of the family of coronaviruses that infect humans. Enhanced surveillance and further investigation are ongoing. (Funded by the National Key Research and Development Program of China and the National Major Project for Control and Prevention of Infectious Disease in China.)

Emerging and reemerging pathogens are global challenges for public health. Coronaviruses are enveloped RNA viruses that are distributed broadly among humans, other mammals, and birds and that cause respiratory, enteric, hepatic, and neurologic

199

diseases. Six coronavirus species are known to cause human disease. Four viruses — 229E, OC43, NL63, and HKU1 — are prevalent and typically cause common cold symptoms in immunocompetent individuals. The two other strains — severe acute respiratory syndrome coronavirus (SARS-CoV) and Middle East respiratory syndrome coronavirus (MERS-CoV) — are zoonotic in origin and have been linked to sometimes fatal illness. SARS-CoV was the causal agent of the severe acute respiratory syndrome outbreaks in 2002 and 2003 in Guangdong Province, China. MERS-CoV was the pathogen responsible for severe respiratory disease outbreaks in 2012 in the Middle East. Given the high prevalence and wide distribution of coronaviruses, the large genetic diversity and frequent recombination of their genomes, and increasing human–animal interface activities, novel coronaviruses are likely to emerge periodically in humans owing to frequent cross-species infections and occasional spillover events.

In late December 2019, several local health facilities reported clusters of patients with pneumonia of unknown cause that were epidemiologically linked to a seafood and wet animal wholesale market in Wuhan, Hubei Province, China. On December 31, 2019, the Chinese Center for Disease Control and Prevention (China CDC) dispatched a rapid response team to accompany Hubei provincial and Wuhan city health authorities and to conduct an epidemiologic and etiologic investigation. We report the results of this investigation, identifying the source of the pneumonia clusters, and describe a novel coronavirus detected in patients with pneumonia whose specimens were tested by the China CDC at an early stage of the outbreak. We also describe clinical features of the pneumonia in two of these patients.

Methods
Viral Diagnostic Methods

Four lower respiratory tract samples, including bronchoalveolar-lavage fluid, were collected from patients with pneumonia of unknown cause who were identified in Wuhan on December 21, 2019, or later and who had been present at the Huanan Seafood

Market close to the time of their clinical presentation. Seven bronchoalveolar-lavage fluid specimens were collected from patients in Beijing hospitals with pneumonia of known cause to serve as control samples. Extraction of nucleic acids from clinical samples (including uninfected cultures that served as negative controls) was performed with a High Pure Viral Nucleic Acid Kit, as described by the manufacturer (Roche). Extracted nucleic acid samples were tested for viruses and bacteria by polymerase chain reaction (PCR), using the RespiFinderSmart22kit (PathoFinder BV) and the LightCycler 480 real-time PCR system, in accordance with manufacturer instructions.12 Samples were analyzed for 22 pathogens (18 viruses and 4 bacteria) as detailed in the Supplementary Appendix. In addition, unbiased, high-throughput sequencing, described previously,was used to discover microbial sequences not identifiable by the means described above. A real-time reverse transcription PCR (RT-PCR) assay was used to detect viral RNA by targeting a consensus RdRp region of pan β-CoV, as described in the Supplementary Appendix.

Isolation of Virus

Bronchoalveolar-lavage fluid samples were collected in sterile cups to which virus transport medium was added. Samples were then centrifuged to remove cellular debris. The supernatant was inoculated on human airway epithelial cells, which had been obtained from airway specimens resected from patients undergoing surgery for lung cancer and were confirmed to be special-pathogen-free by NGS.

Human airway epithelial cells were expanded on plastic substrate to generate passage-1 cells and were subsequently plated at a density of 2.5×105 cells per well on permeable Transwell-COL (12-mm diameter) supports. Human airway epithelial cell cultures were generated in an air–liquid interface for 4 to 6 weeks to form well-differentiated, polarized cultures resembling in vivo pseudostratified mucociliary epithelium.13

Prior to infection, apical surfaces of the human airway epithelial cells were washed three times with phosphate-buffered saline; 150 µl of supernatant from bronchoalveolar-lavage fluid samples was inoculated onto the apical surface of the cell cultures. After a 2-hour incubation at 37°C, unbound virus was removed by washing with 500 µl of phosphate-buffered saline for 10 minutes; human airway epithelial cells were maintained in an air–liquid interface incubated at 37°C with 5% carbon dioxide. Every 48 hours, 150 µl of phosphate-buffered saline was applied to the apical surfaces of the human airway epithelial cells, and after 10 minutes of incubation at 37°C the samples were harvested. Pseudostratified mucociliary epithelium cells were maintained in this environment; apical samples were passaged in a 1:3 diluted vial stock to new cells. The cells were monitored daily with light microscopy, for cytopathic effects, and with RT-PCR, for the presence of viral nucleic acid in the supernatant. After three passages, apical samples and human airway epithelial cells were prepared for transmission electron microscopy.

Transmission Electron Microscopy

Supernatant from human airway epithelial cell cultures that showed cytopathic effects was collected, inactivated with 2% paraformaldehyde for at least 2 hours, and ultracentrifuged to sediment virus particles. The enriched supernatant was negatively stained on film-coated grids for examination. Human airway epithelial cells showing cytopathic effects were collected and fixed with 2% paraformaldehyde–2.5% glutaraldehyde and were then fixed with 1% osmium tetroxide dehydrated with grade ethanol embedded with PON812 resin. Sections (80 nm) were cut from resin block and stained with uranyl acetate and lead citrate, separately. The negative stained grids and ultrathin sections were observed under transmission electron microscopy.

Viral Genome Sequencing

RNA extracted from bronchoalveolar-lavage fluid and culture supernatants was used as a template to clone and sequence the genome. We used a combination of Illumina sequencing and nanopore sequencing to characterize the virus genome.

Sequence reads were assembled into contig maps (a set of overlapping DNA segments) with the use of CLC Genomics software, version 4.6.1 (CLC Bio). Specific primers were subsequently designed for PCR, and 5'- or 3'-RACE (rapid amplification of cDNA ends) was used to fill genome gaps from conventional Sanger sequencing. These PCR products were purified from gels and sequenced with a BigDye Terminator v3.1 Cycle Sequencing Kit and a 3130XL Genetic Analyzer, in accordance with the manufacturers' instructions.

Multiple-sequence alignment of the 2019-nCoV and reference sequences was performed with the use of Muscle. Phylogenetic analysis of the complete genomes was performed with RAxML (13) with 1000 bootstrap replicates and a general time-reversible model used as the nucleotide substitution model.

Results

Patients

Three adult patients presented with severe pneumonia and were admitted to a hospital in Wuhan on December 27, 2019. Patient 1 was a 49-year-old woman, Patient 2 was a 61-year-old man, and Patient 3 was a 32-year-old man. Clinical profiles were available for Patients 1 and 2. Patient 1 reported having no underlying chronic medical conditions but reported fever (temperature, 37°C to 38°C) and cough with chest discomfort on December 23, 2019. Four days after the onset of illness, her cough and chest discomfort worsened, but the fever was reduced; a diagnosis of pneumonia was based on computed tomographic (CT) scan. Her occupation was retailer in the seafood wholesale market. Patient 2 initially reported fever and cough on December 20, 2019; respiratory distress developed 7 days after the onset of illness and worsened over the next 2 days (see chest radiographs, Figure 1), at which time mechanical ventilation was started. He had been a frequent visitor to the seafood wholesale market. Patients 1 and 3 recovered and were discharged from the hospital on January 16, 2020. Patient 2 died on January 9, 2020. No biopsy specimens were obtained.

Detection and Isolation of a Novel Coronavirus

Three bronchoalveolar-lavage samples were collected from Wuhan Jinyintan Hospital on December 30, 2019. No specific pathogens (including HCoV-229E, HCoV-NL63, HCoV-OC43, and HCoV-HKU1) were detected in clinical specimens from these patients by the RespiFinderSmart22kit. RNA extracted from bronchoalveolar-lavage fluid from the patients was used as a template to clone and sequence a genome using a combination of Illumina sequencing and nanopore sequencing. More than 20,000 viral reads from individual specimens were obtained, and most contigs matched to the genome from lineage B of the genus betacoronavirus — showing more than 85% identity with a bat SARS-like CoV (bat-SL-CoVZC45, MG772933.1) genome published previously. Positive results were also obtained with use of a real-time RT-PCR assay for RNA targeting to a consensus RdRp region of pan β-CoV (although the cycle threshold value was higher than 34 for detected samples). Virus isolation from the clinical specimens was performed with human airway epithelial cells and Vero E6 and Huh-7 cell lines. The isolated virus was named 2019-nCoV.

To determine whether virus particles could be visualized in 2019-nCoV–infected human airway epithelial cells, mock-infected and 2019-nCoV–infected human airway epithelial cultures were examined with light microscopy daily and with transmission electron microscopy 6 days after inoculation. Cytopathic effects were observed 96 hours after inoculation on surface layers of human airway epithelial cells; a lack of cilium beating was seen with light microcopy in the center of the focus (Figure 2). No specific cytopathic effects were observed in the Vero E6 and Huh-7 cell lines until 6 days after inoculation.

Electron micrographs of negative-stained 2019-nCoV particles were generally spherical with some pleomorphism (Figure 3). Diameter varied from about 60 to 140 nm. Virus particles had quite distinctive spikes, about 9 to 12 nm, and gave virions the appearance of a solar corona. Extracellular free virus particles and inclusion bodies filled with virus particles in membrane-bound vesicles in cytoplasm were found in the human airway epithelial ultrathin sections. This observed morphology is consistent with the

Coronaviridae family.

To further characterize the virus, de novo sequences of 2019-nCoV genome from clinical specimens (bronchoalveolar-lavage fluid) and human airway epithelial cell virus isolates were obtained by Illumina and nanopore sequencing. The novel coronavirus was identified from all three patients. Two nearly full-length coronavirus sequences were obtained from bronchoalveolar-lavage fluid (BetaCoV/Wuhan/IVDC-HB-04/2020, BetaCoV/Wuhan/IVDC-HB-05/2020|EPI_ISL_402121), and one full-length sequence was obtained from a virus isolated from a patient (BetaCoV/Wuhan/IVDC-HB-01/2020|EPI_ISL_402119). Complete genome sequences of the three novel coronaviruses were submitted to GISAID (BetaCoV/Wuhan/IVDC-HB-01/2019, accession ID: EPI_ISL_402119; BetaCoV/Wuhan/IVDC-HB-04/2020, accession ID: EPI_ISL_402120; BetaCoV/Wuhan/IVDC-HB-05/2019, accession ID: EPI_ISL_402121) and have a 86.9% nucleotide sequence identity to a previously published bat SARS-like CoV (bat-SL-CoVZC45, MG772933.1) genome. The three 2019-nCoV genomes clustered together within the sarbecovirus subgenus, which shows the typical betacoronavirus organization: a 5' untranslated region (UTR), replicase complex (orf1ab), S gene, E gene, M gene, N gene, 3' UTR, and several unidentified nonstructural open reading frames.

Although 2019-nCoV is similar to some betacoronaviruses detected in bats (Figure 4), it is distinct from SARS-CoV and MERS-CoV. The three 2019-nCoV coronaviruses from Wuhan, together with two bat-derived SARS-like strains, ZC45 and ZXC21, form a distinct clade. SARS-CoV strains from humans and genetically similar SARS-like coronaviruses from bats collected from southwestern China formed another clade within the subgenus sarbecovirus. Since the sequence identity in conserved replicase domains (ORF 1ab) is less than 90% between 2019-nCoV and other members of betacoronavirus, the 2019-nCoV — the likely causative agent of the viral pneumonia in Wuhan — is a novel betacoronavirus belonging to the sarbecovirus subgenus of Coronaviridae family.

Discussion

We report a novel CoV (2019-nCoV) that was identified in hospitalized patients in Wuhan, China, in December 2019 and January 2020. Evidence for the presence of this virus includes identification in bronchoalveolar-lavage fluid in three patients by whole-genome sequencing, direct PCR, and culture. The illness likely to have been caused by this CoV was named "novel coronavirus-infected pneumonia" (NCIP). Complete genomes were submitted to GISAID. Phylogenetic analysis revealed that 2019-nCoV falls into the genus betacoronavirus, which includes coronaviruses (SARS-CoV, bat SARS-like CoV, and others) discovered in humans, bats, and other wild animals. We report isolation of the virus and the initial description of its specific cytopathic effects and morphology.

Molecular techniques have been used successfully to identify infectious agents for many years. Unbiased, high-throughput sequencing is a powerful tool for the discovery of pathogens. Next-generation sequencing and bioinformatics are changing the way we can respond to infectious disease outbreaks, improving our understanding of disease occurrence and transmission, accelerating the identification of pathogens, and promoting data sharing. We describe in this report the use of molecular techniques and unbiased DNA sequencing to discover a novel betacoronavirus that is likely to have been the cause of severe pneumonia in three patients in Wuhan, China.

Although establishing human airway epithelial cell cultures is labor intensive, they appear to be a valuable research tool for analysis of human respiratory pathogens. Our study showed that initial propagation of human respiratory secretions onto human airway epithelial cell cultures, followed by transmission electron microscopy and whole genome sequencing of culture supernatant, was successfully used for visualization and detection of new human coronavirus that can possibly elude identification by traditional approaches.

Further development of accurate and rapid methods to identify unknown respiratory pathogens is still needed. On the basis of analysis of three complete genomes obtained in this study, we *designed several specific and sensitive assays targeting ORF1ab, N, and E regions of the 2019-nCoV genome to detect viral RNA in clinical specimens. The primer sets and standard operating procedures have been shared with the World Health Organization and are intended for surveillance and detection of 2019-nCoV infection globally and in China. More recent data show 2019-nCoV detection in 830 persons in China.*

Although our study does not fulfill Koch's postulates, our analyses provide evidence implicating 2019-nCoV in the Wuhan outbreak. Additional evidence to confirm the etiologic significance of 2019-nCoV in the Wuhan outbreak include identification of a 2019-nCoV antigen in the lung tissue of patients by immunohistochemical analysis, detection of IgM and IgG antiviral antibodies in the serum samples from a patient at two time points to demonstrate seroconversion, and animal (monkey) experiments to provide evidence of pathogenicity. Of critical importance are epidemiologic investigations to characterize transmission modes, reproduction interval, and clinical spectrum resulting from infection to inform and refine strategies that can prevent, control, and stop the spread of 2019-nCoV.

Before I hand you over to professional analysis of this paper by Patrick Quanten I will highlight here one simple observation.
"Although our study does not fulfill Koch's postulates,"
Even in their own words the paper did not fulfill Kock's Postulates. The big question is though; did it fulfill any of those postulates, including the most important, the isolation of the virus itself?

The Illusion of Virus Isolation - Patrick Quanten MD

Modern sterile laboratories where extremely clever people perform extremely complicated tasks are impressing the population, producing jaw dropping statements about something as complex and sinister as life itself. The tasks they perform are so complicated that each person only performs a specific action within an entire chain of events. The technology involved requires one person to be trained to the highest possible level to perform only one of those steps. They become expert employees on one detail of the entire sequence. This is certainly the case in laboratories where viral experiments and research is being conducted. Everybody simply performs a task that they have been trained for without actually understanding the entire process. The entire process is hidden from plain view – you wouldn't understand it anyway! – and within the walls of the laboratory complex the entire process is only revealed to their employees on a 'need-to-know' basis. This is the perfect setup to perpetuate mistakes without anybody being in a position to ask relevant questions about the working method or the reasoning behind the working method.

Let's follow the process of virus isolation as the industry describes it to us. Let's cast our critical eye upon their words and actions. It's a rotten job, but somebody has to do it!

First of all, we need to understand what they are looking for. A very important thing they are looking for is a genetic code sequence, which they claim belongs to a virus. There are two types of genetic coding sequences, DNA and RNA. What's the difference?

We will pick out some important differences that are relevant to the story of the isolation of a virus. DNA is a double helix molecule, while RNA is a single strand molecule that is much shorter. DNA is responsible for storing and transferring genetic information and cannot leave the cell nucleus, while RNA directly codes for amino acids and acts as a messenger between DNA and ribosomes (a structure outside of the nucleus) to make proteins. In other words, RNA can be found everywhere within the cell compound, both in the nucleus as well as in the cytoplasm. DNA is self-replicating, while RNA is a transcript of a small portion of the DNA, single stranded, and cannot replicate itself. There are three types of RNA of which mRNA is by far the most common. It stands for messenger RNA because the transcript of a short part of the DNA sequence is in fact 'a message' that will be delivered to the ribosomes of the cell, where cells produce proteins. In other words, mRNA delivers the instructions from headquarters (the DNA inside the cell nucleus) to the factory (outside of the cell nucleus) for the production of materials.

Let's now follow the steps of the process that lead to the isolation of the virus as described by the industry.

> *Bronchoalveolar-lavage fluid samples were collected in sterile cups to which virus transport medium (VTM) was added. The VTM that is urgently required needs to support viral replication, as well as other routine diagnostic approaches.*

The transport medium needs to support viral replication! Why? Not just stop the breakdown of the genetic code, but actually encouraging replication, multiplication of genetic coding material. The use of virus transport medium has been introduced because virus samples degrade – no genetic code can be found within any sample - very quickly unless they are stored at ultralow temperatures or in liquid nitrogen. The RNA parts quickly fall apart unless you are able to instantly freeze the lot. A way around this is to use chemicals. However, the function of these chemicals (VTM) is not 'to freeze' the sample but to replicate the RNA sequence that may be present within the sample.

The commonly used VTM's are saline solution, phosphate-buffered saline (PBS), or foetal bovine serum (FBS).

- In the *Journal for Virological Methods* (November 2022) they published the result of a comparative study which showed a saline solution not to be an adequate viral transport medium.

- All tests on a phosphate-buffered saline solution, as well as on the saline solution of the previous paragraph, have been done under laboratory conditions. RNA sequences have been replicated multiple times before adding the solution, otherwise no RNA can be found within the samples. It also turns out that storage temperature needs to be very low (around 4°C) in order to still produce positive test results for 'viral' RNA.

- In June 2020, a study was published entitled *'The impact of viral transport media on PCR assay results for the detection of nucleic acid from SARS-CoV-2 and other viruses'* by P.D. Kirkland and M.J. Frost (Virology Laboratory, New South Wales, Australia). They concluded the following: ... *Coronavirus RNA was rapidly destroyed in the commercial transport media. ... Collectively these data showed that the commercial viral transport media contained nucleases or similar substances and may seriously compromise diagnostic and epidemiological investigations. ... Recommendations to include foetal bovine serum as a source of protein to enhance the stabilising properties of viral transport media are contraindicated. ... The inclusion of foetal bovine serum presents a biosecurity risk for the movement of animal pathogens and renders these transport media unsuitable for animal disease diagnostic applications. While these transport media may be suitable for virus culture purposes, there could be misleading results if used for nucleic acid-based tests (looking for genetic codes – my clarification). Therefore, these products should be evaluated to ensure fitness for purpose.*

- Foetal bovine serum is the most widely-used growth supplement for cell culture media because of its high content of embryonic growth-promoting factors. When used at appropriate concentrations, it supplies many *defined and undefined* components that have been shown to satisfy specific metabolic requirements for the culture of cells. FBS is a complex mixture of biomolecules that includes growth factors, proteins, trace elements, vitamins, and hormones. These are important for the growth and maintenance of cells in vivo and in culture. Hence, the collected virus samples are added to a cell culture with the sole purpose of increasing the virus production by those cells, increasing the viral genetic sequence.

After having been manipulated by the transport medium and the conditions in which the samples have been held, these samples arrive at the laboratory.

Samples are then centrifuged to remove cellular debris. The supernatant is inoculated on human airway epithelial cells.

The supernatant is to all intents and purposes the extracellular fluid. This contains everything the cells have expelled. The cellular debris is in the supernatant, and what they call 'the cellular debris' that centrifuging is removing is in fact intact cells. They no longer want the old cells from the transport medium. They simply want the fluid that contains the waste products of the cells. This supernatant, the cellular waste, is then mixed with human cells.

Prior to infection, apical surfaces of the human airway epithelial cells were washed three times with phosphate-buffered saline.

Phosphate-buffered saline solution is a toxic environment for the cells. They use the phosphate-buffered saline to stop the cells from bursting, which basically stops the cells from displaying a disease. However, they have a number of potential disadvantages. Phosphates inhibit many enzymatic reactions and procedures that are the foundation of molecular cloning. This includes cleavage of DNA by many restriction enzymes, ligation of DNA, and bacterial transformation. So the DNA can no longer separate and initiate cell division. This conflict leads to the genetic coding of the DNA double helix of the cells to break into pieces in a desperate attempt to function 'normally'.

After a 2-hour incubation at 37°C, unbound virus was removed by washing with 500μl of phosphate-buffered saline for 10 minutes. Human airway epithelial cells were maintained in an air–liquid interface incubated at 37°C with 5% carbon dioxide. Every 48 hours, 150μl of phosphate-buffered saline was applied to the apical surfaces of the human airway epithelial cells, and after 10 minutes of incubation at 37°C the samples were harvested.

They keep 'washing' the cells with phosphate-buffered saline and then collect the cellular waste they have extracted from the cells. The poisoned cells are being prevented from bursting so they keep 'washing' out cellular bits of rubbish for quite a long time.

> *RNA extracted from bronchoalveolar-lavage fluid and culture supernatants was used as a template to clone and sequence the genome. ... Specific primers were subsequently designed for PCR, and 5'- or 3'-RACE (rapid amplification of cDNA ends) was used to fill genome gaps from conventional Sanger sequencing.*

Added to the supernatant, before 'the search' for the viral genome begins, are some specific primers for genome sequencing. Their function is to complete the full set of the coding they are searching for from the moment it detects something that resembles the template. In other words, the procedure produces a number of exact sequences, set out by the researchers, out of bits that have some similarity with the sequence one wants to find. The total number of these *corrected sequences* results in a positive 'identification' of the viral RNA.

Following this procedure from sample taking to replication of genome sequences it must be obvious that cellular debris plays a major part in the obtained results. Cells are added to the samples at various stages of the procedure and extracellular fluid is being collected for examination, which contains everything the cells expel, including bits of their own DNA structure, a process that is being enhanced by the process of chemical manipulation the researchers perform. Poison a cell and it begins to show signs of wavering function and specific debris will start to show itself.

In the end one 'identifies' small genetic sequences, bits of RNA, of which the origin is unknown and of which many have been given a helping hand in order 'to get it right'. It is also impossible to say if the 'identified' sequences were actually present in full within the examined fluid, besides the fact that the sample was taken a long time ago under precarious conditions and then transported to the laboratory under questionable conditions. What one has 'identified' this way cannot scientifically be linked to anything that possible was present within the original sample. Hence, the origin of the RNA sequence is scientifically unknown and therefore cannot be named as the RNA sequence belonging to a specific virus. The RNA sequence of the virus has not been isolated, nor has it been identified. Scientifically it looks much more like *the creation of a RNA sequence* in a few obscure steps.

The same conclusion must we come to with regards of the electron microscopic pictures that are taken both from the supernatant and from the epithelial cell culture. On these pictures one 'identifies' certain shapes as being typical for a specific family of viruses. However, there is no scientific way to link those shapes on the picture to the RNA sequence obtained. Truth is, we don't know where the RNA sequence comes from and we don't know where the shapes on the picture come from. Neither do we know if there is a connection between either of these, even if we for a moment contemplate the possibility that both are what viral experts say they are.

Another theory, which does take into account the findings of the laboratory research, and which can possibly explain both the RNA sequences and the shapes on the pictures, goes as follows.

When a cell becomes ill and begins to malfunction it may become a problem so big that the genetic coding system becomes overwhelmed. In a frantic effort to rectify the function of the failing cell the DNA sends out multiple messages, mRNA, which the cell factory is mostly unable to carry out. The cell fills up with redundant mRNA, many of which are replicas as the genome of the cell is desperately trying to get the *message across*. Unfortunately it isn't working. In an effort to still organize the inner workings of the cell, it tries 'to bag up' these mRNA bits so they wouldn't get locked into the factory system, blocking whatever is left of the function of that factory. The cell deteriorates, fills up with 'unheard' messages and eventually dies, releasing all these bagged up RNA sequences into the extracellular fluid.

And how does this version of the story hold up against scientific knowledge?

In the first place, science tells us that life is a continual interaction of energies. The physical part of life is formed out of an energy field and the way life functions and evolves is a direct result of these interactions. Disease then becomes an imbalance within that field, which manifests itself in the function, and later on equally in the structure, of the cell, of the organ, of the organism.

The scientific germ theory confirms this sequence of events. It states that the disease comes first and is later followed by the appearance of micro-organisms within the cellular debris the disease has caused. So micro-organisms do not cause an infectious disease but they are the result of the already existing disease.

Following this scientific knowledge a virus, which is nothing but a short RNA sequence within a simple protein membrane, would become a result of the disease and not the cause. It would appear inside the cellular debris, not entering the cell from the outside. Indeed, a scientific theory already exists stating that what has been called viruses are also known as endosomes, small protein bags with a bit of RNA inside them. These small intracellular bags first make an appearance, in very small numbers, within a functional cell. They also have been photographed attached to the cell membrane and in the extracellular space, where they are called exosomes. The scientific theory states that genetic cellular debris is bagged up inside the cell and made ready for expulsion. From endosome to exosome. From a rubbish bag in your kitchen to the same rubbish bag outside your front door, ready for collection. Experts confirm that endosomes (exosomes) are

214

indistinguishable from viruses. 'Indistinguishable' means *not able to be identified as different.*

This would explain why young fresh cells are constantly being added to the procedure of viral isolation. Without the cells, one would not have any short RNA sequences in the sample, bearing in mind that one needs to add a transport cell medium to the sample immediately. In the laboratory, one then changes the living conditions of cells – they are constantly being 'washed' – which makes them malfunction, the precondition for the production of genetic debris.

Taking that debris to start the search for a predetermined sequence may result in *the finding* of that particular sequence, greatly enhanced by the fact that you 'fill in the gaps'. The machine looks for copies of the RNA sequence entered and anything that remotely looks like it is counted and 'corrected'. It does not *identify* the found sequence as anything particular. It is a short RNA sequence. That is all. That is not identification'. When I find a shoe of a certain shape and size, I should not state that a six foot two, grey haired, Irishman was here some time ago. Let alone I begin to tell you what he was doing while he was here! RNA sequences are a normal part of every living cell and can be found in and around every living cell. And as long as I can't isolate an entire intact virus from which I can extract the full RNA I cannot scientifically make any statement regarding the origin of the found RNA, nor its function, nor can I say anything about the bubble that I believe contains the very same RNA.

As the procedure we have described is the standard procedure used to identify all viruses you may with confidence conclude that no virus has ever been isolated or identified. This conclusion has been confirmed by many scientific studies and reviews as the HIV hoax clearly has revealed. Science has exposed the floors within the virology research on many occasions, including the false claim about the isolation of the covid-virus. However, the media, and with it the only 'scientific' information you will hear about, does not mention this. As it is part of the industry it needs to ensure the official narrative remains the only one that is heard by the public. It's the official narrative that counts, not the truth.

Let's not bother with science when we can make some money!

MORE DOCTORS OF TRUTH

Dr Stephan Lanka is a former virologist who now prefers to simply refer to himself as a biologist. Similar to Patrick he has been challenging the scientific world as to the nature of these alleged viruses for many years.

> "All claims about viruses as pathogens are wrong and are based on easily recognizable, understandable and verifiable misinterpretations ... All scientists who think they are working with viruses in laboratories are actually working with typical particles of specific dying tissues or cells which were prepared in a special way. They believe that those tissues and cells are dying because they were infected by a virus. In reality, the infected cells and tissues were dying because they were starved and poisoned as a consequence of the experiments in the lab."

> "... the death of the tissue and cells takes place in the exact same manner when no 'infected' genetic material is added at all. The virologists have apparently not noticed this fact. According to ... scientific logic and the rules of scientific conduct, control experiments should have been carried out. In order to confirm the newly discovered method of so-called 'virus propagation' ... scientists would have had to perform additional experiments, called negative control experiments, in which they would add sterile substances ... to the cell culture."

– Dr Stefan Lanka, The Misconception Called Virus.

> "Virologists have never isolated a complete genetic strand of a virus and displayed it directly, in its entire length. They always use very short pieces of nucleic acids, whose sequence consists of four molecules to determine them and call them sequences. From a multitude of millions of such specific, very short sequences, virologists mentally assemble a fictitious long genome strand with the help of complex computational and

statistical methods. This process is called alignment. The result of this complex alignment, the fictitious and very long genetic strand, is presented by virologists as the core of a virus and they claim to have thus proven the existence of a virus."

"Virologists who claim disease-causing viruses are science fraudsters and must be prosecuted".

– Dr Stephan Lanka

The results of a so far unpublished paper by Dr Lanka 'Lanka S. Preliminary results: Response of primary human epithelial cells to stringent virus amplification protocols (unpublished'). April 2021" can be found in the booklet *'Breaking The Spell: The Scientific Evidence for Ending The COVID Delusion'* by Dr Tom Cowan at www.drtomcowan.com. The results of this preliminary control experiment clearly show that when the medium of a cell culture increases in toxicity (adding more antibiotics) and is reduced in nutrition (reducing bovine calf serum) a cytopathic effect (CPE) appears. This happens even though no pathogenic virus was added to the culture. So regardless of whether pathogenic virus is added or not the result shown is the same cytopathic effect, backing up completely the statement that the grey blobs, seen in electron microscopic photos, that the whole pathogenic virus story is built on, are actually cellular debris that has been pushed out in a form of house cleaning and damage limitation by the cell itself.

Dr Andrew Kaufman MD and Dr Tom Cowan MD with Sally Farron Morell MADr Andrew Kaufman MD and Dr Tom Cowan MD with Sally Farron Morell MA are challenging the USA medical science community in pretty much the same way. This is part of their statement, similar to what other brave doctors have now stated. It will take many more brave doctors to come out and speak this truth to make a difference but the first dominoes are now falling. This truth is what will free us from this invisible attack that is controlling our lives. The whole basis of the lockdown is a PCR test that nobody knows what it's testing for, except some fragments of genetic material all based on a picture of a blob from an electron microscope. It may seem incredible that this is the truth and yet so many 'experts' cannot see it at all but hopefully this will be explained later on when we go into the power of beliefs and how they control our perception. Clearly thousands of doctors around the world are not knowingly lying to the public, they just cannot see what is there, hidden in plain sight.

Statement On Virus Isolation (SOVI)

- Found at www.andrewkaufmanmd.com

Isolation: The action of isolating; the fact or condition of being isolated or standing alone; separation from other things or persons; solitariness.

(Oxford English Dictionary)

The controversy over whether the SARS-CoV-2 virus has ever been isolated or purified continues. However, using the above definition, common sense, the laws of logic and the dictates of science, any unbiased person must come to the conclusion that the SARS-CoV-2 virus has never been isolated or purified. As a result, no confirmation of the virus' existence can be found. The logical, common sense, and scientific consequences of this fact are:

the structure and composition of something not shown to exist can't be known, including the presence, structure, and function of any hypothetical spike or other proteins;

the genetic sequence of something that has never been found can't be known; 'variants' of something that hasn't been shown to exist can't be known;

it's impossible to demonstrate that SARS-CoV-2 causes a disease called Covid 19.

Sally Farron Morell, MA,   Dr Andrew Kaufman, MD
Dr Tom Cowan MD

Dr Sam Bailey and Dr Mark Bailey from New Zealand have been questioning the whole pandemic story from the beginning. Many well-constructed videos and resources can be found at drsambaliey.com including the free paper *A Farewell To Virology (Expert Edition)*. Dr Mark Bailey.

An extract from 'Settling the Virus Debate' - Statement 14 July 2022

> "Perhaps the primary evidence that the pathogenic viral theory is problematic is that no published scientific paper has ever shown that particles fulfilling the definition of viruses have been directly isolated and purified from any tissues or bodily fluids of any sick human or animal. Using the commonly accepted definition of 'isolation', which is the separation of one thing from all other things, there is general agreement that this has never been done in the history of virology. Particles that have been successfully isolated through purification have not been shown to be replication-competent, infectious and disease-causing, hence they cannot be said to be viruses. Additionally, the proffered 'evidence' of viruses through "genomes" and animal experiments derives from methodologies with insufficient controls"

The whole statement is a challenge by 20 qualified professionals to the scientific world to prove the reality of pathogenic viruses.

> "If the virologists fail to obtain a satisfactory result from the above study, then their claims about detecting 'viruses' will be shown to be unfounded. All of the measures put in place as a result of these claims should be brought to an immediate halt. If they succeed in this first task then we would encourage them to proceed to the required purification experiments to obtain the probative evidence for the existence of viruses".

> "It is in the interest of everyone to address the issue of isolation, and the very existence, of alleged viruses such as SARS-CoV-2. This requires proof that the entry of morphologically and

biochemically, virus-like particles into living cells is both necessary and sufficient to cause the appearance of the identical particles, which are contagious and disease causing".

"We welcome your support and feedback for this initiative"

During the pandemic Dr Sam was given no option but to take her videos down from YouTube, videos that were challenging the entire virus debate. They can still be found though on her website and this courageous couple continue to go with the truthful scientific investigations, sacrificing their own medical careers in the process. At the time of writing this book, Dr Sam is being threatened with losing her medical license in New Zealand after already losing her television career as a public figure in matters relating to health. With a clear decision to pursue truth and morality, this I am sure will be water off a duck's back and probably, similar to Dr Jane Donegan, a relief.

THE FIRST WAVE

Italy

The virus was first confirmed to have spread to Italy on 31st January 2020, when two Chinese tourists in Rome tested positive. One week later an Italian man repatriated back to Italy from the city of Wuhan, China, was hospitalised and confirmed as the third case in Italy.

Lombardy

The alleged outbreak in Lombardy came to light when a 38-year-old Italian tested positive in Codogno, a commune in the province of Lodi. On 14th February, he felt unwell and went to see a doctor in Castiglione d'Adda. He was prescribed treatments for influenza. On 16th February, as the man's condition worsened, he went to Codogno Hospital, reporting respiratory problems. Initially there was no suspicion of COVID-19, so no additional precautionary measures were taken, and allegedly the virus was able to infect other patients and health workers. On 19th February, the wife of the patient revealed he had met an Italian friend who had returned from China on 21st January, who subsequently tested negative. Later, the patient, his pregnant wife and a friend tested positive. On 20th February, three more cases were confirmed after the patients reported symptoms of pneumonia.

Thereafter, extensive screenings and checks were performed on everyone that had possibly been in contact with or had been near the infected subjects. It was subsequently reported that the origin of these cases had a possible connection to the first European local transmission that occurred in Munich, Germany, on 19th January 2020.

Doctors in Codogno stated that the 38-year-old patient led an active social life in the weeks before his illness and potentially interacted with dozens of people before spreading the virus at their hospital.

An interesting story, but one that cannot be proven.

On 22nd February, the government announced a new decree imposing the quarantine of more than 50,000 people from 11 municipalities in Northern Italy. The quarantine zones are called the Red Zones and the areas in Lombardy and Veneto outside of them are called the Yellow Zones. Penalties for violations of the quarantine rules ranged from a €206 fine to three months of imprisonment. The Italian military and law enforcement agencies were instructed to secure and implement the lockdown.

March 9th in the evening, Conte announced in a press conference that all measures previously applied only in the so-called 'red zones' had been extended to the entire country, putting approximately 60 million people into lockdown. Conte later proceeded to officially sign the new executive decree.

Source: analysis by *Istituto Superiore di Sanità* on partial set of data.

Confirmed COVID-19 cases in Italy by gender and age 26/5/2020

Classification	Cases		Deaths		Lethality
	Number	(%)	Number	(%)	(%)
	230,811	(100.0)	31,676	(100.0)	(13.7)
Male	106,035	(45.9)	18,744	(59.2)	(17.7)
Female	122,535	(54.1)	12,932	(40.8)	(10.4)
Above 90	18,602	(8.1)	5,415	(17.1)	(29.1)
80-89	40,532	(17.6)	12,980	(41)	(32)
70–79	33,141	(14.4)	8,562	(27)	(25.8)

60–69	30,880	(13.4)	3,259	(10.3)	(10.6)
50–59	41,435	(18.0)	1,109	(3.5)	(2.7)
40–49	29,942	(13)	273	(0.9)	(0.9)
30–39	17,934	(7.8)	62	(0.2)	(0.3)
20–29	12,933	(5.6)	12	(0.0)	(0.1)
10–19	3,442	(1.5)	0	(0.0)	(0.0)
0–9	1,919	(0.8)	4	(0.0)	(0.2)
n/d	51	(0.0)	0	(0.0)	(0.0)

Information from an article in Bloomberg:

*Italy Says 96% of Virus Fatalities Suffered From Other Illnesses –
Tommaso Ebhardt and Marco Bertacche May 26, 2020.*

Italy Coronavirus Deaths
Percentage of patients by prior illnesses

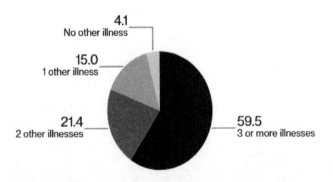

Source: Italian National Health Institute, May 21 sample of 3,032 deceased

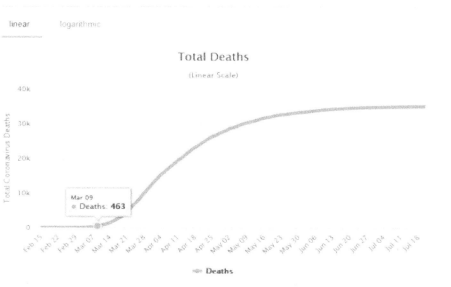

Notice the sharp rise in coronavirus deaths occurring *after* the strict lockdown, a common theme as we shall see later on. It is also worth noting that the vast majority of deaths were elderly people and that children didn't seem to be affected at all. The main points to make about the data are that 'cases' just mean a positive result obtained by a meaningless, non-diagnostic, test. The people who were actually dying were mainly the elderly with underlying health conditions. As for the graph showing the sharp rise in 'COVID deaths', that too doesn't really tell you much as we know after lockdown mass testing began and with a random test like PCR the more you test then the more positives you will produce.

The centre of the outbreak was Lombardy, a region with a population of about 10 million people, in the industrial centre of Italy and well known for its pollution, being some of the worst in Europe. It is also worth noting that Italy has an elderly population, which will become a major factor in what was happening, especially when we look into the UK and Sweden care home deaths.

The Bloomberg article, which gets data from Italy's ISS Health Institute, also shows just 1.1% of fatalities were from people under 50 years old. Though the average age of positively tested cases was 62 years old, the average age of the deceased was 80 years old. It showed furthermore that 30% of the positively tested were under 50 years old and 57% of fatalities were 80 years old. The connection with pre-existing medical conditions turned out to be 68% for high blood pressure, about 30% for diabetes and 28% for heart disease.

The Telegraph Online, March 23rd 2020, Professor Walter Ricciardi, scientific adviser to Italy's minister of health said:

> "the way in which we code deaths in our country is very generous in the sense that all the people who die in hospitals with the coronavirus are deemed to be dying of the coronavirus."

> "On re-evaluation by the National Institute of Health, only 12 per cent of death certificates have shown a direct causality from coronavirus, while 88 per cent of patients who have died have at least one pre-morbidity - many had two or three."

So, again, why is the medical thinking just to blame a virus when clearly there were many factors involved? With the ageing population in Italy and all the other health issues playing a part in becoming ill, it was something that was bound to happen one day to a large proportion of the elderly. It seems that this potential for a health crisis was manifested via the fear, hysteria and protocols making me suspect that this area of Italy was pre-chosen for the start on an 'outbreak'. Again, we saw the horrific pictures of hysteria, control, panic and death raging in Italy coming out of the mainstream news, all blaming it on this new novel virus from China, which was on a mission to destroy us all. Again, where was the calm and rational holistic thinking?

A common theme is the medical profession saying that the rise in deaths started with the lockdowns because they caught the virus just at the right time, and if it wasn't for the lockdown timing, things would have been worse. Great to have a story you don't need to prove, fear propaganda is enough, and even more incredible that this non-alive, non-moving virus seems to coordinate its attack just at the time of lockdowns and not before. The 'virus' then spread to Spain and we saw similar data and scenes, including lockdowns and rising 'cases' and 'COVID deaths'. The people of the UK were waiting for the inevitable declaration.

Terrorism Act UK 2000

Terrorism: interpretation

(1) In this Act "terrorism" means the use or threat of action where—

a) *the action falls within subsection (2),*

b) *the use or threat is designed to influence the government [F1or an international governmental organisation] or to intimidate the public or a section of the public, and*

c) *the use or threat is made for the purpose of advancing a political, religious [F2, racial] or ideological cause.*

(2) Action falls within this subsection if it—

d) *involves serious violence against a person,*

e) *involves serious damage to property,*

f) *endangers a person's life, other than that of the person committing the action,*

g) *creates a serious risk to the health or safety of the public or a section of the public, or*

The Enemy Has Landed

GOV.UK, 31/1/2020

Chief Medical Officer, Professor Chris Whitty, statement about *cases of novel coronavirus in England.*

> "We can confirm that 2 patients in England, who are members of the same family, have tested positive for coronavirus. The patients are receiving specialist NHS care, and we are using tried and tested infection control procedures to prevent further spread of the virus".

> "The NHS is extremely well-prepared and used to managing infections and we are already working rapidly to identify any contacts the patients had, to prevent further spread. We have been preparing for UK cases of novel coronavirus and we have robust infection control measures in place to respond immediately. We are continuing to work closely with the World Health Organization and the international community as the outbreak in China develops to ensure we are ready for all eventualities."

On 12th March, there had allegedly been 596 cases and ten deaths from the 'deadly virus'. Boris Johnson, UK Prime Minister marched through the huge doors and onto the podium to greet the press and address the nation live on television to announce:

> "This is the worst public health crisis in a generation ... and I must level with you and the British public, more families, many more families, are going to lose loved ones before their time."

We were being repeatedly told that "at all stages we have been guided by the science, we will do the right thing at the right time" coming from Mr Johnson, again, and of course Matt Hancock. Then the Chief Scientific Advisor Sir Patrick Vallance estimated *"that the UK was four weeks behind the trajectory of the crisis in Italy and that the peak might not come for 10-14 weeks running into June."*

Dr David Halpern is the chief executive of the government-owned Behavioural Insights Team, known as the 'nudge unit', and a member of Whitehall's Scientific Advisory Group for Emergencies (Sage) and also co-authored a government document titled 'MINDSPACE':

> *"If the virus spreads as modelling suggests it will, government advisers believe some hard choices will need to be made about how to protect groups that are more vulnerable to the disease – particularly the 500,000 older people in care homes and those with respiratory conditions."*

> *"There's going to be a point, assuming the epidemic flows and grows as it will do, where you want to cocoon, to protect those at-risk groups so they don't catch the disease. By the time they come out of their cocooning, herd immunity has been achieved in the rest of the population."*

> -Dr David Halpern

> *"The thing about a new virus is, of course, nobody has antibodies ready-made to it. The virus is having a field day; the desire will be to infect as many people as it can."*

> -Deputy Chief Medical Officer Jenny Harren:

> *"The virus is having a field day; the desire will be to infect as many people as it can."*

> - UK Deputy Chief Medical Officer Jenny Harren

So, again, repeating that this virus is *'new'*. We don't have the required antibodies to protect us – antibodies the WHO know don't mean 'protection' - and the virus has a 'desire' – a virus with a wish list is truly 'novel' - to 'infect' as many people as it can'. So the general message is that they are using the 'best available science' and that we need to be afraid, to be very afraid. Many of us will die and basically, there is nothing we can do except run and hide and hope for the best. The enemy is coming, the invisible beast whose only reason to live ((though it's not actually alive) is to kill human beings with its insatiable appetite. This message was put out by the government and their array of medical and scientific 'experts' and was repeated without any investigation whatsoever by all the mainstream press and media. No health advice was given and we were told we were all potential victims of this monster.

16th March 2020 - Imperial College COVID-19 Response Team

Report 9: Impact of non-pharmaceutical interventions (NPIs) to reduce COVID-19 mortality and healthcare demand

Extract taken from introduction:

'The COVID-19 pandemic is now a major global health threat. As of 16th March 2020, there have been 164,837 cases and 6,470 deaths confirmed worldwide. Global spread has been rapid, with 146 countries now having reported at least one case. The last time the world responded to a global emerging disease epidemic of the scale of the current COVID-19 pandemic with no access to vaccines was the 1918-19 H1N1 influenza pandemic'.

The report talked about three options.

- The first option was no action and no change in public behaviour with *an estimated 81% of UK and US population infected with 510, 000 deaths in UK and 2.2 million in the US.*

- Second option was mitigation *with an estimated 250 000 deaths in UK and 1.1-1.2 million deaths in the US.*

- The third option was suppression. It is not clear from the report what the estimated number of deaths would be if suppression was chosen, but Azra Ghani, a member of the Imperial team, was reported to have said that suppression *"might bring total deaths down to about 20,000 if they were observed strictly".*

Extract taken from summary:

'The global impact of COVID-19 has been profound, and the public health threat it represents is the most serious seen in a respiratory virus since the 1918 H1N1 influenza pandemic. Here we present the results of epidemiological modelling which has informed policymaking in the UK and other countries in recent weeks. In the absence of a COVID-19 vaccine, we assess the potential role of a number of public health measures –so-called non-pharmaceutical interventions (NPIs) – aimed at reducing contact rates in the population and thereby reducing transmission of the virus. In the results presented here, we apply a previously published microsimulation model to two countries: the UK (Great Britain specifically) and the US. We conclude that the effectiveness of any one intervention in isolation is likely to be limited, requiring multiple interventions to be combined to have a substantial impact on transmission. Two fundamental strategies are possible: (a) mitigation, which focuses on slowing but not necessarily stopping epidemic spread – reducing peak healthcare demand while protecting those most at risk of severe disease from infection, and (b) suppression, which aims to reverse epidemic growth, reducing case numbers to low levels and maintaining that situation indefinitely. Each policy has major challenges. We find that that optimal mitigation policies (combining home isolation of suspect cases, home quarantine of those living in the same household as suspect cases, and social distancing of the elderly and others at most risk of severe disease) might reduce peak healthcare demand by 2/3 and deaths by half. However, the resulting mitigated epidemic would still likely result in hundreds of thousands of deaths and health systems (most notably intensive care units) being overwhelmed many times over. For countries able to achieve it, this leaves suppression as the preferred policy option'.

The report ended by saying:

> 'We therefore conclude that epidemic suppression is the only viable strategy at the current time. The social and economic effects of the measures which are needed to achieve this policy goal will be profound. Many countries have adopted such measures already, but even those countries at an earlier stage of their epidemic (such as the UK) will need to do so imminently'.

> 'Our analysis informs the evaluation of both the nature of the measures required to suppress COVID-19 and the likely duration that these measures will need to be in place. Results in this paper have informed policymaking in the UK and other countries in the last weeks. However, we emphasise that is not at all certain that suppression will succeed long term; no public health intervention with such disruptive effects on society has been previously attempted for such a long duration of time. How populations and societies will respond remains unclear'.

It turns out this 'expert', Neil Ferguson, is basically a mathematician in a white coat. He doesn't seem to have looked into the historical conditions of the 1918 pandemic and had based all his models on an invisible enemy called a virus, transmitting a disease from one person to another. He also seems to have no knowledge of the human experiments conducted by the Public Health Service and the US Navy we showed earlier, where it was shown not to be possible to infect any volunteers with flu from ill patients, no matter how hard they tried.

To be clear about these computer-generated models, what you get out depends on what you put in. Crap in, crap out. The 'R' rate is from a computer-generated model based on germ/viral theory which we already know is not only far from being correct but has actually been proven to be wrong. Let's take a look at the history of this man who was chosen as the team 'expert' to give us the best information and advice on how to deal with the coming threat.

Professor Neil Ferguson

Imperial College epidemiologist, Neil Ferguson worked on the disputed research that sparked the mass culling of eleven million sheep and cattle during the 2001 outbreak of foot-and-mouth disease.

In 2002, Ferguson predicted that between 50,000-100,000 people could die from exposure to BSE (mad cow disease) in beef. In the UK, there were only 178 deaths from BSE.
In 2005, Ferguson predicted that up to 200 million people could be killed from bird flu. Only 282 people died worldwide from the disease between 2003 and 2009.
In 2009, a government estimate, based on Ferguson's advice, said a 'reasonable worst-case scenario' was that the swine flu would lead to 65,000 British deaths. In the end, swine flu killed 457 people in the UK.
(Worldwide the WHO reported only 18,449 deaths from swine flu as of 1/8/2010.)

So while all the time the government tells us they are being led by the 'best available science', they take advice from a man with a track record like this. Is this incompetence, stupidity or, again, something more sinister? The above data is the official data to come out regarding these alleged viral outbreaks. To be clear though, the figures are totally meaningless as we have already shown that viruses are not contagious disease causing agents. The main point is that this was a man who, even if their theory on viruses was correct, had a very poor track record in predicting outcomes of infectious epidemics. Yet this man is given the most important job of our time, of predicting the danger of this invisible enemy coming to get us all. Exactly the thing he has shown to be totally incompetent of.

Remember Tony Blair giving us the best available science of 'weapons of mass destruction', advice that led to the massacre of hundreds of thousands of innocent Iraqis and the total destruction of a nation? A man that to this day is still allowed a political voice and mercilessly pushed the COVID-19 vaccine.

Remember doctors promoting and prescribing thalidomide? Again, they were giving the 'best scientific advice' they had and look how that turned out!

Remember being told the ice caps are going to melt, the polar bears will all die, the world will be flooded and England will be like the Mediterranean? Well that was thirty years ago and they are still pushing it now. Strange they never put that big yellow thing in the sky part of their calculations. And by the way, the polar bears seem to be doing just fine and I'm still waiting for the Mediterranean climate we were promised. Another scientific model not based on reality.

So, with just ten deaths confirmed by a test that could not find a virus even if it existed, we go into lockdown. Locked up safely in their homes the fearful public then started to watch the show unfold minute by minute, hour by hour, update after update with the scary numbers on the screen to keep the fear factor in control.

As you will see, the massive spike in deaths occurred *after* lockdown. Again, as you will see, this is a common theme. So we go to war, or at least the politicians and their 'medical experts' tell us to prepare for war. Our glorious leaders giving us permanent updates of how the enemy is attacking and, I'm not sure about you, but the whole drama with politicians dramatically coming through doors to address the nation was like watching Hitler, or any other dictator, taking the stand to address the masses. We were given a vision of Boris Johnson being a new Winston Churchill. Of course, a nation at war and in emergency conditions gives politicians a free-for-all in taking our freedoms away in the name of protecting us. We started to see mass Orwellian doublespeak being used to perfection and then the masses started banging their pots and pans.

Scary stuff, and I'm not talking about the virus.

From GOV.UK website:

Status of COVID-19

> *As of 19 March 2020, COVID-19 is no longer considered to be a high consequence infectious disease (HCID) in the UK.*

> *The 4 nations public health HCID group made an interim recommendation in January 2020 to classify COVID-19 as an HCID. This was based on consideration of the UK HCID criteria about the virus and the disease with information available during the early stages of the outbreak. Now that more is known about COVID-19, the public health bodies in the UK have reviewed the most up to date information about COVID-19 against the UK HCID criteria. They have determined that several features have now changed; in particular, more information is available about mortality rates (low overall), and there is now greater clinical awareness and a specific and sensitive laboratory test, the availability of which continues to increase.*

> *The Advisory Committee on Dangerous Pathogens (ACDP) is also of the opinion that COVID-19 should no longer be classified as an HCID.*

> *The need to have a national, coordinated response remains, but this is being met by the government's COVID-19 response.*

> *Cases of COVID-19 are no longer managed by HCID treatment centres only. All healthcare workers managing possible and confirmed cases should follow the updated national infection and prevention (IPC) guidance for COVID-19, which supersedes all previous IPC guidance for COVID-19. This guidance includes instructions about different personal protective equipment (PPE) ensembles that are appropriate for different clinical scenarios.*

On the 23rd March 2020, four days after COVID-19 was declared to be no longer a high-consequence infectious disease, the UK went into lockdown, not quarantine, but the prison term of lockdown was used. So let's be clear, when 'COVID-19' was considered to be a high consequence infectious disease life went on as normal. When it was declared to no longer to be a high consequence infectious disease we go into lockdown. These clear contradictions were a regular feature of the show.

"From this evening I must give the British people a very simple instruction – you must stay at home."

– Boris Johnson, after allegedly 6,030 cases and 359 deaths from 'COVID-19'.

The Prime Minister announced that the police will now have the power to fine people if they leave their homes for any reason other than the following:

- Shopping for basic necessities

- One form of exercise a day – either alone or with members of your household

- Medical need or to provide care help vulnerable person

- Travel to work – but only if necessary and you cannot work from home

- You should not be meeting friends. You should not be meeting family members who don't live in your home. You should not be shopping except for essentials.

- If you don't follow the rules, the police have power to enforce them including with fines. (Something later declared to be unlawful.)

- Police have also been given extra powers, stopping motorists to check if their journeys are essential.

- We will stop all gatherings of more than two people in public and stop all social events.

For me personally, whilst the whole nation was running around buying toilet rolls and running for cover, I went home and had a cup of tea. Remember the film *'Carry On Up The Kyber'* when the fort was being bombed and the officers were just in the dining hall having dinner with their wives, all dressed up and going on as though nothing at all was happening? That is the British way. When the brown stuff hits the fan. just sit down and have a cup of tea. The British solution to many a problem, or just the best thing to do when there is nothing else you can do.

Here are some examples of madness in the first few weeks. The madness, though, is still continuing to date.

Police screaming at people in the street in London, "Go home. You're killing people."

Police putting a black dye in a lake at an isolated beauty spot in Yorkshire after they filmed and shamed a woman together with her child walking her dog in the middle of nowhere with her child.

Police stopping and fining people in their cars just for being on the road or even for just walking to work. Something they had no right to do.

Police setting up road blocks to stop people to ask why they are out of their homes.

Police being asked to go into supermarkets to check that what people were buying was all essential stuff.

Police arresting a woman for doing yoga on a bench alone in a London park.

Police telling people on beaches or in parks or even outside their own homes to go in; *it's the virus,* you know.

The list for police stupidity and order following could go on and on.

There were people at home ranting on social media or shouting out of their windows about someone outside their house or across the street walking his dog and stopping to talk for someone. There was the general consensus they were putting us all in danger.

For years people have been whingeing about teenagers in groups out on the street, taking part in anti-social behaviour. Now they are complaining about social behaviour. Now social behaviour becomes a killing machine. Let's all behave like good citizens and be total anti-socials!

The great toilet roll crisis, I've still no idea what that was about.

We were told it was all about 'flattening the curve' and 'taking the pressure off the NHS'.

Then all the mad, insane guidelines like, you can visit your mum and dad but only one at a time in separate rooms and ten minutes apart. Oh, and please 'don't sing or shout'. All the things you can do and the things you can't, even in your own home, all the contradictions, all the nonsense which we were told was being 'guided by the best science'. Guidelines changing almost every day. No one really knowing what was going on. Different rules in England, Wales, Scotland and Northern Ireland. Please never forget 'love holes' and mask wearing sex advice with 'safe sex positions'. A total shambles, but it was an organised chaos. Chaos creates confusion, confusion means no one can see what is really happening, this way people can be easily controlled. Out of the chaos must come the order and the order was to be *the new normal*.

Coronavirus Act 2020

Extracts from 'SCHEDULE 21 PART 2 Powers relating to potentially infectious persons in England'

Powers to direct or remove persons to a place suitable for screening and assessment

6

(1) This paragraph applies if, during a transmission control period, a public health officer has reasonable grounds to suspect that a person in England is potentially infectious.

(2) The public health officer may, subject to sub-paragraph (3) —

(a)   direct the person to go immediately to a place specified in the direction which is suitable for screening and assessment,

(b)   remove the person to a place suitable for screening and assessment, or

(c)   request a constable to remove the person to a place suitable for screening and assessment (and the constable may then do so).

(3)   A public health officer may exercise the powers conferred by this paragraph in relation to a person only if the officer considers that it is necessary and proportionate to do so —

(a)   in the interests of the person,

(b)   for the protection of other people, or

(c)   for the maintenance of public health

(4)   Where a public health officer exercises the powers conferred by this paragraph, the officer must inform that person —

(a)   of the reason for directing or removing them, and

(b)   that it is an offence —

(i)   in a case where a person is directed, to fail without reasonable excuse to comply with the direction, or

(ii)   in a case where a person is removed (by the officer or by a constable), to abscond.

7

(1)   This paragraph applies if, during a transmission control period—

(a)   a constable, or

(b)   an immigration officer in the course of exercising any of their functions, has reasonable grounds to suspect that a person in England is potentially infectious.

(2)   The immigration officer or constable may, subject to sub-paragraph (3) —

(a) direct the person to go immediately to a place specified in the direction which is suitable for screening and assessment, or

(b) remove the person to a place suitable for screening and assessment.

(3) An immigration officer or constable may exercise the powers conferred by this paragraph in relation to a person only if the officer or constable considers that it is necessary and proportionate to do so —

(a) in the interests of the person,

(b) for the protection of other people, or

(c) for the maintenance of public health.

(4) Where an immigration officer or constable exercises the power to direct or remove a person under this paragraph, the officer or constable must inform that person —

(a) of the reason for directing or removing them, and

(b) that it is an offence —

(i) in a case where a person is directed, to fail without reasonable excuse to comply with the direction, or

(ii) in a case where a person is removed, to abscond.

(5) An immigration officer or constable must, before exercising the powers conferred by this paragraph, consult a public health officer to the extent that it is practicable to do so.

Part 10 interested me – "*impose other requirements*" – so vague it is a permission slip to do anything.

10

(6) A public health officer may —

(a) require the person referred to in paragraph 8 to be screened and assessed, and

(b) impose other requirements on the person in connection with their screening and assessment.

Remember, it was a PCR test for a non-existent viral pathogen that was deciding how much freedom you had and how much power PHE had over you and your body.

It is an absolute must that everyone should be read this 'act'; and never forget it. It is pure medical tyranny. Where is the 'law of consent' here? Basically all rights over your own body are gone and you and your children can be whisked off anywhere they choose. With all the new rules and guidelines to be enforced, how could it possibly be done by the police force alone? Easy, get the people to police themselves. Schools were teaching children before the lockdown to tell everyone at home to stop touching their faces, even to shout, "*Face!*" at their parents when they did. These 'educated' children, Hitler Youth, would enforce policy on the parents. The rest would be done by being a 'good citizen' and by telling on your neighbour. Add to that, people in fear shouting at non-conformers in the street. So the sheep would sheep themselves.

As psychologist Professor Jordan Peterson stated, "*you probably would have been a Nazi too*", when talking about how Nazi Germany came about and why it was all backed by the majority of the public and men in uniform just 'doing their job'. We have the script of George Orwell's '*1984*' in full flow with plenty of Aldous Huxley's '*Brave New World*' social engineering thrown in for good measure.

Then surprise, Boris Johnson 'gets it'. This disease whose main symptom was a persistent dry cough. He addressed the nation, telling us of his trial with the illness and without even coughing once. hmmmm! After a touch-and-go illness, 'nudged' away from public view, we'll just have to take their word for it, our glorious leader came back with more energy for the war than ever. More energy to tell us what we can and cannot do. It may seem to many that comparing the government propaganda to being war-like is over the top, but given that now we know the military are being used to actually monitor the population they are sworn to protect, we need to ask, who is the enemy here?

Enter the 77th Brigade

> *"We are a combined Regular and Army Reserve unit. Our aim is to challenge the difficulties of modern warfare using non-lethal engagement and legitimate non-military levers as a means to adapt behaviours of the opposing forces and adversaries."*

So the British Government is joining forces with the British Army to *'adapt behaviours of the opposing forces and adversaries'*. The obvious question here is, who are the *'opposing forces and adversaries'* and what *'behaviour'* needs adapting? Well, considering behaviour is controlled by beliefs – we will come to that later – the question should be, what beliefs are deemed dangerous by the British Government concerning the 'corona pandemic'?

> *"Some of the ways we help"* are *"Collecting, creating and disseminating digital and wider media content in support of designated tasks."*

So it seems clear they are an intelligence unit scanning social media and the like with *'designated tasks'* in mind. So, again, what information are they looking for that would highlight people as possible *'adversaries'*? When targeted, where does this information go? And what is the next step against these *'adversaries'*?

Well, it's clear they are working with government on the information surrounding the 'corona pandemic'. Therefore it would then be clear they are looking for information to find people who do not believe in the government narrative. People who, through research, have come to different conclusions to those put before them. This would suggest that these are the *'adversaries'* they are looking for, us.

Also part of what they do under *Human Security* is:

"Human Security puts the emphasis on security of the people and their social and economic environment rather than focusing on security of the state."

Doesn't it seem strange to you that a unit in the British Army which is claiming to protect the people and their social and economic security, is actually being used by British politicians who are taking all the freedoms away from the British people? In the process, they are not only destroying but reconstructing all the social interactions and putting into place rules that will no doubt destroy the economy and bankrupt the nation?

Under *"news and events"* they show us more of their activities:

"Dispelling rumours. Don't believe everything you read elsewhere, if you want to check what the Army is doing for COVID-19 check here and our social media channels on Twitter, Facebook, LinkedIn and Instagram."

So they are actively engaging in social media to push the government line and to see who is out there with alternative opinions. If these alternative opinions are so wrong and dangerous then why not have a full public debate and let us see all this 'fake news' for what it is? They avoid every direct confrontation and debate so the real fake news will not be exposed. Why would you take that 'risk', if all you need to do to secure your position of power is to brand certain information as *fake* in order for the public 'to know' what is fake?

Just a look at what happened in Victoria, Australia, where people's Facebook pages were being monitored and people were being arrested or harassed because of their posts questioning the official narrative. If peoples questions were so wrong surely we could have all seen it for ourselves. This all comes down to control of information and therefore control of truth which leads to control of behaviour.

"The Army's priority remains to protect the UK public in these unprecedented times."

So by protecting us they mean they are making sure we think *'the right way'*. I don't think the enemy has landed. I think it was here all along.

WELCOME TO ORWELLIAN BRITAIN

The Chaos Continues

The following graph put together by UKColumn News with data taken from the ONS show an eight-year cycle of deaths. Notice that the large spike just after lockdown happened was later than in previous years and that there was the usual normal winter spike just before. Why the extra spike? Well, going on from the previous information this certainly backs up the idea that this massive sharp rise in excess deaths was not a natural phenomenon and that the suggestion that the lockdown was in some way involved needs to be investigated further. It was certainly not caused by a 'novel new virus' as we have already shown.

The next graph also from the UKColumn shows how the huge spike in deaths happened after the lockdown. So beyond doubt there were actual excess deaths, and not just 'COVID deaths' that did not affect the average deaths for that time of year. We had real provable excess deaths and whilst the media were blaming it all on a virus I felt it was best to look into the circumstances that had changed at the lockdown. To be clear all data shown to us claiming 'COVID deaths', 'cases' and 'R rates' were all psychological tools to keep people in fear and confused, and that they did.

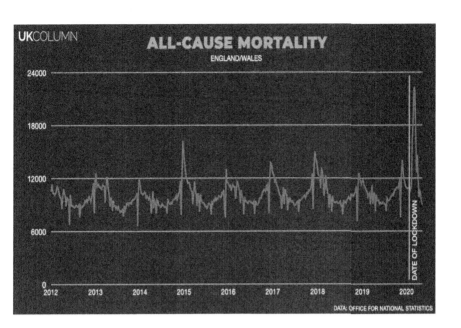

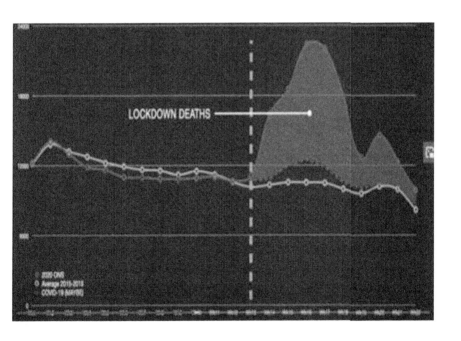

The ONS stated:

"Of the deaths involving COVID-19 that occurred in England and Wales in March to May 2020, there was at least one pre-existing condition in 90.9% of cases; this is a similar level to that shown in March and April 2020."

Conditions such as ischaemic heart disease, chronic pulmonary disease, diabetes, chronic kidney disease, chronic neurological disorder, dementia, asthma, rheumatic disorder, learning disability or autism and receiving treatment for mental health conditions.

So it seemed people with already underlying health conditions were mainly the ones dying.

It was well known doctors were putting down 'COVID-19 'as cause of death even if it was just suspected. I personally know of one lady who lost an elderly relative early in the crisis who tested negative but was still put down as a 'COVID-19' death. So if someone died of cancer, but at death tested positive for 'covid', it was allowed to be also counted as a 'COVID-19' death. This was the standard procedure for anyone dying of a long-term illness or even old age – we all die eventually. If 'COVID-19' was symptomatically present then it was also put on the death certificate, artificially inflating COVID-19 deaths, even though the symptoms of 'covid' are indistinguishable from those of the common cold and flu. I also know of one lady who had at least fifteen years of illness and breathing issues, wheelchair bound and other health issues and in her seventies who was said to have died of 'COVID 19'.

Let's be clear, one of the symptoms of dying, in fact the main and last symptom, is lack of breath. But 24 hours a day we got the ever increasing death rate of 'COVID-19' ripping through society via government updates and shamelessly repeated through the mainstream media. And again, nothing said about boosting your system with fresh air, supplements, sunlight and deep breathing. In fact again these are the things the lockdown policies were taking away from people. Just run and hide and hope and pray it doesn't get you and your loved ones. I personally know another lady who with well over a decade of health and breathing issues passed away and of course it was put down as 'COVID'.

Mask Madness

On the 24th July 2020, just a couple of days after Michael Gove saying they were not going to mandate masks, the self-proclaimed 'right and honourable' Mat Hancock announced: *"Face coverings to be mandatory in shops and supermarkets from 24 July"*.

The reason:

> *".. the death rate of sales and retail assistants is 75% higher among men, and 60% higher among women than in the general population. So as we restore shopping, so we must keep our shopkeepers safe."*

This statement, though, did not come with any science to back it up. I guess we'll have to take their word for it, like when they said *'bus drivers are dropping like flies', and* they said it so it has to be true. It should be clear by now that when they want to pass some legislation it doesn't matter at all that they haven't got any science to back it up, just pass the new rules and they'll make it up as they go along or find a study soon enough. Irrespective of whether there are another thousand studies that say the opposite. The only data they want is what backs up their story. Worth noting is that even the WHO had no studies to back up mask wearing but it was politically driven and not scientific. In fact, early on when questioned about 'protection' by wearing masks in public places, the WHO stated that there was no evidence that suggested any benefit would be forthcoming from such a rule. Mask wearing was only 'thought' to be useful within very specific surroundings such as operating theatres.

Again, note how they play with our minds, something we will be

247

going into more. They say no, then they do it anyway. This creates the confusion they want. At the height of 'the pandemic' in the UK there were very few people in my local area wearing masks despite the fact that many people had died. But when the government announced it was a new needed measure, even though deaths were falling rapidly, the people who before had no interest in mask wearing were now convinced, not by facts, but by fear. So now it becomes the best thing to do.

We now had a society split into the socially responsible mask wearer and allegedly the arrogant and selfish non-mask-wearer. And with Police Chief Cressida Dick stating,

> "My hope is that the vast majority of people will comply, and that people who are not complying will be shamed into complying or shamed to leave the store by the store keepers or by other members of the public,"

It became clear we were going to be played off, one against the other. More divide and conquer. This woman is a disgrace and should be fired on the spot and charged with inciting violence or at least unlawful harassment.

Many doctors have stated that using masks as a blocking mechanism for viral particles is 'like putting a chain mail fence up to protect against mosquitos'. Totally useless! Especially when we know these viral particles they speak of are just cellular debris and do not cause illness.

And as for the safety aspect, well, the UKColumn News 12th August 2020 showed that there had been no government risk assessment at all. It doesn't take a rocket scientist to see that restricting your own breathing cannot be good for your health. You are limiting the amount of oxygen you can take in and not allowing all the waste air out so you breathe in your own waste. Clean air in, dirty air out, that is what your breathing is about, and forcing back in what has just come out as waste is pure madness. I'm gobsmacked at the number of people who have been taken in by this madness. As a friend told me, "it's mandated self-harm".

It shows a lot about the level of evil controlling society, and sadly even more about the lack of critical thinking within society. It should be clear that mask wearing is a psychological exercise to take away our power, individualism and humanity and is an outer portrayal of obedience to the State. The long-term effect will not just be the breathing issues but the mental health problems caused, especially for the young ones. Imagine a baby seeing its parents most of the day as mask wearers. This will disconnect and confuse them and affect their psychological and emotional development. But one man's symbol of slavery can also be sold to another's as a symbol of their caring, selfless, virtuous nature. Belief does control perception as we will see later.

Clean Hands Please

Again, do we really need a discussion of why it is bad to put toxic hand cleansers on your hands multiple times a day?

More madness, and remember the skin is the body's biggest detoxification area so it opens up to let things out; this means it is also open to things going in, and toxic hand sanitizer going in simply cannot be good. It would be easy to look up scientific data on this but come on, folks, if you need scientific data for this then there is no hope. Sure, public health measures and hygiene were some of the things that caused the massive drop in infectious disease BEFORE vaccines, as we have seen, but wash your hands after the toilet and after work with soap and water and I think you'll live a long life.

I work outside and sometimes, away from towns in the country-side, I have my 'pee bushes', where after I may blow my nose after then eat my butties – we don't say sandwich in Manchester – after working all day with dirty water, I'm still alive and I never get ill and I don't think I'm that special. We are creating a nation of nervous hypochondriacs who feel under threat all the time and it is going to end in a lot of mental illness and anxiety.

I'd prefer to stay sane with my dirty hands.

Summer on the Beach

Here in Cornwall, South-West England, when lockdown finally broke (for those who followed the rules) and we got the much-needed tourist money, people were very fearful of what might happen. Well, it turns out two million 'infected' tourists from the UK 'hotspots,' packing the beaches and the small Cornish towns actually made us healthier than ever. Yes, they put our deaths below average even with the 'deadly virus' being brought in from all round the country.

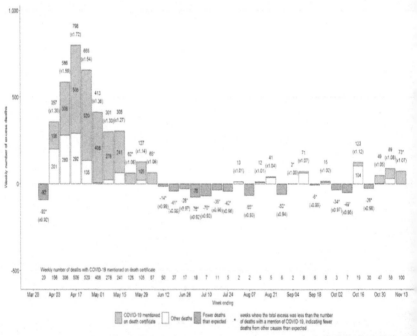

Weekly excess deaths by date of registration, South West

Source: Public Health England analysis of ONS death registration
Note: deaths registered on 20/21 March 2020 are not disp...

Notice the huge spike from the first lockdown and the slight drop below average deaths in the busy summer, then the slight rise again as lockdown restrictions came back. Despite this data, Cornwall Council continued to push the closing of tourism until the 'second wave' was under control. I have no idea what data they are looking at to make the statement that tourists are putting us at risk when, in contrast, it seems that closing down Cornwall pushes the deaths up.

One healthcare assistant, Shelley Tasker from Treliske Hospital Cornwall, publicly resigned outside Truro Cathedral, a stunningly brave act from someone who could not live a lie. She stated she had basically been 'twiddling her thumbs' through the 'pandemic'. Although slated in the local media and on social media, all she stated was fact checked during a special interview with UKColumn and shown to be correct. The crime she had committed was speaking the truth, a truth that affected the reputation of the worshipped NHS and their 'hero' workers on 'the front line'. This was something the public could not allow.

This is a freedom of information reply from Royal Cornwall Hospitals where Shelley worked:

FOI Ref:11938

"From the 01st January 2020 to 24th November 2020 the Royal Cornwall Hospitals Trust had one deceased patient who tested positive for Covid 19 and had no pre-existing health conditions."

Again, this backs up what she had been saying and the fact that despite the packed Cornish summer, nothing actually really happened. It also shows that the ones who were dying of 'COVID' were people who all, bar one, who had underlying health conditions.

The police who were out and about as usual in the 'war zone' did not seem to be at all affected by the 'deadly virus'. They did though seem to be harassing innocent people all day long looking for excuses to fine them. With a long summer of protests in London with police charging and attacking peaceful, maskless people shouting for their freedom back, and dealing with some not so peaceful government approved protestors for *Black Lives Matters*, you would have thought the police would have been dropping like flies.

Freedom of Information Request Reference No: 01.FOI.20.014369

"How many police officers have died in the frontline in England, Scotland and Wales due to Coronavirus this year? This can be statistics provided in a table format and should include a category for ethnicity.

The reply came back

"Please note that this response is in relation to MPS officers only, we do not hold data for the whole of the UK.

I have been advised that there have been no deaths of frontline officers in relation to the coronavirus."

One example of big 'change' in the NHS is the massive reduction in beds over the last twenty years. Every winter, for as long as I can remember, we see front-page headlines of the NHS being over-stretched, in fact we are always being told that the NHS is ALWAYS under pressure. And yet with a growing population we have seen a reduction in beds of about 77,000, approximately 30%. The following graph shows a drop from about 240 000 to about 162 000. I can understand reductions due to efficiency, better management and moving more people into community care but this enormous drop is far beyond those reasons, especially as stated with a growing population. Remember that with 'Exercise Cygnus' supposedly preparing the country for public health emergencies you would not expect such a huge drop in beds.

The lockdown measures included the massive undertaking of building at fast speed the Nightingale Hospitals and despite the media fear propaganda they were not even used. It did though create a great fear spectacle, backed up by military on the streets and even fully uniformed military going to schools in military vehicles. Again the theme of being under attack and at war with an invisible enemy was thrown onto the minds of a terrified populace.

This was an organised, conscious agenda (at the top level) to put massive pressure on the NHS. With a huge reduction in beds in a growing population and daily fear propaganda creating an environment for more illness, the claim of doing this to 'protect the NHS' is simply absurd. Insanity and absurdity though seemed to be the theme of the whole lockdown.

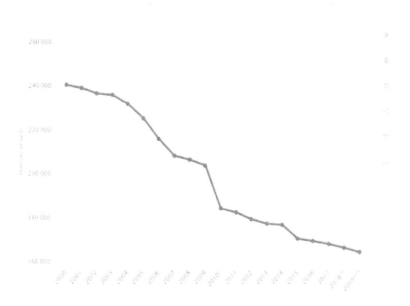

Hospital beds in the UK from 2000-2019. Source – statista.com

This was *'The First Wave'* in the UK. We will now take a look at some simple data for some other countries. The main issue is who was dying, how many and why.

USA

I could easily do a long chapter on the USA but the only relevant data is; who was dying, how many and in what circumstances? It's all run by Dr Fauci with his connection to Bill Gates. Dr Fauci was on the Leadership Council for the Gates Vaccine initiative. The link between them is very clear, as is his connection to another scandal, namely HIV, when again the PCR test was used as a diagnostic tool.

From the CDC 21/2/21:

Comorbidities and other conditions

Table 3 shows the types of health conditions and contributing causes mentioned in conjunction with deaths involving coronavirus disease 2019 (COVID-19). The number of deaths that mention one or more of the conditions indicated is shown for all deaths involving COVID-19 and by age groups. For 6% of these deaths, COVID-19 was the only cause mentioned on the death certificate. For deaths with conditions or causes in addition to COVID-19, on average, there were 3.8 additional conditions or causes per death

Taken from the CDC website dated 24/2/21

2020/2021	All Sexes	0-17 years	204
2020/2021	All Sexes	18-29 years	1,684
2020/2021	All Sexes	30-39 years	5,030
2020/2021	All Sexes	40-49 years	13,482
2020/2021	All Sexes	50-64 years	70,160
2020/2021	All Sexes	65-74 years	103,451
2020/2021	All Sexes	75-84 years	133,557
2020/2021	All Sexes	85 years and over	151,344
2020/2021	All Sexes	All Ages	478,912

So again, a very clear picture of people dying with comorbidity and advancing age as major contributing factors. And remember again, the 6% who died with no known health issues were found positive with a completely meaningless test in diagnostic terms. The UKColumn also reported the difference between lockdown states and non- or less-lockdown states and it was the lockdown states that seemed to be worse affected. The picture clearly shows once again that these 'COVID' deaths were affecting the aged and already weak. I am starting to see a pattern here.

One of the main questions is: was there actually a rise in the death-rate?

It's ok pushing numbers of COVID deaths, but did it result in excess deaths or was it just a reclassification of deaths that were happening normally? As pathogenic viruses do not exist then if there was a noticeable rise in the death-rate then it must be down to other factors, possibly including the lockdown measures.

Here we can see that there was in fact a noticeable rise in the death-rate in 2020 and 2021. Something did happen and it was not a virus.

Death rate in the United States from 2011 to 2021
(in deaths per 1,000 inhabitants)

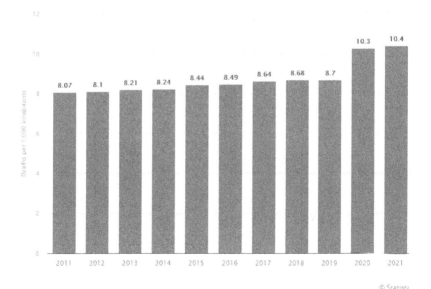

© Statista

Peru

On 15 March 2020, President Martín Vizcarra announced a country-wide lockdown, closing borders, restricting domestic flights, and forbidding non-essential business operations, excluding health facilities, grocery stores, pharmacies, and banks. Peru imposed one of the earliest and strictest lockdowns in Latin America, before the UK and some other European countries. The county's borders were shut, curfews were imposed, and people could only leave their homes for essential goods. But 'infections' and deaths started to massively rise to rise.

According to Wikipedia-

> 'The second full day of quarantine on 17 March saw citizens being required to fill out an online form to obtain permission to leave home. The military patrolled the streets of Lima to enforce this, and people were not allowed to walk together. At 8 pm that night through an organized effort, Peruvians and residents in Peru went out to their balconies and windows to applaud the front-line workers such as doctors, the Peruvian Armed Forces, market shop owners, and National Police of Peru to applaud their efforts during the pandemic.The next day on 18 March, the government tightened the measures of quarantine, implementing a curfew from 8 PM-5 AM where citizens are not allowed to leave their home.'

So people were going out at 8 p.m. to their balconies and opening windows to applaud the front-line workers. Now where have we heard that before!

On 19 March, the Peruvian Ministry of Health (MINSA) was briefed about the first death related to the disease, a 78-year-old man. Peru is an interesting case for me as I have spent about two years there living in Lima and the Amazon capital of Iquitos, two of the most affected areas. I know of the living conditions and the environment and it is easy for me to see why the deaths occurred only after lockdown.

When the lockdown began, men were allowed out only twice a

week to shop and exercise. Women also twice a week but on separate days. Mask wearing was compulsory at all times outdoors and at one point it was a double mask. With many people living in small apartment rooms, many with shared bathrooms, few of the large population of Lima having outside garden space and still a hot time of the year, it is not difficult to see that this could have an adverse effect on health. In Iquitos, with the all-year-round hot and humid climate, and again, many people living in houses with no gardens (surprisingly, in a large jungle town but that is how it is structured) and very unsanitary conditions in Belen by the river with, again, mask use, then why would it be a surprise people were getting ill? Add to this a tendency for Latin people to be easily pushed into group think and herd mentality, something the politicians use to great effect during elections, then this was always a recipe for fear and for conditions that were bound to create a public health disaster. But rather than looking into the government lockdown measures and wondering why nothing happened before the lockdown, the propaganda came out that it was people's fault for not obeying the rules and that despite all the deaths the government got it right.

Wed 20 May 2020 The Guardian-

> "Peru's response was right on time," said Elmer Huerta, a Peruvian doctor and trusted broadcaster on public health matters for Latin American audiences. "It was the first country in Latin America to respond with a lockdown."

> "But the problem was people's behaviour," he said. "The fact that on the eighth week of confinement you have thousands of people who are positive [for Covid-19] means that those people got the virus while the country was in lockdown – which means they did not respect the law."

As you can see according to worldometers there was not one single death from 'COVID-19' before the lockdown. The same pattern emerges again.

Total Coronavirus Deaths in Peru

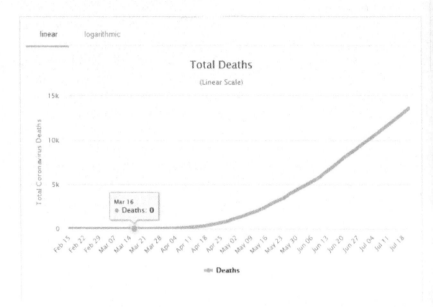

The most important figure though is actually how many people died, overall deaths, irrespective of the cause of death. The following graphs show clearly there was a large increase in mortality during the lockdown.

The death-rate had been in a slow decline before 2020 then you can clearly see a sharp rise in 2020 and 2021. These figures show not only a sharp increase in the death-rate during the first year of lockdown when the controls were more severe, but also the long lasting effects of the continued lockdowns. Many areas came out of the strictest lockdown measures on July 1 2020, but they were introduced again on Jan 31 2021 due to 'an aggressive second wave'. Peru was known to be a country that did not invest massive amounts into their healthcare system despite having Latin America's lowest debt-to-GDP ratio before 'the pandemic' began. This lack of healthcare infrastructure and masses of fear, panic and lockdown restrictions causing massive harm could only mean disaster. With adults having a legal obligation to look after their parents in Peru, (not actually a bad thing in some ways) they

258

do not have the massive care home system like we do in the West. But still elderly and weak people as usual would be the ones first affected.

The next graph (p260) shows actual deaths compared to the expected average of the previous few years. The dotted line being what would have been expected. The graph, from the Peruvian Ministry of Health, looks a bit odd in that it seems to show a sharp rise in deaths at about early March, though official data states the first 'COVID' death was announced on March 19 but that could be down to the presentation of the graph. All reports though seem clear that nothing was really happening in Peru until the lockdown. Even their own figures, which separated 'Official Covid-19 deaths ' from 'other excess deaths' clearly show the huge impact that the lockdown was having on mortality. Again, as we have already scientifically established 'SARS-CoV-2' was never isolated and contagious disease causing agents named viruses have never been found. This now shows you the real effect the strictest lockdown in the world was having on its population.

Following graph from statista

Peru: Death rate from 2011 to 2021

(in deaths per 1,000 inhabitants)

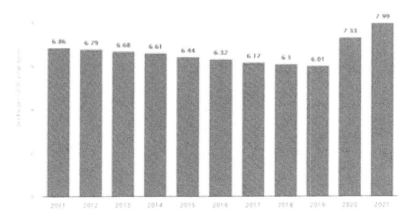

259

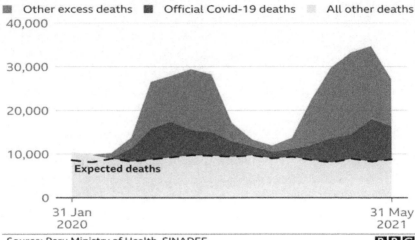

Total deaths in Peru compared with average
Deaths per month before Covid redefinition on 31 May 2021

■ Other excess deaths   ■ Official Covid-19 deaths   ■ All other deaths

40,000

30,000

20,000

10,000

Expected deaths

0

31 Jan
2020

31 May
2021

Source: Peru Ministry of Health, SINADEF   BBC

Sweden and Norway

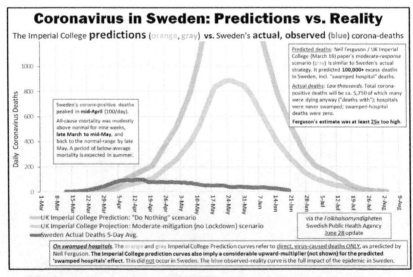

Coronavirus in Sweden: Predictions vs. Reality
The Imperial College **predictions** (orange, gray) **vs.** Sweden's **actual, observed** (blue) corona-deaths

Predicted deaths: Neil Ferguson / UK Imperial College (March 16) paper's moderate-response scenario (gray) is similar to Sweden's actual strategy. It predicted **100,000+** excess deaths in Sweden, incl. "swamped hospital" deaths.

Actual deaths: Low thousands. Total corona-positive deaths will be ca. 5,750 of which many were dying anyway ("deaths with"); hospitals were never swamped; swamped-hospital deaths were zero.

Ferguson's estimate was at least 25x too high.

Sweden's corona-positive deaths peaked in mid-April (100/day). All-cause mortality was modestly above normal for nine weeks, **late March to mid-May**, and back to the normal-range by late May. A period of below-average mortality is expected in summer.

Daily Coronavirus Deaths

UK Imperial College Prediction: "Do Nothing" scenario
UK Imperial College Projection: Moderate-mitigation (no Lockdown) scenario
Sweden Actual Deaths 5-Day Avg.

via the *Folkhälsomyndigheten* Swedish Public Health Agency June 28 update

On swamped hospitals. The orange and gray Imperial College Prediction curves refer to direct, virus-caused deaths ONLY, as predicted by Neil Ferguson. **The Imperial College prediction curves also imply a considerable upward-multiplier (not shown) for the predicted 'swamped hospitals' effect.** This did not occur in Sweden. The blue observed-reality curve is the full impact of the epidemic in Sweden.

https://swprs.files.wordpress.com/2020/07/sweden-projection-reality-june-28.png

The previous graph is showing what would have happened in Sweden going by Neil Ferguson's 'expert 'method in predicting disease patterns. As was well reported, Sweden was one of those countries that did not go into lockdown. The public health authority did ban gatherings over 50 people, closed high schools and universities, and advised people to keep a safe distance. But basically they let them get on with life and told them to use their own common sense. We had the whole of the world's governments and media announcing their arrogant and cavalier approach to this 'deadly virus'. People sat back and looked for the coming disaster, very similar to what happened in Leicester in 1885.

What happened? We'll let the data tell us.

Graph of number of 'COVID-19' deaths in Sweden in 2020 by age groups as of 17th July.

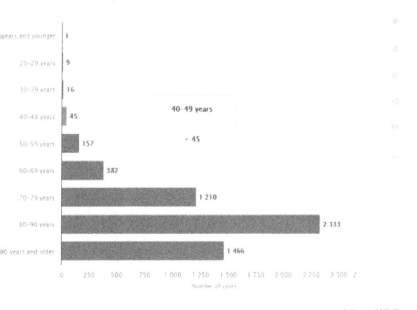

As you can see, 'COVID' deaths seemed to be hitting the elderly really hard. We know though that 'Covid' doesn't actually mean anything in real life but it does show that at least symptomatically it seemed that the elderly were showing signs of this alleged disease and dying. To get a clearer picture though we need to know if these were excess deaths or just normal deaths classified as 'COVID'.

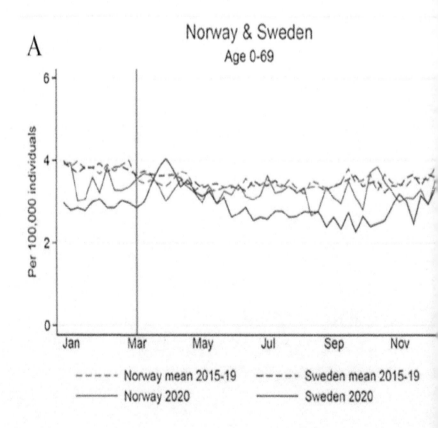

As you can see that when comparing Sweden with Norway in the
0-69 age group nothing much really happened in comparison to
what would have been expected normally. The graph shows 0-6
persons per 100 000 individuals so any small deviation in reality is
not significant at all. Things then in both countries seemed to be
as normal. No pandemic here then.

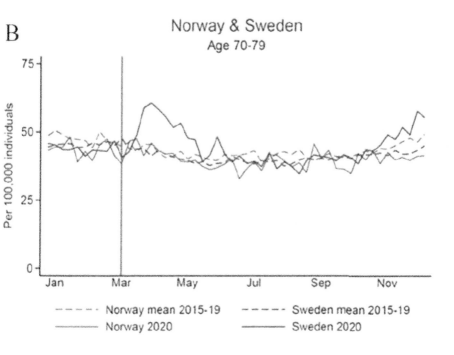

B

Norway & Sweden
Age 70-79

Per 100.000 individuals

- - - - - Norway mean 2015-19   - - - - - Sweden mean 2015-19
———— Norway 2020   ———— Sweden 2020

Here in the age group 70-79 with now the graph showing 0-75 per
100 000 individuals, a deviation from the normal could possibly
mean something. As we can see,Norway did not seem to deviate
from the expected curve where as directly after lockdown in
Sweden there was a sharp rise in deaths to show a clear curve of
excess deaths. In other words, there were a number of excess
deaths. This would indicate something out of the expected
normal in the real world and it would warrant an investigation.

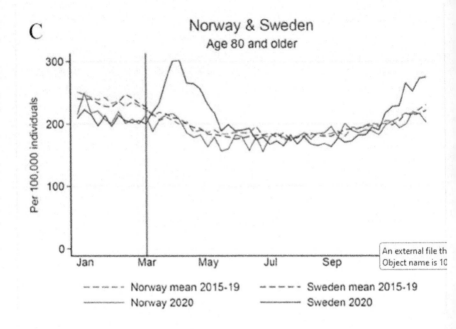

Norway & Sweden
Age 80 and older

- - - - - Norway mean 2015-19   - - - - - Sweden mean 2015-19
———— Norway 2020   ———— Sweden 2020

And here again in the age group 80 and over we see a similar graph except this time the numbers of the left are 0 – 300 individuals per 100 000 meaning any deviation from the mean would be quite significant. Again we see not much change at all in Norway but a very significant sharpe rise at lockdown in Sweden showing mass excess deaths.

https://www.ncbi.nlm.nih.gov/pmc/articles/PMC8807990/

The main things to look at are the measures Norway and Sweden took with regards to the lockdown. Norway put forward strict lockdown measures on the population whilst it is well known that in Sweden people were basically told to take care, use common sense but basically get on with life.

On 10 March 2020 in Sweden health care staff working with risk groups, including nursing homes, were asked not to work if they had any symptoms of respiratory infection. Relatives of elderly were advised to avoid unnecessary visits at hospitals and in facilities for elderly, and never visit if there were any respiratory symptoms. So on top of the measures being taken inside care homes the elderly were now being limited with contact from outside.

On the 31st March Sweden introduced its care home policies, including a ban on visits.

Norway it seemed was putting more care into the elderly as they saw these as the vulnerable and susceptible. More care to them seemed to mean more *protection*. Sweden seemed to take a UK style approach with the elderly, in that more isolation and less care equated to the idea of more protection. An extract from this article *Elderly care during the pandemic: Norway and Denmark stand* out may give us some clues.

> *Gautun points out that there may also be other reasons why Norway fared so well.*

> *"Norway stands out in that we have, to a large extent, transferred tasks from the specialist health service and hospitals to the municipal health and care services. We have competent municipalities that are used to adapting quickly and carrying out new tasks."*

> *"This means that the nursing homes have relieved the hospitals during the pandemic. Compared with other countries, Norway also has more nurses on staff at elderly care institutions, as well as nursing home physicians who visit the homes regularly."*

> https://www.oslomet.no/en/research/featured-research/elderly-care-during-pandemic-norway-denmark-stand-out

Many care home workers in Sweden were coming forward to criticise regional healthcare authorities for protocols which they say discourage care home workers from sending residents into hospital, and prevent care home and nursing staff from administering oxygen without a doctor's approval, either as part of acute or palliative (end-of-life) services.

As reported by the BBC, 19th May 2020:

Coronavirus: What's going wrong in Sweden's care homes?

"They told us that we shouldn't send anyone to the hospital, even if they may be 65 and have many years to live. We were told not to send them in," says Latifa Löfvenberg, a nurse who worked in several care homes around Gävle, north of Stockholm, at the beginning of the pandemic.

"Some can have a lot of years left to live with loved ones, but they don't have the chance... because they never make it to the hospital," she says. *"They suffocate to death. And it's a lot of panic and it's very hard to just stand by and watch."*

Mikael Fjällid, a Swedish private consultant in anaesthetics and intensive care, says he believes *'a lot of lives'* could have been saved if more patients had been able to access hospital treatment, or if care home workers were given increased responsibilities to administer oxygen themselves, instead of waiting for specialist COVID-19 response teams or paramedics.

So it is clear that what went wrong in Sweden nearly all took place in care homes and with the elderly in the community despite the Swedish authorities saying that shielding risk groups was its priority.

"We did not manage to protect the most vulnerable people, the most elderly, despite our best intentions."

– Prime Minister Stefan Löfven

It is clear from the data that if it wasn't for the massive mistakes in policies, set out to protect the vulnerable which resulted in a major cause of many premature deaths of those very same people, then Sweden would have breezed through all this, and all without a lockdown, no masks and no economic suicide. The data has shown that the number of 'COVID' deaths is about the same as the excess deaths for that period, excess deaths that can be blamed on the policies in 'care homes' alone.

Despite this clear data, the world medical scientific community and world governments continue to ignore these findings in fear maybe of opening up a Pandora's Box of lies, deceit and an unscientific basis to force lockdown policies and treatments on confused and afraid people.

Japan

Japan, like Sweden, did not introduce any hard lockdown at all or even go with the mass testing. They did order a state of emergency and people and non-essential businesses were asked to stay at home but there were no penalties for not doing so. Allegedly, Japan has more elderly people per capita than anywhere else in the world, and very densely populated cities. This, you would expect to be the perfect breeding ground for this 'deadly virus'. When looking at the data, though, it seems hardly anything at all has happened. In fact, if you look at the deaths allegedly from 'COVID', it doesn't seem to have raised the average deaths expected at all. Remember, an average is just that and slightly above and below is also perfectly normal. Only a real large spike would suggest something out of the normal which did not happen.

With a population of around 126 million and around 38 million in Tokyo alone, you would certainly think any 'deadly virus' would have a field day, especially within the elderly population. But it didn't happen, and in fact, if it wasn't for the testing then it could easily be said nothing at all out of the ordinary would have been noticed. This, like Sweden, is a problem for the people pushing the official narrative and it will be interesting to see what happens in the near future. Though declaring over 74,000 'COVID' deaths, the overall death rate did not seem to be affected by this. You can see below that there was not much movement at all and, in fact, there was a slight decrease from the previous year. This is clear evidence of more reclassification of death from other illnesses to 'COVID'.

When the overall death rate does not change significantly, while at the same time the number of deaths related to one specific disease is peaking, then the only scientific explanation can be that a number of deaths were simply renamed. Numbers are shifting from one column of *suspected causes of death* to another. This is not a public health problem. This is simply a medical classification problem.

(in deaths per 1,000 inhabitants)

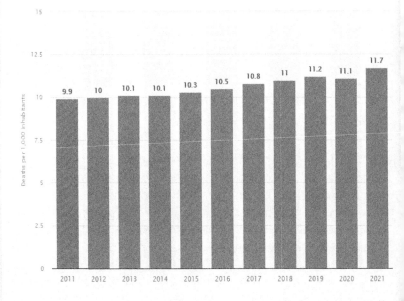

© Statista 20.

DEATH BY LOCKDOWN

Thanks to Ann Leyshon for her research and writing on this most important chapter.

As explained in the previous chapter, there was a sudden rise in excess deaths for all the countries studied only after lockdown was enforced. Additionally, when you look at how the UK compared with the rest of the world, the results are indeed shocking. As data has shown, the UK had the second highest deaths per million in the world.

The British Medical Journal had also written a paper requesting the urgent address of the fact that only a third of the thousands of excess deaths seen in the community in England and Wales could have been explained by 'COVID-19'. Another study has found that the majority of those hospitalised were those who were completely self-isolating as instructed and not going out at all.

Even 'The Guardian' newspaper reported that there were almost 10,000 unexplained extra deaths among people with dementia in England and Wales in April according to official figures that have prompted alarm and raised questions about the severe impact of social isolation on people with the condition.

So what is going on?

So what had caused the sudden spike in deaths only after lockdown and such huge discrepancies in excess deaths between countries? This is clearly about lockdown and even more so, the lockdown policies implemented. To properly appreciate the complexities involved, each area will need to be looked at individually.

Care Home Deaths

By far the biggest impact in Europe of this pandemic was within the care home system. The countries with the highest death rates ALL had a policy of isolating the elderly in these facilities as opposed to ongoing and normal care within communities and families. Around 50% of the deaths occurred within this area.

It is widely acknowledged that the vast majority of those who allegedly died with "COVID-19" had at least one serious comorbidity and were over 65 years old with more than 83% over 70. The deaths have occurred almost exclusively among those who were approaching, or already receiving, end-of-life care. It would appear that these deaths within care home facilities were effectively hastened. How could this have happened? What was implemented that could have possibly achieved this result?

The following policies were implemented at the beginning of lockdown in order to 'protect the NHS':

1. NHS England decided not to allow specified groups of vulnerable patients to be admitted to hospital. This meant not treating those over the age of 70, who displayed normal vital signs, and any who had supposedly elected not to be resuscitated, regardless of their health condition.

2. Vulnerable and older people both in care homes and within the community were pressured to sign "do not attempt resuscitation" (DNAR) notices. Additionally were numerous reports of these being completed en masse without the older person's consent in care settings, automatically excluding vulnerable people from hospital treatment.

3. Further, the guidance advised that vulnerable people should not be taken to Accident and Emergency departments unless approved by a clinical adviser, thereby increasing the delay in treatment during the vital golden hour. This caused considerable concern amongst health professionals.

While these policies were implemented, all care home visits from family and loved ones were suspended. Residents were isolated and confined to their rooms, routine care and therapies were withdrawn, as was the ability to go outside and exercise. An often unfamiliar skeleton staff remained who were often barely able to attend to basic needs. This kind of treatment and confinement would highly likely lead to the development of serious life-threatening illnesses and terrible health and mental outcomes. Reduced mobility could cause an elderly person to become constipated and this may push up on the diaphragm and cause atelectasis or cause them to vomit and aspirate leading to pneumonia. Confinement may have caused them to develop urinary retention and UTI, secondary to constipation, and become bedbound, causing more time in a prone position and development of basal collapse of the lungs and again, atelectasis and pneumonia. Just the fact that they had reduced mobility may even mean they spent more time in bed or just sitting, which again, is enough to cause chest infection/pneumonia.

The Mail Online on the 12th July 2020 headlined:

"Did care homes use powerful sedatives to speed Covid deaths?"

They show that through the month of April, out-of-hospital prescription for the drug midazolam, a powerful sedative that can be used to relieve anxiety, pain and stress and if enough is used can provide total sedation to dying patients, went from the average of 15,000 to 38,582, more than double.

They quote retired neurologist Professor Patrick Pullicino as stating:

"Midazolam depresses respiration and it hastens death. It changes end-of-life care into euthanasia." He also said, "Midazolam depresses respiration and it hastens death. It changes end-of-life care into euthanasia."

So the question is, what was happening in the care homes that was creating such anxiety, stress and pain? And was midazolam being used in the manner of the infamous "Liverpool Care

Pathway", prematurely ending patients' lives?

A small French study labelled what they found as *"confinement disease"*. The April paper concluded that more than 24 deaths at a long-term care facility, that staff believed were due to the virus were actually from hypovolemic shock, a life-threatening condition caused by a rapid loss of blood or fluids. The victims had been confined to their rooms for days with no assistance eating or drinking due to low staff numbers and a lack of personal protective equipment.

More than a month after Shoshana Padro's Toronto nursing home closed to visitors, her daughter Lenore got news that she was barely eating or drinking and was on the verge of death. Lenore Padro had been worried about how her mother would manage without extra help at mealtimes. The 79-year-old, who had dementia and needed to be spoon-fed, always ate more when her daughter or private caregiver visited and had time to coax her to take another bite. The elder Ms. Padro, who twice 'tested negative' for the 'coronavirus', died on April 28th. Her health had previously been stable, and her daughter believes she died of dehydration or starvation.

Heather Keller, who researches nutrition and ageing at the University of Waterloo, said long-term care residents who eat in their rooms don't consume as much, especially those with cognitive impairments, who lose out on the important social cues they would otherwise get in the dining room. *"That's a big part of this, is the lack of that social connectedness at meal times that stimulates food intake for older adults,"* Prof. Keller said.

Ralf Leswal is haunted by worries that his wife, Karen, who had Huntington's disease, wasn't properly cared for in her final weeks. He used to spend hours every day caring for her at Orchard Villa, her nursing home in Pickering, Ont, including slowly feeding her so that she wouldn't aspirate her food. Ms. Leswal allegedly contracted COVID-19 and died on April 30th. *"I wonder, did my wife actually die of COVID or did she die of neglect?"* he said.

"People, we're hearing, are really not eating. Not everyone, but there's a real concern," said Laura Tamblyn Watts, chief

executive officer of CanAge, a national seniors advocacy organisation. *"It's incredibly dire."*[1]

Other staff at care homes reported that residents confined to their rooms and forbidden to have visits from loved ones were giving up on life and 'fading away'. *"The virus won't be the killer of these people, it's the distress and fear of not seeing family that is doing it,"* **s**aid one carer who asked to remain anonymous but who reported her concerns to the Care Inspectorate in Scotland.[2]

So while susceptibility to illness was greatly increased, medical support was almost completely withdrawn, even GP support. Although staff members in nursing homes are medically qualified, this is not the case in the majority of care homes or among those providing community care. They are reliant upon primary care advice and intervention from their local GP. But the lockdown regime virtually removed GP support from care settings and the community and instead people were reliant on telephone consultations instead. There were zero visits.

Alzheimer's UK have many testimonies to illustrate just how devastating these actions were on their website, here is just one:

After 53 years of marriage, separation is very hard. Tony's wife, Sheila, was diagnosed with Alzheimer's disease in 2017 and currently lives in a care home. Following their enforced separation because of coronavirus, Tony shares how the lockdown has affected them, and a new poem.

> *"Before the coronavirus lockdown, I would make daily visits to the care home. Sheila always greeted me with a big smile, a kiss and a hug. I miss this very much. Blowing kisses via a video link is not the same."*
>
> *"I am losing some of the 'good days' left to us."*

---

[1] https://www.theglobeandmail.com/canada/article-what-happened-when-families-were-blocked-from-long-term-care-homess/
[2] https://news.knowledia.com/CA/en/articles/isolated-uk-care-home-residents-fading-away-say-staff-and-families-fadb09a57eeb438bf1a4b8e87fc6eb8dfe385504

The poem he was inspired to write for his wife, *'Painted Lady Summer'* – Tony Ward, is for public view on the Alzheimer's UK website and tells a sad yet beautiful tale.

"Between May and September 2019, over 10 million Painted Lady butterflies migrated from North Africa to Northern Europe – a once in a decade phenomenon."

Gavin Terry, head of policy at Alzheimer's Society, said that isolation can be devastating as family members and friends often play a crucial role in maintaining the health of people with dementia by bringing them meals, taking them out regularly to exercise and keeping people socially engaged. Withdrawing this support can cause people to rapidly go downhill, he said. *"We're hearing that some people are 'just giving up' or 'switching off' and not eating or drinking,"* he said.

The article on Friday 5th June in The Guardian Online headlined: *"Extra 10,000 dementia deaths in England and Wales in April"* stated:

> *"Aside from coronavirus, in April there were a further 9,429 deaths from dementia and Alzheimer's disease alone in England and 462 in Wales. That number is 83% higher than usual in England, and 54% higher in Wales."*

Clearly there was much concern about the policies being forced upon them. On May 7th 2020, in response to Boris Johnson's comment on the 6th May when he said he *"bitterly regrets"* the coronavirus crisis in care homes – and the government was *"working very hard"* to tackle it, Gavin Terry stated:

> *"We haven't seen any evidence to suggest that deaths in care homes are slowing down, and any other implication would be dangerously complacent. In the past month, we know that the number of people who have died in care homes is twice the average; in the last week alone we saw the death rate rise by 30%. And it is not only deaths due to coronavirus that we fear - we are concerned there will be a sharp rise in deaths due to dementia, not least because of the*

impact of isolation, when the full figures are known."

People with dementia, who make up about two-thirds of the long-term care population, are particularly vulnerable. Many need partial or full feeding assistance, which takes time that staff don't always have. Changes in routine, such as being confined to their rooms because of an *outbreak*, often cause confusion and worsen symptoms. Two-and-a-half months after restrictions were put in place, family members and seniors advocates stated there had been preventable deaths from dehydration and other residents were wasting away without the help of relatives and the private caregivers they relied on at mealtimes. The loss of extra assistance comes as many facilities struggle with severe staffing shortages.

William Laing, the author of the new analysis on excess deaths among care home residents, said their treatment was *"a scandal which is just emerging."* He said he believed a series of failings were behind the high number of excess deaths: *"At the peak of the crisis, there were widespread reports of normal medical support simply being removed from care homes,"* he said. *"Ambulances would not turn up to take emergencies to hospital, since capacity had to be kept clear for Covid cases."*

Martin Green, chief executive of Care England, has commented,

> *"the true scale of the coronavirus crisis 'burning through' care homes may never be known".* He said in a scathing attack on the government's 'herd immunity' policy: *"I saw letters from GPs sent to care homes saying 'we will not be doing consultations, we will not be sending people to hospital'. I think there's a real issue that lots of people just were denied access to hospital."*

If the intention was to protect the most vulnerable, it is ludicrous to imagine that the cumulative effect of these policies didn't lead to early mortality among the most vulnerable. The lockdown regime was utterly devastating to the health of the very demographic it was supposedly designed to 'keep safe'.

I know of one lady who could not see her husband for the last week of his life because he was isolated in a 'care home'. They had been married for 67 years.

Hospital Deaths

Regular rules and best practices for treating respiratory and influenza-type diseases ceased to be applied because of 'COVID-19' and instead new protocols were implemented with the focus being on minimising the spread of *the virus* rather than the best interests of the patient. One of these was the routine use of ventilation for suspected COVID patients and this was heavily promoted in the media and the supposed shortage of ventilators widely publicised. What was not publicised, however, was that this is an incredibly invasive and often deadly procedure involving a highly toxic cocktail of drugs and other interventions and that this was not the usual treatment method for patients presenting with symptoms of respiratory distress. A subsequent study in New York found that 80% of those ventilated died when ordinarily a death rate of 20% would have been expected.

Another protocol for treating 'COVID-19' featured in The Lancet and touted as the 'model treatment':

Here, the 50-year-old patient was given high doses of cortisone; methylprednisolone 600mg; moxifloxacin, a very strong antibiotic; a DNA gyrase inhibitor; Lopinavir and Ritonavir (both protease inhibitors from AIDS treatments); and finally at the end another broad-spectrum antibiotic. This would be a highly toxic mix with interferons with immunosuppressive effects.

The patient, who was not in a risk group, unsurprisingly died.

Erin Marie Olszewski, a frontline nurse in New York reported publicly on this, going as far as saying she felt that these patients were being 'murdered' by a general lack of care, over vigorous diagnosing of 'COVID-19' and the ventilation used to treat them. Her story very much aligned with that of other doctors and nurses in the UK who have come forward or posted to social media, and who confirmed some of the worst aspects of these new protocols that were causing avoidable deaths. She went on to write a book about her experience in hospital during the crisis:

'*Undercover Epicenter Nurse: How Fraud, Negligence, and Greed Led to Unnecessary Deaths at Elmhurst Hospital*'. This gives us a good insight into her experience.

> "*You've got doctors and nurses that, at that point, just didn't care because everybody was going to die anyway so what's the point? And then you have everybody on a ventilator. So, these patients can't even speak for themselves. They're at the hands of whoever is taking care of them.*"

Legally doctors are always on the safe side if they do 'everything' that is recommended. If the patient then dies, they have committed no error. If they haven't adhered to the recommended protocol and the patient dies, then they have a problem. Remember the first law, 'do no harm'. Combine this top-down, non-scientific approach, with the forced use of DNRs, financial incentives, and it is easy to see how the fear could have escalated and made the whole situation incalculably worse.

For anyone doubting this could happen, The British Medical Journal published a study where they estimated that iatrogenic death (death caused by medical examination or treatment) was the third leading cause of death in the US. There is no reason to think that this is not also the case in the UK especially with the hysteria seen both in diagnosing and then in treating 'COVID-19' particularly in the beginning where the pressure to follow the standardised protocols will have be even greater.

Lastly, the following uncomfortable truth must also be considered. It has been previously and widely alleged in the media that NHS doctors have been prematurely ending the lives of thousands of elderly hospital patients because they are either difficult to manage or to free up beds. In the current crisis, where beds were considered a particular premium and recovery from 'COVID-19' unlikely, just how many elderly patients, without a proper analysis of their condition and who could have lived longer, were placed on an 'assisted death pathway' rather than given routine care? We already know that to free up space in hospitals, elderly patients were discharged into care homes to effectively die.

Community Deaths

Aside from receiving DNAR notices through the post, the most vulnerable in the community were also sent letters telling them to stay at home to 'protect the NHS'.

Not only did ambulance response times increase exponentially, access to hospital treatment was actively deterred and community healthcare and GP support was withheld. Just like in care homes people had to get used to telephone consultations instead of examinations and home visits, hugely increasing the risk to the most vulnerable. Not to mention that for the same reasons as in care home facilities, those in the wider community who now found themselves isolated, terrified and without support, would have also had their susceptibility to illness immeasurably increased.

Being terrified of either contracting the virus or overwhelming the NHS had the effect of drastically reducing emergency admissions and in week 14 there were 100,000 less than in the same week the previous year! At a time when the increase in stress levels was huge, there was a 40% reduction in hospital attendances for heart attacks. People with acute need for cardiovascular treatment (including strokes) were not going to hospital as they otherwise would. There was also a substantial reduction in referrals for acute coronary syndrome as well as reports of people presenting late with complications due to having a heart attack, something that was never normally seen.

Around 170,000 people die every year from cardiovascular disease in the UK so a 40% reduction in callouts, along with substantially lower referrals would likely represent a huge proportion of these excess deaths.

Dr Sonya Babu-Narayan, Associate Medical Director of the British Heart Foundations, said:

"During the lockdown, A&E presentations for heart attacks and strokes dropped by more than half. This resulted in a huge increase of deaths in the home."

Professor Stephen Westaby (a leading heart surgeon) stated:

"We could see thousands of deaths from heart disease and cancer over the next six months. Their families will never forget this. Neither China nor Italy stopped treating these conditions despite the chaos there earlier this year. It's bizarre."

Conclusions

The evidence is clear that it was the lockdown itself that caused ill health and death. If the response to a public health crisis is to withdraw healthcare from those who need it the most, a spike in mortality is the only possible outcome. Not only are those affected by 'the disease' (showing symptoms of illness) more likely to succumb to' it', but increased mortality from every other comorbidity is hard wired into that lockdown policy.

Rather than blaming an unproven virus it was these lockdown measures that accounted for the strong correlation between the imposition of healthcare-limiting lockdowns and sharp increases in mortality.

And so I believe that's the mechanism by which they accelerated the rate of death of immune-deficient fragile people who would have died in the many weeks and months later, eventually in a natural way but instead they accelerated their deaths by doing this.

-Ann Leyshon

As I stated on Feb 6 2020 *"there is nothing going around the world except fear and hysteria"*. As I knew the science of so-called infectious disease was not what we have been told it seemed clear to me that if 'they' wanted to create a pandemic then something would have to change in the environment. Declaring a pandemic and simply reclassifying all normal deaths as 'COVID' would not be enough. 'They' needed excess deaths to sell their story. It was very clear to me how this would happen even before deaths started to rise. I had been warning of 'Medical Fascism' for years and with my understanding of what allopathic medicine does it was clear 'they' would use protocols ingrained into the minds of the medical staff to cause the excess deaths they needed and elderly, weak and vulnerable people were an easy target. It was murder by government policy, or 'DEMOCIDE'.

A Death We Should Never Forget

During a rally in Truro, Cornwall sometime in 2021, arranged to create awareness of the coming cashless society and digital slavery, I met fellow Cornwall resident Debi Evans, a former NHS nurse and now researcher for UKColumn News. Debi introduced me to a lady, Elena Vlaica, a registered general nurse, who recounted to me the story of her husband's death. The one thing I can say was that I was listening to a woman in a deep state of shock and total disbelief at the ordeal she had been put through, and continues to suffer from, from a profession that claims to be looking after our health. Sadly from my own experience and understanding of how things work it was of no surprise, yet it still shocked me, the callousness of the behaviour of the people who we trust to look after us in times of need. This case is the tip of a very large ice-berg in terms of the tyranny that took place during lockdown world-wide and the absolute definition of the Democide I am talking about. Please, if you can, listen to the interview in the link and demand not only that justice is done but that this medical tyranny never happens again.

This is a Debi Evans article regarding Elena's horrific experience with the NHS. The article is linked with the interview attached.
https://www.ukcolumn.org/video/no-time-to-grieve-death-by-pathway

No Time To Grieve: Death by Pathway
Friday, 16th September 2022

While our attention focuses on the tragic accounts of those who have been injured as a result of Covid-19 injections, another wicked act has been happening right under our noses in plain sight of thousands, perhaps millions of others: a deliberate culling of our most vulnerable.

When Elena Vlaica RGN called an ambulance for her soulmate and partner Stuart when he became breathless and unwell, she trusted the NHS to look after him and return him to her better. She was not to have known that this one innocuous call for help would mean his final journey from their home alive.

Stuart was in his early fifties and had had a mild stroke a couple of years previously. Although life was not quite the same as before the stroke, Stuart and Elena still enjoyed a happy active life, and Stuart's family, children and grandchildren were regular visitors.

Elena first contacted UK Column months ago to tell us how her beloved soulmate, who was unvaccinated for Covid-19, had within days of admission been consigned to death, as an End-of-Life Care Plan was implemented without consultation with the family or indeed Stuart himself.

The notorious Liverpool Care Pathway, a pathway to death, was ostensibly abandoned in 2014 after being deemed inhumane, but appears to have been resurrected at the start of the 'pandemic' in early 2020 in many hospitals and care homes across the U.K.

PCR + unjabbed = death

On admission to the Royal Cornwall Hospital Trust, and having been diagnosed as having Covid-19 on the dubious strength of a PCR test, Stuart was left isolated, scared and separated from those he loved. Elena describes how she had to communicate with him through a phone screen and watch him cry as he desperately begged to return home, where he felt safe.

Despite begging the medical teams to continue with a course of antibiotics, he was deemed 'terminal', and as such was immediately started on a Midazolam and morphine protocol, with all of his regular medications abruptly withheld (including the antidepressant Citalopram, which it is well known patients should be slowly weaned off).

Elena knew that the combination of these two drugs— morphine, an opioid, and Midazolam, a benzodiazepine— would kill him, and instructed doctors not to use it. No-one in their right mind would give a respiratory depressant (inhibitor of breathing) to someone who was struggling to breathe.

Unable to visit, Elena was alone and reliant on Stuart's sisters, who were allowed to visit only sparingly. The family discovered, to their horror, that not only was Stuart being slowly sedated and starved into an early death, but he had tried to escape on more than one occasion, only to find he was shackled to the bed by a catheter bag tied to the bedframe.

Elena describes in this interview how "we know Midazolam is torture like waterboarding" and how an NHS employee killed Stuart while Elena held him. Elena, who was born in Ceaușescu's Romania, adds that "they have done a brilliant job on the propaganda".

Not a one-off

The harrowing events of what happened to Stuart in hospital are mirrored across the country. Accelerated end-of-life care plans are being rolled out at pace and by stealth. This is the frightening fruit of a policy of making seemingly anyone with a job in the care sector—regardless of grade or qualification—learn how to 'certify a death' in a half-hour e-tutorial. Yes, the training is online and takes 30 minutes.

Elena tells UK Column of her and her family's dogged determination in fighting for Stuart's life, and subsequently for truth and justice, and how they have all coped since losing him.

She sets out how relatives had to navigate red tape to try to raise awareness urgently in others; there was no time to grieve. That was the cruellest blow of all—mourning denied. It turned out to be impossible to obtain a post mortem (autopsy).

Far from giving up, Elena has returned to nursing where she is allowed to (she is restricted in her duties, as she is unvaccinated) to educate her colleagues and to do her best for her patients. Did she want to return? No; but she felt she had to, in order to help those left behind. She explains how, on numerous occasions, doctors have consulted her for guidance as to how care should proceed in some very sick patients. Her recommendation is always the same: "Let's wait and see; antibiotics and nebuliser first, and then we will reassess". No panic, no rush; just kindness and time.

More Elenas

How many lives have Elena and others of like mind in her profession saved that we don't know about? The quiet saviours in our care homes should be encouraged and thanked for all they are doing to protect some of our most elderly and vulnerable. Many of the most conscience-stricken have already left the healthcare system, but not all. Elena has decided not administer Midazolam and morphine to any patient, and has even refused to update her qualifications

283

over this principle. She vows that no-one else will go through what her darling beloved went through; not on her watch.

We thank Elena and her family for allowing us to share their story, and those doctors, nurses and carers still in the background who are applying Elena's attitude.

As we watch our most vulnerable and elderly jabbed with the new 'bivalent' Covid-19 booster, we can only pray there are many more Elenas in our midst to educate those in the medical profession about what they are doing. Every care home and hospital ward needs an Elena. Do No Harm; tender loving care for all patients.

Death From Anxiety

Imagine for a moment an individual who suffers from anxiety, watches all the media and government updates on the 'deadly virus', believes everything and goes into total fear, fight or flight, except there is nothing visible to fight and nowhere to run to. It is quite possible for a person suffering from anxiety that he/she could go into a panic state and it affects their breathing'. "I've got it, I'm sure I've got it". Then imagine calling an ambulance; they arrive ready for the next *virus case*, your breathing is difficult and they rush you straight to the 'COVID' ward. You arrive into the 'war zone'; people with masks on everywhere ready to deal with another victim and your anxiety now goes through the roof. "Am I gonna survive?" is going through your mind. You are put on the protocols in place and they see your breathing is getting worse and not better; this in turn makes your stress worse and breathing even more difficult. You are then put on a ventilator and after that it is in the hands of God.

This is a scenario that is possible and could be caused by fear, anxiety and stress alone, brought on by the politicians, "experts" and the media constantly telling us we need to be afraid of this invisible enemy coming to get us all. No *virus* needed in this scenario to explain the symptoms. This would have been bad enough to deal with for a fairly healthy person. Now image you already have health issues and are elderly and vulnerable.

Getting to the truth would mean an individual investigation into all excess deaths and 'COVID deaths'; that obviously would be very difficult to do and would still not give us an absolute truth about each individual death but as we have already scientifically ruled out one single cause, a virus, then the lockdown and all that went with it must of clearly had a massive impact on the excess deaths. What is clearly known about fear and anxiety is that it lowers what they call the immune system response. Evolution has created a fight-or-flight reaction to danger; when that happens our energy goes away from our inner body, where our main cleansing happens, and to the outer muscles so we can use the extra energy to escape the danger. This means normal immune function is almost stopped to get us out of danger but returns quickly after the danger has been evaded without much effect on the body. This should be a short-lived scenario but when we are put under permanent, chronic stress then we go into a permanent low level of fight or flight and the extra anxiety restricts our breathing as we can't relax. Over time this will seriously affect your health, especially if you already have on going issues. Your mental and emotional state will affect how your body functions in what we have already called Holistic thinking. How the body works is not rocket science, really, just simple common sense.

"Insanity is doing the same thing over and over and expecting different results."

– Albert Einstein

:

SECOND WAVE OF MADNESS

Remember in *Event 201* it was predicted that:

> "65 million people dead in the first 18 months. The outbreak was small at first and initially seemed controllable but then it started spreading in densely crowded and impoverished neighbourhoods of mega cities. From that point on the spread of the disease was explosive. Within 6 months cases were occurring in nearly every country."

So if it seemed that the first wave was really mainly caused by the lockdown itself then what would this second and possibly massive larger second wave be caused by?

Well, the lockdowns did not go away, except in Sweden where they were never present in the first place, don't let the world forget that one. They were here to stay whether they destroy life as we know it or not and regardless of the physical, emotional and economic harm they were doing.

In Victoria in Australia they announced a state of emergency could be in place for 18 months with just 430 'COVID deaths' to date and only 517 in the whole of Australia. Yes, and that 517 includes the state of Victoria. We had people being dragged out of their cars after the windows were smashed by police just for not wanting to talk. A pregnant woman being man-handled and taken from her home in custody, basically kidnapped, for posting non-approved information on social media. iT was very clear to see that the government and police of Victoria were totally out of control, had lost the plot completely, and Victoria was now a vicious police state that had turned on the people they were supposed to serve and protect.

It was clear this was being driven by psychopathy and an insane, illogical belief that they were all going to die unless the government took complete control. The police, repeating the line that the **'public must comply'**, still sends a shiver down my spine.

The second wave then it seemed would be created by months of people wearing masks and breathing in dirty air; by the time winter comes around when our bodies can struggle anyway due to the colder weather, less sunlight and less outdoor exercise, it was for sure that many people would suffer even worse than normal to cope and would become ill and probably have breathing issues.

Then we have what Matt Hancock announced in the UK as the *'biggest flu vaccine programme ever'* pushed on the population; a flu vaccine that has zero evidence of being effective anyway and is well known to have a side effect of the flu itself. I personally know people who have the flu vaccine and get the worst flu ever, yet the nurse tells them that 'if it wasn't for the vaccine they would have probably died'. No science to back that statement up but the people trust in them and they lap it up and queue up the next flu season to go through the whole thing again.

Then we have the normal flu season which can take tens of thousands of lives by itself. Can you see how all these things could be easily put down as the second wave? Add to that the same lockdown policies that will be repeated again despite massive failings the first time round and you can see globally where the 65 million deaths they predicted (hoped for) could come from if the people went into total fear and compliance.

In reality the 65 million deaths they predicted, again hoped for, did not materialise even with all the data fiddling and protocols. On writing this book august 2023 we have officially 6,911,466 'COVID deaths' worldwide. Still the fear of putting out a big number is what sticks in people's minds and they know this. EVENT 201 was meant to be seen by people so they could play their mind games of fear and confusion.

The flu is well known to be a powerful detox by a system under a lot of stress. Remember when we suppress, or ignore, a mild acute symptom like the common cold then this will not allow a body clear out hence we see what is known as the flu. In the winter when the cold weather, lack of sunshine and more puts us all under pressure our bodies have to work harder to stay in balance.

In nature it's a time when the old and weak succumb to the pressure and pass away. As we are nature too then this also happens to us, the old and weak will be put under more pressure than the rest of us and many will not survive. With the extra pressure of lockdowns and toxic injections then the number under pressure will increase.

Peru has proven beyond doubt the damage of the lockdown and mask wearing. My sister-in-law had 'COVID', Feb 2021, except it was pneumonia and probably caused by the mask wearing, lockdown, fear and the rest of the protocols. Her recovery plan from the medical profession was antibiotics and to stay in her room alone, isolated, without sunshine, until she was better. The debate is over, it is very clear; lockdown kills and as with Sweden had shown (protect and shield policy aside), just getting on with life saves lives.

After a summer of empty hospitals but with the alert still high, because of 'cases', we came into late autumn/winter. In fact, if you even wanted to pursue their flawed science of 'herd immunity' then summer would have been the perfect time to go for it as it is a time of the year when we all come in contact due to more outside group activities due to improved weather during the summer months. This way deaths and illnesses would be low and we would all have 'herd immunity' by winter when we know our systems are low and vulnerable. This would make sense and the coming winter disaster could be avoided, and just maybe our economy would survive. Why was this policy not pursued? Not that I believe in herd immunity but I am trying to use their understanding of disease to base an argument on their science. But as we have seen many times during this 'crisis' the science keeps changing and now 'herd immunity' is not possible as you can get 'COVID' more than once.

Truth is, they had no plan, because the plan was the no-plan plan. The plan was to keep us controlled by fear with the new 'cases' until winter was upon us. But they had lied, the curve had been flattened and there was no pressure on the NHS, in fact it's having a summer timeout as the hospitals were empty. The show was over and it was time to go back to living, or that's what the public thought.

We saw, as expected in the UK, the big flu vaccine programme and the lockdown measures being increased. Again, we saw the rise in deaths occurring at a time when the normal 'flu season' would have started and yet as by magic, the normal flu seemed to have disappeared and been replaced by 'COVID'. Reclassification at its best!

"The second wave could kill 85,000", but it was safe to send your kids back to school.

> *"The evidence is overwhelming that it is in the interest of the wellbeing and the health of children, young people, pupils, to be back in school rather than missing out any more ... So, it is the healthy, safe thing to do."*
>
> – Boris Johnson

This is not politicians doing their best under difficult circumstances; this is very well thought out social destruction on a massive scale. So we had Johnson and Hancock still enforcing controlling laws, mandated masks in public, and now masks being pushed in schools. It was safe but keep distancing, it was safe but the threat was still there, it was safe but many are going die in a *second wave*, it was safe but wear a mask, it was safe but wash your hands, it was safe but keep apart but at the same time go to school, it was safe but...

So now with schools closed down, because apparently it wasn't safe after all, the deaths started to rise.

Whether you believe in the unproven virus theory of disease or not is not relevant to the policy of destroying the ability for people to survive. To lock down the whole world and stop productivity was mass murder and I hope the people wake up to this fact sooner rather than later. Humanity needs to see that the governments are not our friends and instead of bringing in policies to make our lives better and protect our natural freedoms they are actively bringing in policies to create hell on earth. This cannot be by accident, stupidity or ignorance.

The two following graphs are taken from UKColumn News as I know they take their national data from the ONS and their sources are always official. The first graph shows a sharp rise in deaths with the introduction of the COVID vaccine. The second graph shows clearly the movement of a 'second wave' which Sweden seemed to follow. So again, i expected a rise in excess deaths due to the lockdown measures, especially in care homes and a coming COVID vaccine created in record time.

Remember again, the most important aspects of health are clean air, sunshine, exercise, clean water and maybe most important, family and friends. It could be easily said that to prepare for this *second wave* all the vital components of a healthy life were taken away and on top of that the constant fear. Even an obvious supplement of vitamin D wasn't on the table. Again, no health measures, only fear measures. Then with the rollout of the experimental COVID vaccines it didn't look good.

The UKColumn created a special page on their website with the data direct from *the MHRA yellow card scheme* for reported *COVID vaccine adverse reactions and deaths*, more on this later.

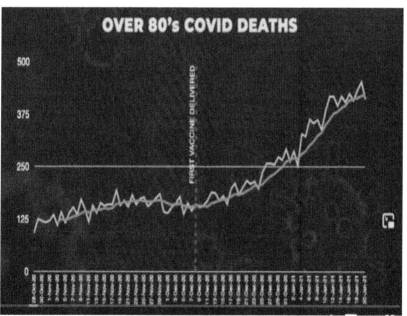

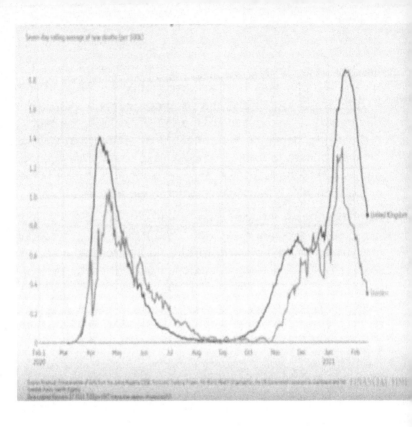

Seven-day rolling average of new deaths (per 100,000)

So the obvious correlation with the vaccine rollout and rise in over 80s deaths is clear. The connection does not mean cause and obviously other lockdown factors in care homes as mentioned above means this wasn't unexpected at all. This correlation alone should have required the stopping of the experimental vaccine rollout until a full investigation is done, especially as the MHRA had already started reporting their 'expected' COVID vaccine deaths and adverse reactions and we were still only in February 2021. This was not incompetence; it was murder, pure and simple. There is no way the self-proclaimed 'leaders' and 'experts' are so stupid they could not see this coming. The ignorant non-thinking order followers on the ground were 'just doing their jobs' but it must be clear that at the top of the power tree people knew exactly what was happening.

Again, to 'save the NHS' during the 'second wave' we see the same tactics.

"Fury at 'do not resuscitate' notices given to Covid patients with learning disabilities"
– The Observer Online, Sat 13th Feb 2021

> *"People with learning disabilities have been given do not resuscitate orders during the second wave of the pandemic, in spite of widespread condemnation of the practice last year and an urgent investigation by the care watchdog.*
>
> *Mencap said it had received reports in January from people with learning disabilities that they had been told they would not be resuscitated if they were taken ill with Covid-19.*
>
> *The Care Quality Commission said in December that inappropriate Do Not Attempt Cardiopulmonary Resuscitation (DNACPR) notices had caused potentially avoidable deaths last year."*

The pattern was the same again; we had closed the country and wrecked the economy and the lives of people and children's education for nothing. The full-year pattern of excess deaths in Sweden follows the UK due to care home policies, yet the lives and economy, and more importantly mental health, of the free general public in Sweden had not been destroyed. Yet again, it was the vulnerable and elderly who took the brunt of government policies, medical protocols and treatments.

The last real question is, do the deaths add up to the worst *plague* since the great Spanish flu? This is what the public are being told but as usual, most people just read the big headlines, take that as truth and yet as we know the devil is always in the details.

Mortality in the UK

As we have established, the only figure that can be relied upon is the deaths. How bad was this pandemic? The figure out for England and Wales for 2020 is 608,002 deaths. We were told the worst deaths since the *Great Spanish Flu* a century ago. Well, if you just take a simple number like that and blow it up in the mainstream media knowing that most people just read headlines then that is a very powerful figure.

An obvious thing to state would be the large population rise since those times so death rates give far more information than just a simple number of deaths. In 1976, the year of the great drought, some 599,000 people died in England and Wales, not too far off 2020 deaths and with obviously a smaller population. And yet I remember that summer of water shortages and hot sun without a care in the world. Certainly I don't remember any government or media frenzy telling us to fear for our lives and masses of people dying. I do remember lots of fun playing football in the park and Manchester United losing a dramatic FA Cup final. I guess if this were to happen today it would be put down as 'death due to climate change', which is an actual diagnosis starting to be used. The climate is something we will go into more detail later.

On the following image the left hand side shows the actual number of deaths in the hundreds of thousands. The right hand side shows the deaths as a death-rate per 1000.The crude number of deaths seemed to peak in 1976 then take a slow downturn before rising again in about 2010. So basically ups and downs are quite normal. The death-rate seemed to be on the slow decline since about 1961 when it started to rise slightly again in about 2010 showing a similar pattern. The death-rates, rather than crude death numbers, give us a better understanding of what is going on as it takes into account population rise and fall.

2. Long-term trends in mortality

The charts below show the number of deaths and the crude death rate in different parts of the UK, in each year from 1961 to 2017.

MORTALITY IN THE UK

1961-2017

England and Wales

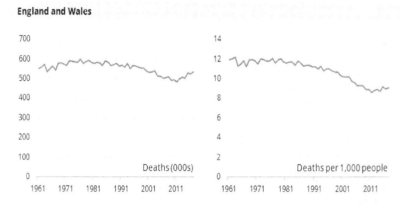

So if we now go to the ONS data for the last thirty-one years, the data shows there were 14 years with a higher 'crude mortality rate' for England and Wales than in 2020. For the 'age-standardised mortality rate' there were 19 years with a higher rate. As you can see it certainly had not been an exceptional year when comparing with the period between 1960-1980 when deaths-rates were much higher. Numerically though it had been high. When you take off what must be, in my opinion, thousands if not tens of thousands of lockdown deaths from various factors, then the question must be asked. Has anything unusual actually happened at all?

Year	Number of deaths	Population (Thousands)	Crude mortality rate (per 100,000 population)	Age-standardised mortality rate (per 100,000 population)
2020	608,002	59,829	1,016.20	1,043.5
2019	530,841	59,440	893.1	92
2018	541,589	59,116	916.1	965.
2017	533,253	58,745	907.7	965.
2016	525,048	58,381	899.3	966.
2015	529,655	57,885	915	993
2014	501,424	57,409	873.4	95
2013	506,790	56,948	889.9	985
2012	499,331	56,568	882.7	987
2011	484,367	56,171	862.3	978
2010	493,242	55,692	885.7	1,017.1
2009	491,348	55,235	889.6	1,033.8
2008	509,090	54,842	928.3	1,091.

2007	504,052	54,387	926.8	1,091.80
2006	502,599	53,951	931.6	1,104.30
2005	512,993	53,575	957.5	1,143.80
2004	514,250	53,152	967.5	1,163.00
2003	539,151	52,863	1,019.90	1,232.10
2002	535,356	52,602	1,017.70	1,231.30
2001	532,498	52,360	1,017.00	1,236.20
2000	537,877	52,140	1,031.60	1,266.40
1999	553,532	51,933	1,065.80	1,320.20
1998	553,435	51,720	1,070.10	1,327.20
1997	558,052	51,560	1,082.30	1,350.80
1996	563,007	51,410	1,095.10	1,372.50
1995	565,902	51,272	1,103.70	1,392.00
1994	551,780	51,116	1,079.50	1,374.90
1993	578,512	50,986	1,134.70	1,453.40
1992	558,313	50,876	1,097.40	1,415.00
1991	570,044	50,748	1,123.30	1,464.30
1990	564,846	50,561	1,117.20	1,462.60

MHRA

This from the website

The Medicines and Healthcare Products Regulatory Agency regulates medicines, medical devices and blood components for transfusion in the UK.

We are the regulator of medicines, medical devices and blood components for transfusion in the UK.
We put patients first in everything we do, right across the lifecycle of the products we regulate. We rigorously use science and data to inform our decisions, enable medical innovation and to make sure that medicines and healthcare products available in the UK are safe and effective.

Our responsibilities are to:
- *ensure medicines, medical devices and blood components for transfusion meet applicable standards of safety, quality and efficacy (effectiveness)*
- *secure safe supply chain for medicines, medical devices and blood components*
- *promote international standardisation and harmonisation to assure the effectiveness and safety of biological medicines*
- *educate the public and healthcare professionals about the risks and benefits of medicines, medical devices and blood components, leading to safer and more effective use*
- *enable innovation and research and development that is beneficial to public health*
- *collaborate with partners in the UK and internationally to support our mission to enable the earliest access to safe medicines and medical devices and to protect public health*

On 23/10/2020 'Ted-tenders electronic daily: Supplement to the Official Journal of the EU' published details of an already negotiated contract by the Medicines and Healthcare Products Agency (MHRA) given to Genpact (UK) Ltd, London, who were the only organisation who put in a bid for the tender. The dispatch of the notice was given as 19/10/2020, yet the contract was awarded to the company on 14/9/2020. So basically the contract was not put out to tender as it was a done deal before it was even published due to 'reasons of extreme urgency'.

(https://ted.europa.eu/udl?uri=TED:NOTICE:506291-2020:TEXT:EN:HTML&tabId=1)

Short description:
The MHRA urgently seeks an Artificial Intelligence (AI) software tool to process the expected high volume of Covid-19 vaccine Adverse Drug Reaction (ADRs) and ensure that no details from the ADRs' reaction text are missed.
Total value of the procurement (excluding VAT)
Value excluding VAT: 1,500,000.00 GBP

Type of procedure

Explanation:

For reasons of extreme urgency under Regulation 32(2)(c) related to the release of a Covid-19 vaccine MHRA have accelerated the sourcing and implementation of a vaccine specific AI tool. 					*Strictly necessary — it is not possible to retrofit the MHRA's legacy systems to handle the volume of ADRs that will be generated by a Covid-19 vaccine. Therefore, if the MHRA does not implement the AI tool, it will be unable to process these ADRs effectively. This will hinder its ability to rapidly identify any potential safety issues with the Covid-19 vaccine and represents a direct threat to patient life and public health. Reasons of extreme urgency — the MHRA recognises that its planned procurement process for the SafetyConnect programme, including the AI tool, would not have concluded by vaccine launch. Leading to an inability to effectively monitor adverse reactions to a Covid-19 vaccine.*

Events unforeseeable — the Covid-19 crisis is novel and developments in the search of a Covid-19 vaccine have not followed any predictable pattern so far

So, from the very start it was accepted by the MHRA there would be an 'expected high volume of Covid-19 vaccine Adverse Drug Reaction (ADRs)'. Historically the MHRA has accepted that it only gets somewhere between 1% - 10% of adverse vaccine reactions and deaths reported via the 'yellow card scheme'. There could be various reasons for this but the main reason I feel would be that not too many people even know the reporting scheme exists. Another reason would be reluctance for doctors to advertise or suspect a vaccine reaction due to the education engraining in their mind-set that vaccines are exceptionally safe; a view shared by the majority of the general public. The defence of the MHRA was that due to the expected blanket roll-out on the population of the covid vaccine, which would entail tens of millions of doses, it would be normal to expect more yellow cards being reported than with other vaccines, which have no-where near the uptake.

Here is an extract from a letter to Debi Evans of UKColumn News from the MHRA.
(https://www.ukcolumn.org/article/mhras-letter-to-debi-evans-we-didnt-use-our-ai-tool-to-assess-yellow-card-data-on-covid)

> *"With respect to the anticipated volume of suspected adverse drug reaction (ADR) reports for the COVID-19 vaccination programme, this was estimated from a number of previous vaccination campaigns. We acknowledged that actual numbers of reports would be dependent on various factors including the number of doses administered and use of concurrent treatments (for instance to manage fevers). Our past experience with other new immunisation campaigns is that we tend to receive a single Yellow Card report per 1,000 doses administered and so we prepared our surveillance systems on that basis. It is important to note that a report of a suspected side effect is not proof that the vaccine caused it but a suspicion of this by the reporter."*

The statement does make one thing clear though: vaccines are not safe! Despite politicians repeating the 'safe and effective' mantra they then made it clear that the vaccine makers would not be liable for any adverse reactions or deaths. I'm not sure what definition of 'safe' these people were using but as usual it seemed like more Orwellian double speak. There is an 'accepted risk' with vaccines, so it is disingenuous to state they are safe.

On 28/09/2022 the UKColumn published their final numbers of their 'COVID-19 Vaccine Analysis Overview' where they had taken data from the covid vaccine yellow card scheme at the MHRA. (https://yellowcard.ukcolumn.org/yellow-card-reports)

Total reports   464,058
Total reactions   1,517,612
Total fatalities   2,272

Close to half a million individual people reported an adverse reaction with on average of just over three reactions per person. If we give the benefit of the doubt to the MHRA and say the higher number of 10% was reported we still have nearly four and half million people adversely affected. If we then go to the reported deaths and again give the more conservative 10% reported, we would get over 22,000 deaths. Yes, as stated by the MHRA, these are just reports and not proven to be caused by the vaccine - correlation does not equal causation - but the reports would have to be based on something. I, due to my work, come into contact with many people on a daily basis and I can say for certain that many of the people I know who took the vaccine soon afterwards became ill, many for a prolonged period of time. All but one seemed to be able to connect the fact they were fine before the vaccine and ill after, yes just one, and none of them filled in a yellow card or even knew the scheme existed. I managed to tell one person about the yellow card scheme after he started having eye problems post-injection and he did fill in the yellow card but only after I had told him the scheme existed. Most people I spoke to who had taken the vaccine and shortly afterwards came down ill were convinced by the *'positive test'* they had taken that they had *'covid'*. "If it wasn't for the vaccine it could have been a lot worse" This was repeated to them by the medical professionals after having seen the 'positive test'.

They are mind controlled into believing vaccines are safe and consequently were also convinced their patients had had a lucky escape and that their miracle vaccine had actually saved them. The fact they were fine and healthy before the vaccine seemed not relevant or did not even enter their field of awareness. To get a compensation payment you have to be at least '60% disabled' and have what they call 'severe disablement'. And despite the £1,500,000 contract for an AI system to monitor the *'expected high volume of Covid-19 vaccine Adverse Drug Reaction'* it seems the high tech system was not even used. Money for nothing as they say, except it was our money they got for nothing. Again, from the letter to Debi Evans.

"We developed a range of resources and technology to support the proactive vigilance of the COVID-19 vaccination programme. The use of artificial intelligence (AI) was one element of that. We take every report of a suspected side effect seriously and we have combined the review of reports of adverse events of special interest with statistical analysis of anonymised clinical records. This specific AI tool chosen for the surveillance of COVID-19 vaccines was due to the potential size and scale of the vaccination campaign. The tool was not used for assessment of Yellow Card data [emphasis added], but to help ensure that all the information from the reporter is well structured to support analysis and subject to robust quality assessment."

And despite the hundreds of thousands of individual reports of adverse reactions and over 2,200 deaths and the fact we know this is under reported, they made this statement that has to make you question what on earth do they feel the word 'safe' means.

"The safety of the COVID-19 vaccines is of paramount importance to us; no new vaccine for children will be approved by the MHRA unless the expected standards of safety, quality and effectiveness are met. Furthermore, as with all vaccines and medicines, their on-going safety is continuously monitored, and benefits and possible risks remain under review. Should a new safety issue be confirmed we will act promptly to inform patients and healthcare professionals and take appropriate steps to mitigate any identified risk and protect public health."

When did the MHRA ever *'act promptly to inform'* anyone at all when the yellow card reports were streaming in? The answer is they did not and neither did the mainstream media, the government officials and the medical professionals. I myself went to my local vaccine centre; it could not have been called a medical centre anymore, when the covid vaccine was first being administered. I walked to the door passing the long line of people waiting for their 'new technology vaccine' to protect them from the enemy. "Lambs to the slaughter", I thought to myself but did not say a word as I knew it would be pointless. Their minds had been made up and anyone even asking them to think it over would be met with anger. I had seen it before. However, I did ask to see the practice manager regarding my research on the 'law of consent'. A few minutes later a masked up doctor came out looking very stressed. I asked him if he was aware of the 'law of consent'. He got very angry and insisted I left the premises. As all GP medical practices are private businesses I had no option but to leave. He rushed back, undoubtedly either thinking of saving all his at risk patients or maybe thinking of the £12.58 per person (later in Nov 2021 £15) jabbed the practice was receiving. Time is money, as they say. That may sound a harsh statement but to be clear GP medical practices are businesses run for profit.

A scheme, which ran from October 2014 to April 2015 and saw GPs being awarded at least £55 to diagnose someone with dementia, saw the number of dementia cases diagnosed jump from 336,445 to 400,700. When the scheme was cancelled the number of cases of dementia fell too. This scheme was pushed by the government who were, in my opinion, finding new customers for the products of their bosses in the corporate world. It was also reported that data for England showed the number of prescriptions for drugs to treat Alzheimer's disease increased from 502,003 in 2004 to three million in 2014. A new diagnosis means a new customer for big pharma and the sad truth is that the people with good intentions, going through medical school, eventually just become drug pushers for the drug companies and vaccine producers.

The CDC on their own website published a link to this under 'Reports of Deaths after COVID-19 Vaccination' (https://www.medrxiv.org/content/10.1101/2022.05.05.22274695v1)

'Reporting Rates for VAERS Death Reports Following COVID-19 Vaccination, December 14, 2020-November 17, 2021'
Setting 'United States; December 14, 2020, to November 17, 2021.'
Results '9,201 death events were reported for COVID-19 vaccine recipients aged five years and older (or age unknown)'.

The fact is many adverse reactions are taking place, some mild some severe. We have a huge rise in heart issues and thousands of deaths are being reported. The response is always the same in that they are only reports and that correlation does not equal causation. This is true but what is the point of having a reporting system if the information coming in is not seen as relevant? What is the point if there is no investigation? Where is the concern if it is acknowledged that only a small per cent of the actual reactions and deaths get reported? How is it possible to persist with the 'safe and effective' stance in the light of all these reports?

For me, this is all part of the game being played, hence I see no need to dig deeper into the damage being done by these vaccines. They are doing damage and that is well known. All the pushback from the mainstream media, medical doctors and

304

scientists and public is focusing attention on the vaccines not being safe and not the fact they are not effective at all against a viral attack, simply because there is no viral attack.

The more time you have spent 'awake' to the manipulation of humanity, the more you see the games within games. The focus of controlled opposition is fronted by Del Bigtree of 'The Highwire' and new hero of the people lawyer Robert Francis Kennedy (RFK). Both have been challenging vaccine safety for many years and there is actually nothing wrong with that. It is something to be respected. Del Bigtree did though, because of pressure from his audience, interview Dr Andrew Kaufman regarding viral isolation. Other heroes of the people, Joe Rogan and Russell Brand, during a recent conversation stated that David Icke is unreliable as he got it wrong over covid when he stated it was caused by 5g. Yes when David Icke first made a statement regarding covid, he did mention he felt it was caused by the radiation coming out of 5g. But within a few weeks he was interviewed on London Real when he explained he had come across the work of Dr Andrew Kaufman regarding virus isolation and he had changed his mind and gone with the new evidence. It was now clear to him that SARS-CoV-2 did not exist and in fact he had seen that the whole viral story was yet another lie. There is no way at all that Rogan and Brand with their money, connections and investigative team behind them would not have known that, especially three years down the line. In fact, Joe Rogan's good friend Patrick Bet David had the courage to interview David Icke and Dr Tom Cowan during 'the pandemic' who both made it clear viral pathogens do not exist; How would Rogan not know of this if they speak regularly? Both Rogan and Brand are still pushing the 'lab leak theory' which is part of the controlled opposition just to keep the idea of a viral attack alive.

The issue of viral isolation, or lack of it, is so clear that there is no excuse anymore, once you have seen the evidence, to pursue the idea of safe vaccines. The real issue is why we are vaccinating at all. The game being played is to keep people within the paradigm of germ/viral theory. As long as the conversation remains within these boundaries then no real positive change can come about. It is the same with the monetary system, climate and the political system in that all arguments are kept within the boundaries of the madness and the manipulators are happy with this. They are literally laughing at us.

Keep believing in germ/viral theory and the need to be protected
Keep believing that when ill the body has gone wrong and needs fixing
Keep believing in the value of currency and the need for it to create wealth
Keep believing in the illusion of owning the land we live on and being able to buy as much as you can with the controlled currency
Keep believing in man-made climate change and the need to fix it
Keep believing politics and all its man-made laws as being real and having to obey them
Keep believing in the idea of an external human authority or a human made organisation having authority over your life
Keep believing in anything except the objective reality of Nature itself and its real laws

Remember those three important questions

- What is it?
- Where does it come from?
- How does it function?

Start asking these questions and you will start to see different realities from the ones you are being presented with and the matrix of control will start to crumble before your very eyes.

Saying that, when a medical intervention imposed upon a population is causing damage, we do need people within the medical profession to speak out. One doctor did speak out though, and it was a man in my own local town of Penzance, Cornwall. A man simply concerned for the health of his patients, something he was contracted and obligated to be concerned about. He was about to get the shock of his life and see his own profession in a totally different light.

Going back to *'duties of a doctor'* here are some relevant reminders.
• *Make the care of your patient your first concern.*
• *Protect and promote the health of patients and the public.*
• *Work with colleagues in the ways that best serve patients' interests.*

Dr David Cartland is, was, a GP in my local town of Penzance. After at first going along with the story of the pandemic, he was not a 'Covid denier', and after taking the first two vaccines Dr Cartland started seeing data and having experiences suggesting the vaccines were causing harm. On Feb 1 2022 Dr Cartland publicly resigned putting a copy of his resignation letter on social media. He then went on to publish an article 'Breaking the Silence About Covid' and has since been a fearless and outspoken speaker of what he believes is a vaccine that is harming and even killing an unknown number of people Here is an extract from his resignation letter.

"It is with regret that I wish to resign from the surgery in my role as GP and from the NHS completely"
"I can leave holding my head held high knowing that I have attempted in so many ways and occasions to raise my concerns about vaccine efficacy, requirement and safety particularly regarding children and healthy adults and many examples of the vaccine causing potential harm to patients."
"I have been astounded by the lack of engagement by colleagues to such concerns and observations and feel as if I have been completely ignored as a concerned professional with valid credentials and experience." –Dr David Cartland

On Feb 9 2020 Dr Cartland posted this quote on social media

"And that right there is why no one speaks out – the veiled threats. Must say though, looking forward to seeing all the safety data presented to me at the GMC to explain away my 'propaganda'. All that defending of ethics too!! And valid consent!! I fear they will throw away the key."

This quote was regarding an article where the Medical Protection Society (MPS) stated

"GPs have been warned that criticising the Covid vaccine or other pandemic measures via social media could leave them 'vulnerable' to GMC investigation"

Here is an extract from, 'Breaking the Silence About Covid'
https://expose-news.com/2022/02/11/breaking-the-silence-about-covid/

"I became a doctor to help my patients, to be their advocate, to help them in their biology, psychology and social circumstances … I will always remember exactly the moment of my graduation when we recited the Hippocratic oath. Part of this powerful oath is a vow. A vow to 'Primum non nocere' - first do no harm … To not recognise, notify or publicise concerns of harm would be contrary to mine and my colleague's oath taken at qualification. I am writing this as a commentary and as a personal reflective piece".

Dr Cartland has now set up his own GP consultation business and is starting on his own long journey of researching holistic and natural health. https://drcartland.com/

He continues to speak out and put forward scientific evidence to back up his stance. With well-known consistent excess deaths continuing in the West, mainly in highly Covid vaccinated countries, he is one of very few medical professionals who even dare to ask why. His latest public statement, 16/9/23, says it all

"The silence from my colleagues literally sickens me"

IT'S ALL A MIND GAME

'Mindspace – influencing behaviour through public policy'
– extracts from the document:
https://www.instituteforgovernment.org.uk/sites/default/files/publications/
MINDSPACE.pdf

> *"Influencing people's behaviour is nothing new to Government, which has often used tools such as legislation, regulation or taxation to achieve desired policy outcomes. But many of the biggest policy challenges we are now facing – such as the increase in people with chronic health conditions – will only be resolved if we are successful in persuading people to change their behaviour, their lifestyles or their existing habits. Fortunately, over the last decade, our understanding of influences on behaviour has increased significantly and this points the way to new approaches and new solutions."*

Why 'social distancing' and not 'physical distancing'?

> *"Influencing behaviour is central to public policy. Recently, there have been major advances in understanding the influences on our behaviours, and government needs to take notice of them. This report aims to make that happen."*

> *"The vast majority of public policy aims to change or shape our behaviour. And policy-makers have many ways of doing so. Most obviously, they can use "hard "instruments such as legislation and regulation to compel us to act in certain ways. These approaches are often very effective, but are costly and inappropriate in many instances. So government often turns to less coercive, and sometimes very effective, measures, such as incentives (e.g. excise duty) and information provision (e.g. public health guidance) – as well as sophisticated communications techniques."*

I recommend for everyone to watch on YouTube 'The Century of the Self' by Adam Curtis. In it he shows how for over a century – actually a lot, lot longer – western governments, again really all governments, have been using their knowledge of psychology to control and guide public behaviour. Edward Bernays, nephew of Sigmund Freud, invented the public relations profession in the 1920s and was the first person to take Freud's ideas to manipulate the masses. He showed American corporations how they could make people want things they didn't need by systematically linking mass-produced goods to their unconscious desires. A very simplified understanding is that many people are driven by their fears and their desires. Ultimately our greatest desire is to freely express ourselves.

So given this knowledge and given that behaviour change is openly being used by the British politicians and the organisations and institutions that are running society, we really need to start to look at what the government want us to think and how they want us to behave. They don't even hide the fact.

A look into the 'MINDSPACE' document should be followed by the 'Behavioural Insights Team' also known as the 'nudge unit'.

On the GOV website it states: *"Behavioural Insights Team is now independent of the UK government"*, meaning it was part of the UK government before.

So, a look to the new website: https://www.bi.team/

> *"We apply behavioural insights to inform policy, improve public services and deliver positive results for people and communities."*

Remember earlier we showed that Dr Halpern is chief executive of the government-owned Behavioural Insights Team, known as the 'nudge unit', and a member of Whitehall's Scientific Advisory Group for Emergencies (Sage) and also co-authored a government document titled 'MINDSPACE'. It is the SAGE team who it seems are running the show and giving the government the 'best available science' which in turn is making the policies which are taking our freedoms away, destroying our economy and destroying our lives. So it is very clear that the government is using psychological techniques on the public. Why?

As we will see next, at the foundation of behaviour is belief. If you can control the beliefs of the population you then control their perceptions, and in turn their behaviour.

Do you remember earlier the words of Boris Johnson after the ridiculous prediction of Neil Ferguson?

> *"This is the worst Public health crisis in a generation" … "and I must level with you and the British public, more families, many more families, are going to lose loved ones before their time."*

> – Boris Johnson, 12th March 2020.

This is what started the biggest psychological experiment the UK has ever seen, but it was just a part of a bigger global experiment; only this experiment wasn't about testing theories, it was about putting them into practice.

'Options for increasing adherence to social distancing measures 22nd March 2020' was prepared for the Scientific Advisory Group for Emergencies (SAGE). The paper was discussed at SAGE meeting 18 on 23rd March 2020. Extracts from document: https://assets.publishing.service.gov.uk/government/uploads/system/uplo ads/attachment_data/file/882722/25-options-for-increasing-adherence-to-social-distancing-measures-22032020.pdf

> *"Perceived threat: A substantial number of people still do not feel sufficiently personally threatened; it could be that they are reassured by the low death rate in their demographic group(8), although levels of concern may be rising(9). Having a good understanding of the risk has been found to be positively associated with adoption of COVID-19 social distancing measures in Hong Kong (10). The perceived level of personal threat needs to be increased among those who are complacent, using hard-hitting emotional messaging. To be*

effective this must also empower people by making clear the actions they can take to reduce the threat)."

"Use media to increase sense of personal threat."

"There are nine broad ways of achieving behaviour change: Education, Persuasion, Incentivisation, Coercion, Enablement, Training, Restriction, Environmental restructuring, and Modelling."

Whatever your opinion is on the illness or why people are dying, it is very clear that the government is manipulating people's perceptions to control behaviour; notice they even used the phrase *'Perceived threat'*. My own local MP had no idea this was going on. Yes, it seems that MPs do not know about the use of psychological techniques being used on the British population by members of the cabinet office to instil fear and control our beliefs so they can make it easier for their policies to be accepted, policies that, again, are destroying the country and people's lives.

In 2017 the WHO published a document: **'Best practice guidance // How to respond to vocal vaccine deniers in public.'**

"This guidance document provides basic broad principles for a spokesperson of any health authority on how to respond to vocal vaccine deniers. The suggestions are based on psychological research on persuasion, on research in public health, communication studies and on WHO risk communication guidelines."

"Prepare three key messages. A person's working memory is responsible for storing visual and vocal in-formation and is strongly restricted in capacity. The audience will not be able to recall or even transfer the provided knowledge when confronted with too much information. Prepare three key messages you really want the public to know and remember."

"Repeat your key messages as often as reasonably possible."

So the message is clear: they see the general public as stupid and childlike. so keep it simple with no more than three messages.

Stay alert – control the virus – save lives.

Hands – face – space.

Or as some members of the public commented.

We're lying – You know we're lying – We know you know we're lying

The War on Information and Truth

"Every record has been destroyed or falsified, every book rewritten, every picture has been repainted, every statue and street building has been renamed, every date has been altered. And the process is continuing day by day and minute by minute. History has stopped. Nothing exists except an endless present in which the Party is always right."
– George Orwell, 1984

People who believe the myths spread by anti-vaccine campaigners "are absolutely wrong", England's top doctor has said. Prof Dame Sally Davies said the MMR vaccine was safe and had been given to millions of children worldwide but uptake was currently "not good enough". In England, 87% of children receive two doses but the target is 95%. The chief medical officer urged parents to get their children vaccinated and ignore *"social media fake news"*.

"A number of people, stars, believe these myths – they are wrong," she said. *"Over these 30 years, we have vaccinated millions of children. It is a safe vaccination – we know that – and we've saved millions of lives across the world. People who spread these myths, when children die they will not be there to pick up the pieces or the blame."*

It is interesting that the UK has never achieved full measles 'herd immunity'; 95% for at least the first two vaccines, but we haven't had the mass deaths they say would have. They still push the fear but don't seem to be able to stop and question their own science.

Headlines like:

"Facebook fake news 'war room' should target anti-vaxxers..." – The Telegraph

"Half of new parents shown anti-vaccine misinformation on social media..." – The Guardian

"MPs to investigate resurgence of anti-vaccine movement..." – ITV news online

"Posting anti-vaccine propaganda on social media could become a criminal offence, Law Commissioner says..." – The Telegraph

We have social media fact checkers warning us about posts and Facebook's own checkers blocking posts and YouTube removing people's channels for challenging vaccination and the current narrative on the corona pandemic. Add to this the 77th brigade with its thousands of people working behind the scenes, and as the graphs have shown, it is clear the medical professionals themselves are being misinformed, then we really are in the middle of a war, a war of truth.

A good example is the Wales alleged measles outbreak of 2013:

"For the entire period 1 January to March 31, 2013 there were just 26 laboratory confirmed cases out of 446 notifications: 10 in January, 8 in February."

"And in March just eight cases out of 302 notifications. That is a percentage rate of over-diagnosis and over-notification of 3774 %. Or put it another way 0.027 of notified cases were actually measles – and it is medical professionals who do the diagnosing and notifying. Kind of knocks your faith in the ability of doctors to diagnose a basic childhood illness. And we must

not forget the poor man who died – but no one knows what he died of and three doctors did not diagnose it as measles."

But if you were around at the time of the 'outbreak' you will remember the media pushing out the fear propaganda, especially after the one death; though again, similar to today, it was a death 'with' and not 'of' and all that with an irrelevant test. The media as usual push out the initial fear, but when things calm down and the real figures come out they never go back and set things straight so the public are left with the memory of events like 'the great measles outbreak of Wales 2013' that never really happened in their minds, the fear goes on and the control gets tighter.

Many whistle blowers, doctors, scientists and researchers who are putting their opinions out there for the public are now being censored or even banned from platforms like YouTube and Facebook. You will never see them on the BBC unless the BBC are doing a hatchet job on them to discredit all they say. But truth has to come out, and it will, as hard as they try; the more they censor, the more people question why. I'm not saying who is right or wrong. I have my opinion, yes, but what we need is a full, open debate for all the public to see. After any coup, control of information is the first thing that is done. Have we witnessed the *'corona coup'*?

Weaponising the Weather Forecast

Many of you may have noticed now that every windy day is now classified as having 'strong gusts', every strong wind is a 'gale' and every storm now here in the UK now even seems to have a name. Storms are a normal part of weather in the British Isles; in fact we are famous for changeable, windy wet weather. Every hot day or two now in summer is 'a heat wave' and a week or so without rain is 'a drought'. We don't simply seem to just have weather anymore; it's always the hottest day since this, the coldest day since that, the wettest since this or the driest since that. Weather maps are also showing up dark red for heat which would have justified light red years back. This total psychological attack is to try and convince the sub-conscious minds of the population that we are in times of extreme weather. But one thing many may not notice is how the weather can also be used to push political messages.

On Feb 22 2018 the UK was hit with a storm that was being called by all the mainstream news hour after hour 'The Beast from the East'. As soon as I heard this and that it was being repeated at every news hour I knew something was up. Cold winter storms are normal here and cold winds coming over from Russia are not unusual. I knew that soon something was about to happen and Russia would get the blame, I just did not know what.

In March 2018, Sergei Skripal, a British citizen who used to work as a Russian intelligence officer, and his daughter, Yulia, nearly died after coming into contact with Novichok, a military-grade nerve agent originally developed by the former Soviet Union. Straight away, and without evidence, the UK Government knew who it was and it was no surprise to me that they named Russian President Vladimir Putin. Yes it all became clear; Putin was 'The Beast from the East'. And this storm had paved the way in the minds of the British people to accept Russia, and particularly Putin, as the new enemy number one and crazy tyrant who was a threat not only to the British people, but to the whole world.

You may think that something so simple as a weather forecast could not so profoundly affect the thinking of a nation, but it clearly can. The people high up in government running the show use all the psychological techniques they know of to get us to think 'the right way' before they set off on a new of part of their agenda of control.

If you want to know what the weather is doing from now on, better just wake up and look out of the window.

Lab Leak 'conspiracy'

From day one, in fact as soon as I heard any news coming from China regarding a 'new novel virus', and publicly on Feb 6 2020 on the interview attached on the first page I stated " the only thing going round the world is fear and hysteria". People need to understand that the people who manipulate humanity are the best psychologists in the world. They know that to control behaviour you need to control perception.

There are a great number of 'conspiracy theorists' in the world who are in fact, whether knowingly or not, aiding the controlling elite. When you have serious researchers looking for objective truth, or as near as possible to objective truth, and they are getting too close to that real truth then putting out crazy 'conspiracy theories' is a great way to either ridicule serious researchers, put people off the track or both.

The 'Wuhan lab leak' is one of those controlled conspiracy theories put out there to put people off the scent of the fact that there is no virus at all, natural or man-made. Newcomers to this arena will have their lack of trust in politicians and knowledge that **there is** a global conspiracy to control humanity manipulated to come to the conclusion that there was corruption and a conspiracy, but simply a controlled one 'they' are happy for you to believe in. 'They' simply want you to believe that viral pathogens actually exist so as to persist with their agenda of control via germ theory and contagious disease causing agents. The naive or not fully informed researchers will be happy they have found out 'the truth' and the manipulators are happy because in reality nothing changes and nothing will change. They don't even care if we find out the covid vaccine is causing damage because again nothing changes.

- We can still 'catch' disease off another human hence the social distancing protocols need to be kept and we need to live in fear of a virus, natural or man-made.

- We still need protection and even though the current vaccine is killing and maiming people we now just need a 'safe vaccine'.

The end product is the same whatever people believe. People need to understand that there are games within games. For me if I am unsure as to what is happening I just try and think and ask myself; where does this explanation lead us to and what is the solution it is leading us too? When you gain more experience you will start to see the real wheat from the chaff and the fake news from the real news.

It literally is all a mind game!

Welcome to the biggest psychological operation the world has ever seen. With them clearly wanting to affect our perceptions, and control our behaviour, we will now look into this very interesting subject.

PERCEPTION

The whole battle to control humanity is centered around controlling perception, as it is that perception that controls our behavior. For a more in-depth look into the human condition see 'A Conscious Humanity - Morality, Freedom and Natural Law' – Rob Ryder &Patrick Quanten. Here we will stick to a simple understanding of how and why we behave as we do.

Our minds, via information coming to the brain via the senses, are constantly processing reality in order to respond in an appropriate way. Life, in effect, is the response from your inner world to the incoming information of your outer world, the environment, reality. Everything too in the outer world is a 'thing' also in its own right and also responds to the information in its own outer world. There is only one reality, one energy field, and every 'thing' in it is part of the whole field. This exchange of information and the responses that go with it we call 'cause and effect'. Life essentially is movement and that movement we call behaviour. Without movement there is no life and no consciousness. Our consciousness allows us to be aware of movement so we can observe life. The outside world is what we call objective reality. It actually exists and contrary to the 'New Age Movement' it is not something we created due to our observation. Reality existed before we were born and will continue to exist after we are gone.

"The senses open up the conscious mind. It is the information picked through the senses that will make us aware of the environment, of the reality, but seen in a specific way and that is the way the brain, the nervous system, interprets the incoming information. The brain plays an important part in the conscious mind. It plays no part in the mind itself. The conscious mind works through the matter and is linked to the brain function; the mind is an energy field that just is. The conscious mind is intrinsically linked to an individual. The mind exists without a body." - Patrick Quanten

What we do create though is our own personal experience of reality. We call this our subjective experience, or as Rupert Sheldrake says we 'clothe reality' with our perceptions. Objective reality does control our behaviour to a large extent. Gravity for example means I will fall to the ground if I walk off the roof of a house. If I foolishly decide to walk across the M5 at rush hour chances are natural forces will leave me objectively splattered on the motorway. A huge part of our behaviour though is controlled by how we view objective reality. It's how we view reality that gives it meaning and that meaning will create an appropriate response. The response therefore is always in balance in regard to our perception of the incoming information.

So you have your individual self, a condensed energy field of unique information made up of all your perceptions and beliefs, some inherited and some taken on through experience. Nature and nurture. Information comes in from the outside world whether it is sight, sound, food, energies and more. For life to happen, movement, or behaviour, the information has to *mean* something to the individual so he/she can respond in the *correct* way and that meaning is based on the beliefs of that human. This belief does not have to be factual or even rational. It is just what you yourself believe to be true. Belief and therefore perception is a very individual thing.

A tarantula for example in objective reality is a large spider. What that spider means though to each individual will dictate their response when seeing a tarantula. If you have had bad experiences with a spider or maybe a childhood seeing family members scream at the sight of a spider then the tarantula may be given the meaning of fear. If though you were brought up around spiders and not had any bad experiences then the meaning maybe neutral. An arachnophile is a person who actually loves spiders so they may give the sight of a tarantula the meaning of curiosity or even affection.

Each given meaning will create a response in balance with that meaning. The meaning 'fear' could make a person jump and run away screaming. The meaning 'neutral' could create a simple glance and the person carries on as normal. The meaning 'curiosity' or 'affection' could create a response of a person moving fearlessly towards the spider and even picking it up. All these responses are in balance with how the individual perceives the spider. There is no right or wrong. The spider has a potential to be dangerous but also a potential to be picked up with no problem.

So knowing that people within and around the government have full knowledge of how this works and that for at least a century this knowledge has been used by governments and corporations to control behaviour and even sell products. The obvious question to ask is; How many of your beliefs have been put into your mind by government?

govern - control. ment comes from Latin, mind. Mind Control.

Worldwide politicians and global organisations are forever talking about 'change' and 'vision'.

What 'change' do they mean? What 'vision' do they have for the world and its people? And how will they get from where they are now to that vision? Why do public servants believe they have a right to change behaviour to fulfil their visions when they are here to serve us and not the other way around? I think this is a very dangerous and sinister game to be playing, especially as the vast majority of people have no idea that there is a game being played. It is impossible to live in a free country if all your perceptions are being manipulated to pursue the hidden agenda of criminal politicians.

Priming the mind for a future event is another tactic used.

Dancing nurses, anyone? Go to Vimeo – 'Predictive Programming ~ The 2012 Olympics from the UNITED KINGDOM'.

Jeremy Hunt oversaw the 2012 London event and as of 29th Jan 2020 became Chair of the Health and Social Care Select Committee. Strange coincidence!

St. Corona is also the patron saint of epidemics.

Throughout Feb and March 2020, after watching a programme on Netflix, the next recommended view offered automatically was a film *'Contagion'*, or it may have been *'Pandemic'*, one or the other. I have never watched programmes like these, I just watch comedies or documentaries, but for a few weeks it kept coming up for me to watch, nothing else.

I urge everyone to watch the video of the song *'Where Are Ü Now'* by Justin Bieber. A video aimed mainly at young children. In it, you will find many disturbing images of death, sex and drugs, even aliens and more. Images so fast that you cannot consciously see any of them but if you go slow enough or freeze frame them all will be revealed, even stating 'Bush did 9/11'. I personally don't think he has the brains to organise that one. But anyway, why would you put disturbing images in a video like that knowing young people would see it? Not all will be affected, I know, but as we know the subconscious mind controls most of our life it is very disturbing indeed.

So a lot of things we see may be there to expose stuff going on or maybe to prime our minds. *'The Hunger Games'* films, for example. Are we being warned or primed? George Orwell and Aldous Huxley. Were they whistle blowers or primers of our minds? I suppose it depends how you take the information on an individual level. I have found *'1984'* and *'Brave New World'* helpful for me to understand how we are being manipulated.

In many films you will see all aspects of an agenda, like in James Bond films, and in the Marvel series *'Captain America: the Winter Soldier'* is very revealing.

So we have this onslaught on our minds to control our behaviour. From birth we are actually the coming together of two *mind fields*, or minds with beliefs holding them together. We then develop in the mother's womb, feeding off her emotions and responses so we can have at least an idea of the world we are coming into. Then for the first 6/7 years we just absorb all the incoming information and also the responses of Mother at first and then the surrounding family. These first 6/7 years can then create a human being ready to start to live in the world he/she lives in, but it is only a perception of the world. It is not all the world and some of those perceptions will be valid and some not, but we will start to live our life through those beliefs that will create a perception of the world we live in.

This is the reason they want our children in school as soon as possible. Nothing to do with 'helping mothers back to work'. We have been fooled into believing that being a full-time mother is not a job in itself so the state can get into the minds of our children, hence control their future perceptions and behaviour. Pure 'Brave New World' social engineering massively helped by the far left and hijacked feminist movement who want to 'free' women. Notice it doesn't seem to be about being free to be women, but seems more about freeing women from the natural constraints of womanhood and even to compete with men.

So now we go through life and as we get older we may, if we are lucky, start to challenge our own beliefs and behaviour which in turn can cause turmoil, which is needed to break down false beliefs and open our minds to more possibilities. It seems the best way to do this is really to stop for a while; take a deep breath, and just stop believing in anything and take a look at your behaviour and reactions to life and situations and try to see honestly why you react and behave a certain way. Find out whether certain behaviour is beneficial or holding you back; be honest with your emotional connection to things and start to put back beliefs which you feel are worthy, truthful and beneficial to yourself as an individual.

An old way to do it would be to imagine a needle in a haystack. It would be very difficult to go looking for the needle. The best way would be to throw out what is not the needle, the hay, and eventually what is left must be the needle. If the needle is truth and the hay is the non-truths then it may be a good place to start to throw beliefs away that are false, holding you back, and see what you have left.

Whatever you do, always try be conscious of what you are doing and this way you do not have to be a victim of your subconscious behaviour and can start living a life in control by being conscious of how you feel and behave and why.

The 'Coronavirus Act' was implemented by people based on their perceptions of what was going on and what they were observing. We know perceptions are just that and not absolute truth; we also know we have a government keen on using techniques to control our perceptions and therefore control our behaviour. When this has been done, all amounts of horrors are possible by people *believing* they are doing right.

> "The receptivity of the masses is very limited, their intelligence is small, but their power of forgetting is enormous. In consequence of these facts, all effective propaganda must be limited to a very few points and must harp on these in slogans until the last member of the public understands what you want him to understand by your slogan."
>
> – Adolf Hitler

STAY SAFE – CONTROL THE VIRUS – SAVE LIVES – BIG BROTHER LOVES YOU

One Moment in Time

The following illustration is possibly the most important piece of information regarding the human condition. It shows how we co-create our human experience, This 'moment in time' could be billions of moments per second via the subconscious responses or a process lasting the duration of an event depending on how you look at it. We can have an impact on the reality around us, but we do not create the reality around us. I can cut down a tree and turn it into a table, and therefore create, some furniture, but I cannot create the tree itself. I can have an impact on reality by my own actions and I can also influence the human experience, society, by my behaviour. Please take time to process this graphic and see for yourself if there is any truth in it by observing your own life and the environment around you. Do not take my word as truth.

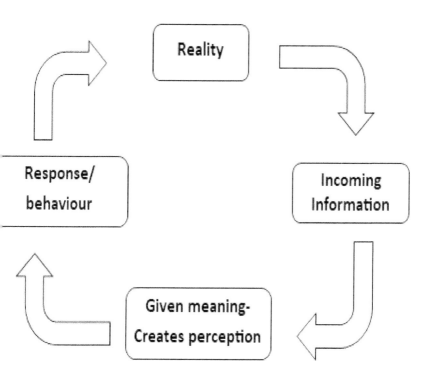

So again, we do not create our own reality, we create our own experience of reality. As our behaviour is actually part of reality then it could be said we are co-creating reality every second of the day. This is of real importance as people are trying to look for solutions to humanities problems. Again the New Age spiritual gurus seem to want to convince people that they, by the powers of their own minds, can manifest anything they desire. I simply do not see any evidence for this or see how that could even work. It goes on the basis that the whole universe exists only for me and is responding only to me. It is not possible for me to prove anything is real or conscious in this universe except my own existence and consciousness. But if I go down the path of the whole of reality is simply my reality then I feel the whole idea of even writing this book becomes pointless.

It certainly seems that other people are real and conscious and that we are sharing this human experience and the reality on this planet, in this universe. The collective human perception creates the collective human behaviour and therefore the collective human experience on this planet. It seems the people who control humanity on this planet understand how the collective experience and reality is created better than all of us. It is time we started to learn the game that's is playing us so we can be free to play the game ourselves.

Reality

The environment around us is what we call reality. It is everything in our field of perception and there is much more that exists outside of our field of perception. Life happens with movement and movement is behaviour. Therefore reality is not a fixed thing but a fluid thing in constant change. Change is the only constant. 'They' know they cannot control reality, the environment, totally. The planet is doing its own thing beyond the control of us mere humans. As we have stated we can have an impact on reality, we can change it and move it around a bit, but on the whole the planet is in control. Even man-made chemicals have come out of nature. Everything is nature and nature existed long before us and will continue long after us.

Incoming Information

What 'they' can control though is how we perceive reality by 'educating' us in what everything means. By taking control of all stages of education, science, government bodies, media and now social media they can feed us a version of reality that will create the behaviour they require to keep humanity enslaved and unaware of its own potential and natural rights. They can spin the incoming information to sell a version of reality that suits their agenda of control. Public relations is basically a sales technique. If you want to sell a worm cake you better put some strawberries and cream on top.

Creating Perception

When 'they' can control to a large extent how we receive the information from the environment then 'they' have great power in putting meaning onto that information for us therefore creating a perception of reality that suits them. For those of us who have a level of consciousness, and distrust of self-proclaimed authority, and have made up our own minds of what reality is and are conscious/aware of our own beliefs we are able to see reality closer to how it really is and therefore respond in a way beneficial for ourselves.

Behaviour

The people who have been sold the version of reality that suits the agenda of the global mafia will now behave in a way that keeps them under control and totally unaware they are slaves. The people who have figured out how this game of life works and have their own version of reality are now in a position to behave in a way that benefits themselves and not the global mafia. This obviously is a danger to the plans for control of all humanity. We now see illusionary rules and regulations made up to control behaviour and fines and punishments put in place for those who dare to think of doing it their own way. In the end, like all criminal gangs, the threat of violence will be used as a last resort. The threat of being kidnapped and pushed into a van and then a prison cell, or even worse, is always there waiting for those of us that chose not to comply. If the threat of government enforcement is not enough, then we also have people fearful of what others might think, the fear of being different, fearful of being our true selves. This is the prison we maintain ourselves with no threat from outside forces.

Reality

As we can see now the short process of 'one moment in time' culminates in the next 'moment in time', back into reality. It is a constant flowing process of life. This is how we co-create our human experience. Nature is doing its own thing and creating the objective reality we live in. We, still a part of nature, are doing our own thing and creating our individual and collective human experience within reality.

If we want to change the human experience it becomes clear we need to start evaluating reality differently and not taking the words of the media, governments and 'expert' scientists as truth. As it is a collective experience then it also becomes clear that to create a better, freer human experience more people need to become aware of how this works and then take the decision to manifest behaviour based on what is right and just, this we call morality. As researcher Mark Passio has clearly stated, the more immoral the people in a society behave the more slavery there will be in that society. The more moral people behave in a society the more freedom will manifest in that society. It's that simple.

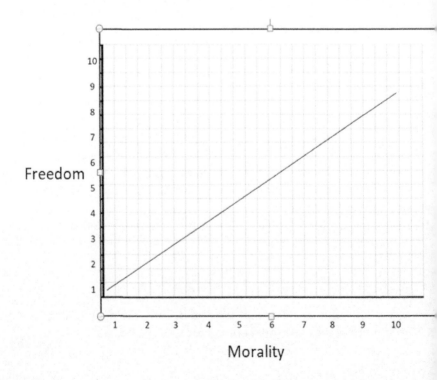

Government is simply the rebranding of the criminal gang to make their crimes 'legal'. It should be obvious by now that governments around the world represent global elite agendas and not the people. It should be obvious that we are here to serve the system and the system is not here to swerve us. The biggest spin of all on reality that controls humanity is the belief in the political system and all the rules and laws that go with it. If you imagine two maps of the world side by side with one a geographical map and the other a political map. The geographical map is where we live and the laws of nature control life. The global mafia have spun the information of reality to make us believe we live in the political map when all it is in reality is a figment of our imagination. The education system and the constant political news on 24/7 is there to reinforce the perception that this political world is real when in fact the only thing that is ever real is nature itself. The world of the political map only becomes *real* when we believe it's real. It's a simple scam, but one that has massive effects in the real world.

If humanity can become aware of the global scam to enslave them by controlling behaviour via controlling perception then that is only half of the battle. We don't all have to agree what reality is, but we need to agree to disagree and allow each other to live in a way that is in balance for that individual without imposing our perceptions on each other. Basically 'live and let live'. Just because we cannot all be friends does not mean we have to be enemies. When the awareness of how we are being manipulated can be seen then it is simply a task of starting to see reality as objectively as possible. When it has been revealed to the audience how the magician did the trick it loses its power and does not work anymore.

SUFFER LITLE CHILDREN

Dr Bruce Lipton when talking about the Romanian orphan children mentioned how many of them turned out autistic. He talked about how they were well nourished physically but were completely malnourished in terms of love, affection and physical touch. Remember we spoke earlier about how a child develops through experience and perceptions based on beliefs. It doesn't take much working out to see the effect on development when there is little physical love or touch.

Humans are social beings and we are meant to hug our kids and each other; it is part of our physical, emotional and social development. The governing bodies of this world have mandated behaviour through a belief of a disease that makes human beings enemies of each other, a baby an enemy to its mother or a mother a danger to her baby.

We have mass autism in the world, behaviour defined by lack of social and communication skills and repetitive behaviours. I know of the history of Dr Wakefield and how he was attacked for giving his own scientific opinion, one that wasn't wanted; whether there was truth in it or not didn't matter. The gut biome and cognitive connection though is well known to science yet he mentioned the V word and he was done for. I do though, know of non-vaccinated autistic children and when we look at the work of Patrick Quanten on the 'formation of a human being', the issues involved become very clear.

Patrick's work takes us through the whole development of a human being from conception to adulthood and it becomes very clear that from conception, even at conception, the perceptions and therefore behaviours of the child are being formed. If a mother and father conceive and have a belief that the world is a very harsh and unforgiving place then that is the information that will form the child. If then throughout pregnancy the mother still sees the world as this terrible place then for the child that is the world he/she is coming into.

In the early years of a child's life the importance of feeling safe is maybe top of the list and the importance of a close physical relationship with close family with freely given and accepted hugs and physical play is also needed to create security and also close bonds. Tickle games are what kids seem to thrive on. If for some reason a child has had a bad start to life physically and emotionally then it is important to help them realise that healthy loving affection is natural thing. Helping bring about a strong trusting bond between child and parents is essential.

Theraplay

Developed in the USA in the 1980s by Phyllis Booth, a scientist, it has become increasingly recognised as highly beneficial in supporting attachment difficulties with parents and children.

The Theraplay Institute

"Theraplay is a dyadic child and family therapy that has been recognized by the Association of Play Therapy as one of seven seminal psychotherapies for children. Developed over 50 years ago, and practiced around the world, Theraplay was developed for any professional working to support healthy child/caregiver attachment. Strong attachment between the child and the important adults in their life has long been believed to be the basis of lifelong good mental health as well as the mainstay of resilience in the face of adversity. Modern brain research and the field of neuroscience have shown that attachment is the way in which children come to understand, trust and thrive in their world."

Core Concepts

"Theraplay uses practitioner guidance to create playful and caring child-adult interactions that foster joyful shared experiences. These activities build attunement and understanding of each other – replicating early relationship experiences that are proven to lead to secure attachment. The interactions are personal, physical and fun – a natural way

for everyone to experience the healing power of being together."

"With the support of the Theraplay practitioner, parents learn to play with their child in a way that establishes felt safety, increases social engagement, expands arousal regulation, and supports the development of positive self-esteem for both the child and the parent."

"Theraplay is useful for a wide variety of children, including those who are withdrawn, depressed, over active, aggressive, have phobias or fine difficulty in socialising. Children with learning disabilities and developmental delays also benefit hugely from theraplay."

– Louise Shuttleworth, Psychotherapist, Clinical Partners UK

The mass behavioural problems with children are now no secret; social anxiety is now the 'new normal'. Many teachers in schools are finding it hard to cope with all the non-academic issues they have to deal with. So knowing all that, why on earth would you completely shut off children from all their social activities? Schools closed, kids' clubs closed, whole families self-isolating in fear. Kids are being told to go completely against their natural instincts which are to physically play and chase and grab each other. I was working near a school when I saw about four young children in the school grounds playing in the bushes; they were about seven years old and having fun like kids do. I thought to myself, after such a long time since seeing this, '*At, last kids playing normally*'. Within about four minutes I heard a woman teacher's voice come over to them and shout, *"Keep away from each other and get out of there."*

It has been said that kids are more likely to die from lightning than from the non-existent 'COVID'. What on earth are we doing to our children's present and future mental health? A child with no issues will certainly struggle with this but imagine a child who already has many difficulties in life; maybe school is the place where he/she can actually be free from stress for a while. What are the long-term consequences of people throwing their irrational fears onto children going to be?

The same reasoning can be given to adults with issues that were previously being dealt with through social meetings or therapies. Let's be clear, the consequences for mental health are going to be devastating and it is total nonsense to suggest that the people behind the lockdown would not know this. It will be interesting to see what the suicide rate for adults with mental health issues who were being locked down and socially isolated will be.

Imagine being created to come into a world like that. Would you want to enter? Having no choice but to enter, would you want to pop out and enter the world with joy and excitement? Or do you think you may have already decided that this world is not for you and maybe your behaviours will reflect that in a way that we would call 'autistic'?

Imagine for a minute the world children are being born and raised in now. What is their family environment like? What is the 'new normal' at school like? What is their perception of the world? Is it a friendly place for adventure or a deadly place we need to survive?

This is complete madness!

When the lockdown measures started to get into schools it was clear this was going to have a massive impact on the mental health of young children. It was in effect a wicked and planned psychological attack on vulnerable children in full knowledge of the temporary and permanent damage it would do. At one point we even had military vehicles going to schools with men in military uniforms all set up for war. When people realise that it was all based on a scam then it will give you some insight of the minds of the people we allow to run our lives.

You would think that parents and professionals around the country would draw a line when it came to the children but sadly, and again not unexpectedly, the children were left as helpless victims to state controlled psychological tyranny.

One lady did speak out though, and again it was from my own local area of west Cornwall. Someone who put her professional role and role as a mother before government tyrannical guidelines and said what needed to be said despite little or no professional back-up.

Sarah Waters is a psychotherapist experienced in working with the effects of abuse, neglect, and childhood trauma. She also specialises in the family therapy and parenting model, Dyadic Developmental Practice (DDP). Sarah is a member of HART (Health Advisory Recovery Team) which is a group of highly qualified UK doctors, scientists, economists, psychologists, and other academic experts who came together over shared concerns about policy and guidance recommendations relating to the COVID-19 pandemic. She is also a member of Therapists For Medical Freedom who are a collective of counsellors, psychotherapists, psychologists and associated therapeutic professionals deeply concerned about the growing use of medical coercion and the loss of civil liberties as part of the international response to managing the COVID-19 pandemic.

Here is the major part of an article Sarah wrote published on the HART website during the madness.
www.hartgroup.org

'Can a Trauma Informed Approach and adherence to COVID-19 guidelines ethically co-exist?'- October 11 2021

An investigation into policies and their traumatic impact on children

Can any therapist, practitioner or organisation that calls itself trauma informed ethically do so if it is adhering to Covid-19 guidelines?

- *Half of 16–25-year-olds said their mental health has worsened since the start of the pandemic.*

- *As many as 10 million people, including 1.5 million children, are thought to need new or additional mental health support.*

- *There has been a 20% increase in babies suffering non-accidental harm.*

- *Two-thirds of domestic abuse victims were subjected to more violence from their partners during lockdown.*

- *There has been a 25% reduction in pre-pandemic learning for primary school children and a 30% reduction for secondary school children.*

What is Trauma Informed Practice?

Trauma informed practice has been a popular concept over the last 10 years, particularly within schools, councils, charities and even police forces. Trainings of between a few hours or a few weeks have been provided, after which trainees have considered themselves trauma informed. While it is acknowledged that some of these practitioners will have undertaken more rigorous and in-depth trauma/child development training, many will have not. Despite the claims by the plethora of trauma training organisations that children and young people's wellbeing, mental health and social/emotional needs are top priority, in a Covid world of unchallenged restrictions can they still claim this to be true?

To put things more into context, a programme, organisation, or system that is trauma informed, as defined by the US Government (also used as the benchmark in the UK):

- *realises the widespread impact of trauma and understands potential paths for recovery*

- *recognises the signs and symptoms of trauma in clients, family, staff, and others involved in the system*

- *responds by fully integrating knowledge about trauma into policies, procedures, and practices*

- *seeks to actively resist re-traumatisation*

Rather than following a prescribed set of policies and procedures, a trauma-informed approach adheres to five key principles:

- *Safety*
- *Trustworthiness*
- *Collaboration*
- *Empowerment*
- *Choice*

The struggle to prioritise children's emotional needs

It was only at the beginning of this century that neuroscientists were able to visibly identify (through fMRI scans) the devastating effects of trauma on children's brains. And only then was it acknowledged by governments who, rather than support families to try to mitigate it happening by investing in early intervention, ploughed their resources into trying to deal with its devastating effects. This strategy however has huge financial and emotional implications, outlined most recently and extensively by the Royal Foundation Centre for Early Childhood set up by The Duchess of Cambridge. The devastating consequences, such as an increased risk of long-term mental health difficulties and the intergenerational repetition of abuse, has already been proven, but persistently ignored, or dabbled in then discarded, such as the Sure Start Initiative launched in 1998. Today Sure Start has dwindled to a shadow of its former self, a reminder of the lack of foresight/care that politicians and councils have around the importance of supporting parents at the most critical point in a child's development – pregnancy and the first 2 years of life.

Numerous psychologists since the 1950's, most notably John Bowlby, have campaigned diligently to reform antiquated and abusive child rearing attitudes and practices, particularly focusing on the very early years in a child's life. Experiences of loss, fear, control, abuse and neglect, often caused by what are now termed 'Adverse Childhood Experiences (ACE's) have been scientifically and irrefutably proven to inhibit the development of children's brains and to negatively affect their emotions, behaviour, relationships and life chances. It is now widely accepted amongst psychologists and psychotherapists that, if children and young people are to thrive, these harmful factors need to be avoided at all costs.

It is also widely accepted that if this has not been possible, these harmful factors need to be fully understood and mitigated in a trauma informed way as children get older. Considering this, those of us in these professions (and others), have felt a huge relief over the last 10 years that children were finally starting to be treated humanely at last. The grim, genetic-deterministic view of human relations seemed to be fading into the past. The greatest contribution that Bowlby and all that have followed him have made to the wellbeing of our culture is the understanding that children are extremely vulnerable but must be resilient to survive. Most importantly, we have learnt that this resilience, in its most damaging form, means adapting in various ways to a hostile environment to ensure this survival.

For the first time in history, the idea that a society's destiny rests upon how it treats its children had scientific foundations and was being acted upon and promoted – at least in schools and other trauma informed organisations. Children's needs were at last being put first and professionals (but unfortunately to a lesser extent parents) were trained to understand, recognise, and promote these needs as, after all, how we treat our children will shape our future. A trauma informed army was born championing the necessity for safety, love, acceptance, connection, close relationships, play, empathy and most importantly – the absence of fear.

337

Then along came Covid 19

And with it a catalogue of guidelines (not laws), taken up at great speed, without any psychological risk assessments whatsoever. All trauma informed knowledge and practice was abandoned as adults, some fuelled by unions, demanded that they were kept 'safe' – despite what this might mean emotionally for the children and young people in their care. A disease that has a median Infection Fatality Rate of 0.05% for under 70-year-olds globally seemed to derail trauma informed practice entirely. There was no mention of how emotionally damaging the measures potentially would be, at all, in the back-to-school trainings (that I attended) provided by numerous child development/trauma 'experts' across the UK. What happened to the trauma informed principles of realising, recognising, responding to, and most importantly resisting trauma inducing practices?

It does not seem to matter that babies, children and young people are having to bear the emotional brunt of a pandemic that mainly affects the over 80's. In fact, it even feels as if some schools relish in masking and segregating their pupils, acting as if the guidelines were in fact law and that they have no choice in the matter. No one can deny that the mental health of the young has been catastrophically impacted over the last year and the question I would like to ask is how can children's emotional needs so easily be set to one side like this? My understanding is that adults are meant to protect children and not the other way around. Why aren't trauma informed practitioners and organisations recognising this devastation and standing up for the children in their care? It is astonishing and heart breaking that children's emotional needs have been so quickly trampled upon and disregarded after the long-fought journey to get these needs recognised.

From new-born babies to teenagers – all are potentially being made to emotionally suffer in their own way. One of the most pernicious and potentially damaging practices that I can see *is the routine wearing of face masks around the very young. Anyone who has done any trauma informed training will know of the Still Face Experiment. It shows the devastating effects, in a very short time, on a baby whose mother stops smiling at it for only a few minutes. A recent discussion paper in The Journal of Neonatal Nursing highlights the difficulty in determining what facial expression a person is exhibiting behind a mask which may present severe challenges for infants and young children. They depend on their parents' facial expressions, coupled with tone and/or voice to regulate their reactions toward others. They advise that health professionals should understand the potential effects of prolonged mask wearing to minimise any potential long-term impact on neonatal development and optimise psychological outcomes for babies, infants, children, and their parents. I have not seen one piece of literature that warns of the dangers of this distressing practice. Everywhere I go, every day I go out, I see evidence that this message is not being passed onto parents by those that are trained to know better.*

Bliss, a charity for babies born premature or sick, have stated that 70% of parents have said they are more likely to have found it difficult to bond with their baby if the neonatal unit where their infant was being cared for had put time limits in place, as part of Covid parent access restrictions . Equally I have heard distressing stories of women being made to wear masks when in labour. Many of us know of the devastating restrictions that were put in place around partners and family being allowed to be with women when they were giving birth, often leaving them vulnerable and distressed. This will have a knock-on effect to the birth and bonding process, which can have lifelong affects. These same women have been denied face to face support after the birth, leading to an increase in Post Natal depression and loneliness. All for a disease that, as of March 2021, sits at no 24 in the UK as the leading cause of death.

Enough has been written in other studies about the numerous detrimental effects, both emotionally and developmentally, on school children over the past year particularly around the wearing of face masks and social distancing. The trauma informed might find it interesting revisiting Steven Porges Polyvagal Theory A subconscious system for detecting threats and safety and what he terms neuroception; a subconscious system for detecting threats and safety. No wonder there is an explosion of psychiatric disturbances, learning difficulties and dysregulated behaviour in children whose nervous systems have been activated by the fear messaging they have been subjected to in schools (and almost every other environment) every day for over a year. And what is the governments answer to this trauma reaction, again with little protest from the trauma informed professionals? Behaviour Hubs – as "parents and teachers know that orderly and disciplined classrooms are best".

Being exempt from facemask use brought its own traumas with it – it is excruciating for a young person or teenager to stand out at school and be different to everyone else. I have heard numerous stories of coercive and bullying behaviour, from teachers and other pupils, against the very few with the strength to stand up for their human rights and not wear a facemask or be invasively tested every week. The list of indignities goes on and on – with the lateral flow/PCR testing pantomime throwing up enormous efficacy, safety, and ethical considerations. Children's and young people's lives and education are being continuously disrupted by a flawed system that seems to fish for positives amongst this age group and cause misery and loss of income for the adults in their lives. The indignity of being tested and the potential dangers from the ethylene oxide used to sterilise the tests again are ignored or deemed worth the risk so that adults can feel safe and damn the effects on the children.

Conclusion

Considering the authorities and organisations that have implemented the Government's suggested Covid-19 guidelines and medical interventions for young people impulsively, without risk assessment, reflection, or critical analysis; I wonder if trauma informed practitioners and organisations are denying their experimental nature alongside the potentially long term, harmful, physical, and psychological effects. The long awaited and so warmly welcomed trauma informed world, that championed children and young people's emotional needs, is now, in my opinion, supporting them, in collusion with the government. They are supporting them to adapt to a hostile, fearful, abusive, and hence traumatic environment that inhibits the long awaited healthy emotional development that we have all be waiting for.

- Sarah Waters

I think I will leave this chapter here as it is, enough said.

FOLLOW THE MONEY

"And Jesus went into the temple of God, and cast out all them that sold and bought in the temple, and overthrew the tables of the money changers, and the seats of them that sold doves, And said unto them, It is written, My house shall be called the house of prayer; but ye have made it a den of thieves."

In the book *'Debt Slavery - The Economics of a Banking Mafia'* Rob Ryder, I go into great detail how the economic and monetary system works that is in pave around the world. It is a system deliberately set up to enslave us into an unpayable debt. Here I will give you in its simplest from.

Economy - Management of available resources in terms of the production and consumption of goods and services
Money - Something generally accepted as a medium of exchange, a measure of value, or a means of payment.
Currency - Currency is a medium of exchange for goods and services, money, in the form of paper or coins. In modern times we have numbers on a computer screen, electric currency, that represent the currency and function as money.

The first thing to understand is that all resources on this planet are free and given to us by nature. The energy we have has been given to us also by nature and our imagination to create is maybe our greatest gift. We could choose to use the resources and make all the exchanges we desire without putting any value on it at all, this we would call a 'gift economy'.

During the history of humanity someone decided to place an imaginary value of an item and therefore want something of equal value in exchange, this we call bartering. All things we give a value to and use for exchanges can be considered money whether it be oil, grain, tools and more, in fact anything we give a value to can be called money.

Currency is money in paper form or coins and now digital numbers on a screen. They are supposed to represent the value of productive energy. For example one unit of productive energy should have the equivalent unit of currency representing it so it can be used for exchanges when bartering is not possible. It is, or at least should be, a token representing a unit of productive energy. So if a society produced 100 000 units of productive energy then it would need £100 000 to represent it in the economy. In this way the currency comes into production to support the economy so that exchanges can be made. This currency can all be created for free by the people for the people. This though is not how it works.

Over 97% of currency comes into existence when banks extent credit to customers. Banks do not lend currency, they create it. It is your 'promise to pay' back the credit that brings it into existence. We are actually creating our own credit. It represents our future earnings. So if someone wanted £100 000 to buy a house, a mortgage, they would sign a document promising to pay back £100 000 over, let's say, 20 years. The bank then credits their bank account with £100 000 and also create a separate account with the equivalent debt, currency to be paid back. This is all good and well as £100 000 is created and £100 000 of your future earnings will pay it back and cancel the debt out.

The problem is the bank need to make a profit for providing this service and so charge you interest. This is a sum that can change on a monthly basis depending on the interest rate which is controlled by the central bank. The point is the initial credit of £100 000, new currency, was created. The extra payment or interest, let's say it adds up to £40 00, was never created. This means that there is a debt of £140 000 but only £100 000 in existence to pay it back. As we stated, over 97% of currency comes into existence this way and is totally controlled by the banking system with the central banks, investment banks and high street banks all working together to enslave humanity into unpayable debt. We also have the IMF and World Bank doing it on an international scale. The whole scam is about asset stripping people and nations to 'own the world'.

The high street banks create the money/debt to get people and businesses trapped into an unpayable debt. The central banks control interest rates, have the power to create physical currency as they see fit, and get nations into debt by facilitating loans. When people, companies and nations cannot pay the debt the investment banks come in and buy it all up and therefore get to 'own the world'. The IMF and World Bank and the almost unheard of Bank of International Settlements, BIS, (the mother of central banks) all promote and insist on privatisation as the stipulation on their loans to developing countries. In effect they are creating currency out of thin air and insisting nations give over all their national wealth and resources as part of this loan package. With unlimited access to currency it would be, and is, easy to bribe and corrupt so-called leaders of developing countries with rich resources to sell out their own people. The book 'The Open Veins of Latin America' by Eduardo Galiano summed up in one line the conquest of his continent *"The Spanish had the cow, but it was others who drank the milk"*. Those "others" were the international banking mafia. There was never a British Empire; it was always a City Of London Banking Empire.

Whilst all the media in the West are giving us the impression of Putin being an evil invading tyrant (remember how they spin reality) behind the scenes the IMF, investment banks like Blackrock, Vangard and the rest are all asset stripping the nation of Ukraine with the approval of the 'hero' Zelensky, a puppet bought and paid for by the banking mafia. Please do not fall into the trap of seeing China and the West as enemies or economic competitors. Again, in my book, *'Debt Slavery'*, I show how the Rothschild and Rockefeller banking families went into China decades ago to start off their economic revolution. The same families that are part of Saudi Arabia and the Middle Eastern oil giants. We live totally in a corporate world with corporate laws with the illusion of 'freedom and democracy' in the West to keep the illusion of governments representing people going.

The simple scam of currency creation is actually too simple for most people to believe. Certainly it is too simple for more highly 'educated experts' called economists. Similar to medical doctors they are 'educated' in a certain way that means they will never think outside the box and ask the simple questions. We have the alleged freedom fighters of Del Bigtree and R F Kennedy both asking for 'safe vaccines' without challenging the science behind it. For me when looking into money creation and allopathic thinking, including germ theory, many years ago three simple questions came to mind that I feel are the foundation for any open investigation

- What is it?

- Where does it come from?

- How does it function?

Again in my book *'Debt Slavery'* I have used these three simple questions to unravel the monetary and financial scam mankind are subject too. As with germ theory, when you actually go back to the beginning, the truth is actually quite simple.

As long as we continue not to question the massive debt ALL nations have, and who that debt is owed to, then a financial collapse of huge magnitude is on the cards. When your own mortgage becomes unpayable 'they' then come for what 'they' wanted all along, your house or assets. As nations too have unpayable debts then the natural resources and infrastructure is what the international bankers will be coming for.

'They' will own EVERYTHING and 'they' will be very happy!

The 'Covid' Economy

After the 2008 financial crash, it became clear to me that another, even bigger, crash was on the way. A system built on unpayable debt can only come to one conclusion. I have been keeping an eye on the growing personal, business and government debt around the world waiting for the bubble to burst. When the news started to come out of Wuhan and it was being said 'it' could spread worldwide, I could see the coming together of many global agendas under the guise of a 'pandemic' One of those agendas was the destruction of the financial system. When the governments started printing currency and at the same time shutting down the economy I knew that it was only a matter of time before we saw hyper-inflation. As we know every unit of currency should represent a unit of productive energy. When you print currency and actually stop production there can be only one result as you are devaluing the currency.

The currency, our currency, was given to big pharma in the billions of pounds, dollars and euros as it was given to the big banks in the massive bail outs in 2008. It was simple, legal money laundering from the global mafia governments to the global corporate mafia. The rest of the 'free money' went to the population to stay at home and not work. With the exception of 'essential' workers, the rest of us took a long holiday incarcerated at home and all paid for by government, with our money of course. The thing the majority of people do not understand is the currency the government give us is currency borrowed in our name from corporate institutions. When the oil prices started to rise due to manipulation, not the Ukraine war, I knew hyper-inflation was round the corner. Increasing the currency supply and shutting down part of the economy can result in inflation but when the price of oil and natural resources go up, EVERYTHING must go up, as oil is the basis for the whole world economy. All manipulated by the same people who 'own the world'.

Above all medical science and tech giants had the biggest gain

346

with vaccine manufacturing, producing track and trace systems, PCR test kits, lateral flow test kits, respirators and more all receiving billions during the 'covid economy'. The drug midazolam saw a huge increase in use in care homes killing an unknown number of elderly people. Boris Johnson pledged £330 million per year over the next five years of our money to Bill Gates and his GAVI organisation. So am I right in thinking that the world is giving billions of dollars to fund a project, that will make a product, that will be sold back to the very nations that funded it? Seems like a good business deal to me and not the actions of a rich caring philanthropist. The NHS budgeted £37 billion for the first two years of 'track and trace' to track and trace the British public and not a virus. The UK Government claimed they underspent by £8.7 billion in the first year but as we are talking in billions it's hardly relevant.

The majority of the population are now paying, literally, for the financial decisions made on our behalf three years ago. Now we are seeing rises in interest rates which in effect are just a pay rise for the bankers with the effect of making debt more expensive, harder to pay back, resulting in businesses going bust and people losing their homes. All daylight robbery backed and supported by the governments and the courts and the police who will enforce it all. Again, one big global mafia.

During this time politicians have been shown to be giving massive medical contracts to mates and making a fortune for themselves. But the main thing they have been doing is funding the future infrastructure for the global human prison. They, with our money, have been busy pushing billions into tech companies, medical science, digital tracking systems and more. We are actually paying for the building of our own prison. Does this make you angry? Well it should. Sadly most people are still listening to 'expert' economists telling us there is no other way and …we'll just have to ride it out, "we're in this together" is the common cry from politicians. Only the 'we' does not include you and me. Similar to the 'pandemic,' as Patrick has explained, they are happy for people to argue over details of the story, as long as they don't question the story itself..

It's common knowledge now many politicians made lots of money via their own personal investments in the covid economy. Well if you know where the money is flowing to and you are the one pushing it that way then why would it be a surprise that elite politicians are serving their own wants and needs and not the publics.

'Conflicts of interest among the UK government's covid-19 advisers' – BMJ, 9th December, 2020
> "By July the UK government had signed a coronavirus vaccine deal for an undisclosed sum with GlaxoSmithKline, securing 60 million doses of an untested treatment that was still being developed. In September, media outlets reported that Vallance had £600 000 (€661 000; $800 000) worth of shares in the company."

When asked on LBC radio when he discovered Sir Patrick's personal shareholding, Matt Hancock said: *"Well, I didn't know about it until I read it in the newspapers."*

Our Digital Future

Having already had knowledge of our planned digital currency it was no surprise when they announced that 'COVID' could be passed on by cash. It actually brought a smile to my face as when you actually know their playbook, they don't actually hide it, when things like that happen you can see how they are going to get from one stage to the next. So this was how they were going to try and get rid of cash, or at least get us more accustomed to using digital payments. It was well known amongst some of us that digital currency was the future as it's the only way these weak, pathetic, power-mad clowns can have the total control over humanity that their complete insecurity requires.

The people that run the monetary system know too well it is all an illusion. The greedy, selfish puppets they control may want the money but the people in the know at the top of the tree are after the control. They have sold us a lie about money and currency and made us believe money = wealth. They have created an economic system where economic production depends on the creation of currency, currency they totally control. But control over currency is not enough; they want to control how we spend it. Cash transactions are private and still give a small amount of freedom for people, even if that cash is sometimes hard to come by. BITCOIN successfully primed peoples mind to get on board with digital currency with many people believing it was going to free mankind from the chains of the international bankers.

For me, all along it was a scam, going from form of illusionary wealth to another and totally dependent of the technology that was clearly going to enslave us all. Central Bank Digital Currency (CBDC) will now very soon use this technology to not just control how much currency we have but how we spend it. "Computer says no" is something many people will be hearing in the next few years. They may take three steps forward and two steps back due to public pressure but it still means they have advanced one more step. I personally think their open plan to enslave humanity into digital slavery by 2030 (agenda 2030) is just more mind games to get us to accept our future under their control. I think it will take longer, if they get there, as I feel the real target for the technological enslavement of humanity are the youth now coming out of university who are actually embracing this new technology for its convenience and 'street cred'.

It has been well published that this CBDC will be monitoring our 'carbon footprint 'and will have the ability to be controlled from a central point by the people behind it. If you have broken a rule then the fine will be taken out automatically. It will be able to ration your food intake, so no beef steaks over your allowance. A petrol allowance to limit travelling, everything 'tracked and traced' and monitored. Whilst we continue to believe in the illusion of currency equating to wealth we will continue to be victims of the game.
The digital currency system will also depend on digital I.D.

Looking at the power of the Rockefeller Foundation and Bill Gate's GAVI and Microsoft, we can now put these together with the ID 2020 alliance.

"Alliance partners share the belief that identity is a human right and that individuals must have "ownership" over their own identity"

This obviously goes on the presumption that just being a human being is not identity enough.

"The ability to prove one's identity is a fundamental and universal human right."

"Over 1 billion people worldwide are unable to prove their identity through any recognized means. As such, they are without the protection of law, and are unable to access basic services, participate as a citizen or voter, or transact in the modern economy."

So without an identity they say we have no *'protection of law'*. Since when did we need an identity to access water, grow crops or create energy? Why would anyone want to be a *'citizen'* if in doing so they lose their natural sovereignty and rights? As for voting, again why vote for who is going to control you? I have seen the small villages along the Amazon River and its tributaries being dragged into 'the system' via tempting them with modern technology if in return they take on a Peruvian ID. They are being told it will give them all the rights and privileges of 'the system' when in fact it is simply taking all their natural rights and privileges away and the result is that what was once free they now have to pay for.

What they are really saying is that without a digital ID, one that they will control, you will actually lose all your basic human rights.
From the book *'IBM and the Holocaust: The Strategic Alliance between Nazi Germany and America's Most Powerful Corporation:* Edwin Black

"..detailing IBM's conscious co-planning and co-organizing of the Holocaust for the Nazis, all micromanaged by its president Thomas J Watson from New York and Paris."

So we have another American company, IBM, with very close connections to the Nazis and their Eugenics programme, the same IBM that in 1980 Microsoft formed a partnership with to bundle Microsoft operating systems with IBM computers. Now remember, it is Bill Gates who seems to be at the moment the main man in telling nations and medical authorities what the strategic plan is to cope with the any future pandemic, the same global strategic plan that clearly is resulting in mass early death of the weak and elderly, and as in the case at least in the UK, putting do not resuscitate – DNR – orders on many old, weak and physically and mentally disabled people.

His new 'GERM Team' has proclaimed itself the absolute authority of so-called contagious disease and given itself massive powers. Oh and yes, you were not asked but you will be subject to all of their orders.

> "Here's how a GERM response would work: The team's disease monitoring experts would look for potential outbreaks. Once it spots one, GERM should have the ability to declare an outbreak and work with national governments and the World Bank to raise money for the response very quickly. Product-development experts would advise governments and companies on the highest-priority drugs and vaccines. People who understand computer modeling would coordinate the work of modelers around the world. And the team would help create and coordinate responses, such as how and when to implement border closures and recommend mask use."

The BBC did an interview with Mr.Gates during 'the pandemic' and his face could be seen on a screen the size of a cinema screen, whist the interviewer looked up at him from his distant position, looking like an ant in comparison. Again, the science being used here is psychology and not medical science. We are being given an image of a God like messiah here to save us all. Would you like this man to be given all control via your digital ID and be dependent on him for all your basic needs?

351

Climate Tyranny and the not so Green Economy

"Because of the sudden absence of traditional enemies, "new enemies must be identified."
"In searching for a new enemy to unite us, we came up with the idea that pollution, the threat of global warming, water shortages, famine and the like would fit the bill... All these dangers are caused by human intervention, and it is only through changed attitudes and behaviour that they can be overcome. The real enemy then, is humanity itself."

– Book by The Club of Rome, 1991,'The First Global Revolution'

To build a world-wide, elitist, corporate or communist system, depending on how you look at it, or dictatorship it is a lot easier if you convince the people to build it themselves for their own good. An in your face push to build a police state will have a limited life-span as eventually enough people will see it and in time survival instincts will kick in and they will rebel. 'Freedom and Democracy' is being promoted by the same politicians who have taken all the natural rights off the people they claim to serve, and yet still most people lap it up and think of themselves as so fortunate to live in a society where they have a vote, not knowing that at best, that vote, is just our controllers letting us have an opinion on our slavery to give the illusion of choice. We always vote for who rules over us and not who serves us.

'The perfect dictatorship would have the appearance of a democracy, but would basically be a prison without walls in which the prisoners would not even dream of escaping. It would essentially be a system of slavery where, through consumption and entertainment, the slaves would love their servitudes. "– Aldous Huxley

The green economy has come in to 'save the planet' from humanities mere presence. Everything we do now has a carbon count and a negative impact on the planet, or so we are being told. The solution is all an all-electric smart grid, solar energy, wind farms, approved heating and fuel and ALL human activity needing approval of very rich people who we will never meet. It's just another mind game being played in the same way as the 'viral pandemic'. Tell people their lives are in danger and that if they don't act in a responsible way and trust the 'experts' then their very existence is under threat. This time though it is not just our human existence but the existence of the whole planet. The green economy has come from, and will be controlled by, the banking elite.

> *"Firms that align their business models to the transition to a net zero world will be rewarded handsomely. Those that fail to adapt will cease to exist"*
> – Mark Carney, former Governor at the Bank of England

Mark Carney is an international banker, and even as 'Governor at the Bank of England' he was never a public servant.

Yes, the same International Bankers who have, and still do, fund all sides in wars. War is big business, it is of no consequence to these people how many people are killed and how many lives and societies are destroyed. Add to this the monumental, destructive environmental impact of war then are we seriously to believe these psychopaths care a jot about preserving the environment.

It would take just a few minutes to research the environmental damage being done in Africa, Asia and Latin America to mine all the minerals needed for the electrical smart grid. A few minutes more to see the child slave labour and horrific human rights abuses of the people working to mine this 'green future'. Also, wind turbines cannot be recycled and don't produce much energy anyway and are certainly not 'carbon efficient' The scam of man-made global warming and a coming climate catastrophe is another psychological operation to put people into a state of fear so they can be easily controlled. The mass trashing of the planet, which I myself have witnessed, in the amazon and the man-made toxic chemicals pushed into our environment everyday do not seem to be an issue, but CO2, or the gas of life, is a threat to us all.

I myself have witnessed the trashing of the Peruvian amazon with tonnes of unnatural, and unasked for, man-made products and materials being brought in so they can make 'progress'. In the villages in the amazon EVERYTHING is, was, disposable and biodegradable. Your plate to eat off would have been a banana leaf that you could just drop on the ground and within a short time it would be turned into new soil. With the influx of processed foods and bottles of beer and fizzy drinks and the massive amount of plastic bottles and packaging, again that the people did not ask for but were simply given, they now have the enormous problem of dealing with all this man-made toxic waste. On top of that we have the mining and oil wells that use many toxic chemicals that spill out into the environment. The general population cannot be blamed for this at all. As sad a site as it is they simply throw most of their rubbish straight into the river. They have a natural throw away culture where natures does the recycling for them and it is so ingrained into how they live they do the same with the plastic and other waste. I'm sure outside of Iquitos where we lived there must be a massive landfill dumping all of this waste from the city giving the impression it is being dealt with.

The truth is the problem of plastic should have never come about. Again, we see the Rockefeller family using their massive control over oil to create a useful product that even at the time could have been made out of plant made plastic. Hemp was widely cultivated before it was demonised and given the tag of a drug. Hemp can do everything oil can do and more and without the environmental destruction that goes with it. There was even a car called the 'soy bean car' that was again made out of natural plastics. Imagine ordering your favourite coffee to go and then discarding the hemp cup into a river for the fish to eat. The

354

solution had been around before the problem, but hemp can be grown by anyone and competition is not allowed when trying to build a world of human dependency.

It would take minutes to see that polar bear numbers are going rapidly upwards since the emotional propaganda put out decades ago claiming these beautiful creatures were going to be extinct and it would be all our fault. A few minutes more and you will see that not only are the Maldives not under water, they are actually building new airports. The coral reefs in Australia are blooming. Even here, in a small town on the west coast of Cornwall, we see electronic mind control signs telling us "not to idle air pollution". Yes a small town next to the see where all of a sudden car emissions are a problem. The science of climate change is the same science used by governments to make us afraid viruses. The science of psychology.

The one area of environmental destruction that is easily fixed is regarding consumerism. We are constantly told by politicians and 'economic exerts' about the need to grow the economy. The simple question though is why? Surely an economy is simply about producing goods to benefit the lives of human beings. What they don't tell you is that the economy *has* to constantly grow because it all has a foundation on an unpayable debt and that financial gambling and corruption is how the elite grow their wealth. Research 'electric car mountain in China', 'electric bike mountain China' and 'ghost cities China' to see how insane financial scams backed by banks and governments are creating massive environmental damage and using up the worlds resources for insane money making scams.

To keep the whole insane system going companies need to produce stuff and get it sold and into landfill as quick as possible to keep the conveyor belt of madness going or it literally collapses overnight. Without the unpayable debt, interest, currency could be created for free by countries and communities as a simple representation of their productivity. This way the economy will be based on what we can produce for the benefit of us all instead of what we can produce to pay off the debt. There is one trap 'they' have set for us all though when it comes to solutions in that CBDC in the end could be sold as the people's currency and they could even make it debt free. In the end it is all about control, and if it is controlled by government then this would be a social credit system that would be like a communist system. It may clean up the planet but it will enslave humanity in the process.

The ultimate--problem – reaction – solution.

or as in the case of 'the pandemic'

no problem -- -reaction -- solution.

Whether there is a real problem or not is not important. What is important is to create public fear of a problem so their behaviour can be controlled.

The Open Society Foundations

Another big player we can't really leave out is George Soros; it would need a book alone for his story but we'll focus on now and his Open Society Foundations. As usual he got his multi-billions from investment banking or using a financial system I call 'the economics of a banking mafia'

> "George Soros is the founder and chair of the Open Society Foundations. He has given away more than $32 billion of his personal fortune to fund the Open Society Foundations' work around the world."

With $15.2 billion in the last three decades into:

Democratic Practice

Early Childhood and Education

Economic Equity and Justice

Equality and Antidiscrimination

Health and Rights

356

Higher Education

Human Rights Movements and Institution

Information and Digital Rights

Journalism

As you can see, another rich man's Foundation having massive influence over worldwide policies and social movements, to help push his own 'vision', I'm sure. Where there are activists it's a good bet Soros and his Open Society will be behind funding it.

They are also heavily active in the 'pandemic'.

"Emergency Response to COVID-19" with the current President Patrick Gaspard stating: - Open Society Foundations

> *"But beyond this initial response, it's time to think long and hard about the kind of world we want to live in. For many of us, the pandemic has underlined the challenges to our globalized world, and to the old ways of running our economies, posed by the existential threat of climate change. The current catastrophe also presents an opportunity—an opportunity to push for fundamental changes needed to build societies that are stronger and more resilient in addressing the challenges to come. I assure you that the Open Society Foundations will be an active participant in this search for a better world to emerge from the trauma of our present horror."*

Again, we have a big worldwide problem needing to be solved and the solutions always include a 'change' that comes from these rich philanthropists. So, who has created the "trauma of our present horror"? Could it be the same people who now want to 'transform' society to build a new and improved model for the world and its 'citizens' where we will live in accordance with their 'vision' and be dependent on their system and their 'experts' to the point where freedom of thought will not only be allowed, but not needed?

Let's now take a look at the people who we allow to run our lives.

In Whom we Trust

Boris Johnson was the man who locked down the UK, took all our freedoms away, and used psychology to put the fear of God into everyone. His policies caused the deaths of tens of thousands of people who he claimed to be serving. Are we to believe this man is a decent, honest man doing his best and who really cares about the people of the UK.

Boris Johnson jokes about dead bodies in Libya

'Foreign Secretary Boris Johnson quipped on Tuesday that Libya can become a new Dubai if it can clear the dead bodies away, the latest gaffe by Britain's top diplomat.'

"They've got a brilliant vision to turn Sirte, with the help of the municipality of Sirte, to turn it into the next Dubai," Johnson said. "The only thing they've got to do is clear the dead bodies away and then we will be there."- REUTERS October 3, 2017

Not the words of a decent caring man full of compassion and humanity. The big surprise for me is not that a man who uttered those words whilst being Foreign Secretary later became Prime Minister. In a system as corrupted as ours it's kind of the norm to get promoted for doing bad things. What really leaves me dumbfounded is how quickly people forget those words then vote for a man who clearly does not have one ounce of compassion for other human beings. It is not really an indictment against the system he serves rather than against the people who allow, and even vote, for him to serve over them.

Presently we have Rishi Sunak who is from a billionaire family and could not care less about the people of the UK. I am pretty sure he and his family would have gained from the 'covid economy'. And let's not forget Tony Blair and his 'weapons of mass destruction' lie. A man who pushed for covid vaccine passports and continues now in his well-paid role of pushing global elite agendas.

In the US the man who locked down the country again causing massive death and economic hardship, Donald Trump, is somehow seen as the returning messiah to bring down the 'deep state'. I guess you could at least say Trump was claiming to serve his people. With Joe Biden and his family we now have an actual open criminal cabal running America. Though I don't feel Joe himself is doing much of the organising as he struggles to even create a single cognitive sentence. Both Donald Trump and Bill Gates were both visitors to the infamous 'Epstein Island' Let's be clear, the elite went there to pursue and get away with immoral sexual behaviour or to make business contacts and make deals to expand their business empires.

We know for absolute certainty that at the highest levels of the political system in the West the sexual abuse of children is rife. This is an enormous subject and a massive piece of the world control system. I don't want to go off track here but it is clear that the blackmail of politicians who were involved in scandals with 'small boys' is part of the political control system and a way to get politicians to support particular policies and agendas that serve the global elite and their own agenda of power and control.

Child abuse files lost at Home Office spark fears of cover-up

"A dossier compiled by an MP detailing allegations of a 1980s Westminster paedophile ring is one of more than 100 potentially relevant Home Office files destroyed, lost or missing, it has emerged.

The government faced fresh calls for an overarching inquiry into historical cases of paedophilia as it was revealed that a total of 114 Home Office files relevant to allegations of a child abuse network have disappeared from government records. David Cameron has already ordered the Home Office permanent secretary to look into what happened to a lost dossier given earlier in the 1980s to Leon Brittan, then home secretary, by the campaigning Tory MP Geoffrey Dickens."

-The Guardian Online sat 5 July 2014

'Theresa May oral statement to Parliament on child abuse investigations'.

"Mr Speaker, in my statement today I want to address two important public concerns. First, that in the 1980s the Home Office failed to act on allegations of child sex abuse. And second, that public bodies and other important institutions have failed to take seriously their duty of care towards children".

Home Office and The Rt Hon Theresa May MP Published 7 July 2014

"The investigation found that 114 potentially relevant files were not available. These are presumed – by the Home Office and the investigator – destroyed, missing or not found, although the investigator made clear that he found no evidence to suggest that the files had been removed or destroyed inappropriately".

Here is an extract from a BBC interview with Tim Fortescue who was a conservative whip from 1970-73.

"anyone with any sense, who was in trouble, would come to the whips and tell them the truth, and say, 'Now, I'm in a jam, can you help?' It might be debt, it might be ... a scandal involving small boys, or any kind of scandal in which a member seemed likely to be mixed up in. They'd come and ask if we could help, and if we could, we did. And we would do everything we can because we would store up brownie points ... and if I mean, that sounds a pretty, pretty nasty reason, but it's one of the reasons because if we could get a chap out of trouble then, he will do as we ask forever more ..."
– Trevor (known as Tim) Fortescue

If you want to control someone then bribery is the easiest way. But if you want them to do some really bad things or pass policies that will obviously hurt the nation, but benefit certain others, then blackmail is the way to go. Years back a simple extra marital affair would be suffice to get someone to do your dirty deeds. Then it was homosexuality that seemed to be the tool to blackmail people in power. Nowadays nobody seems to care who is sleeping with whom and doing what, nobody judges the sexual promiscuity and cheating, they are more concerned about the gossip rather than judging. But one line that you would think could not be crossed would be the raping of children. This sickening crime thankfully is still considered by most people the most immoral, perverted, evil act one can do. Yet despite people saying that they still allow the political elite to get exposed time after time with no full investigation or consequences for those involved.

These are just a few examples of the behaviour coming from the people 'in whom we trust'.

CLIMATE CHANGES

Patrick Quanten MD

Does it? Climate is *the description of the long-term pattern of weather in a particular area*. Hence, different areas have different weather patterns and therefore also different climates. And a pattern is *a particular way in which something is done, is organized, or happens*. The seasons form a yearly recurrent pattern in terms of general weather conditions. These conditions may be different in different places on earth but each place has got a yearly weather pattern.

What isn't defined is 'long-term'. So the yearly weather pattern in one particular place becomes the climate of that place over a long period of time. How long? We talk about the Mediterranean climate, the tropical climate, the Scandinavian climate, each declaring a specific weather pattern in a specific area over a longer period of time. The climate is the weather *pattern* and any extremes are simply regarded as a normal part of what makes up 'the average' weather for the region. The actual weather itself is at no moment 'average'. When 'we' talk about the climate in these places, we basically consider what humans have been observing and experiencing in living memory. But the earth itself is much older than the living memory of human beings. So, has the climate in all those places ever been different from what we know it to be right now?

Indeed, it has. There have been at least five major ice ages in earth's history (the Huronian, Cryogenian, Andean-Saharan, late Paleozoic, and the latest Quaternary Ice Age). An ice age is a period of colder global temperatures and recurring glacial expansion capable of lasting hundreds of millions of years. This means that in a lot of places on earth, over a very long period of time, the temperature drops considerably. Outside these ages, earth seems to have been ice-free even in high latitudes; such

362

periods are known as greenhouse periods. The last glacial period began about 100,000 years ago and lasted until 25,000 years ago, a time when humans were around too. I am sure they were burning log fires but they weren't driving motor vehicles. Will they have contributed significantly to the ice age? Or maybe they managed to warm the earth up again and rescued it from self-destruction?

Bullet points to remember:

- The climate in various places on earth has changed dramatically back and forth over a very long period of time. This happened without any human help.

- Taking 'an average' of temperature, wind speed, rainfall and so on, of various places on earth teaches you nothing about the climate in any of those places.

When people talk about 'the earth's climate' it confuses me a bit. There does not exist a climate outside the earth's atmosphere, so why specify it's the earth's climate you talk about? Also, climate is always linked to a particular area, meaning an area *on earth*. However, scientists do consider the very long time period changes resulting in ice ages and in between the global warmer periods. They also have identified the reasons for these massive swings in overall temperatures. The earth's climate system adjusts to maintain a balance between solar energy that reaches the planetary surface and that which is reflected back to space: a concept known to science as the "radiation budget". The energy entering, reflected, absorbed, and emitted by the earth system are the components of the earth's radiation budget. Based on the physics principle of conservation of energy, this radiation budget represents the accounting of the balance between incoming radiation, which is almost entirely solar radiation, and outgoing radiation, which is partly reflected solar radiation and partly radiation emitted from the earth system, including the atmosphere. An energy budget that is constantly changing causes the temperature of the atmosphere to increase or decrease and eventually affect the climate in most places on earth. The effect is the result of the energetic interaction between the earth and its environment.

This is in line with the scientific knowledge that says that every effect we observe is the result of an interaction between the outer and the inner, between the environment and the subject. Effects we are seeing on the earth are the result of the earth's energetic environment, which is mainly influenced by the sun's activity and the energetic state of the earth itself. The sun changes by itself in a cyclic movement and the earth has its own inner energy movement cycle. These two constantly interact and create changing circumstances within the earth's atmosphere and on its surface. One such result is a cyclic cooling and warming of the earth's surface, and the main influencing factor is the radiation from sun, the solar activity cycle.

Bullet points to remember:

- The weather is constantly changing in a cyclic fashion, which changes the climate in various places, which may make the earth as a whole cool down or warm up. The weather is caused by energetic changes to the earth's field.

- The sun's activity is constantly changing in a cyclic fashion, which will change the energetic input into the earth's system, which may make the earth cool down or warm up. It is a major factor in energetic changes occurring within the earth's field.

Question: How is mankind going to stop the climate from changing? Follow-up question: If they succeed, how is that contributing to the balance of the earth's ecosystem which, like everything else in nature, evolves constantly?
The warmer periods in between the ice ages are called the greenhouse periods. I am so glad to be living in one of these

periods! But over the past three decades the greenhouse period we are currently in has become a big problem to some people. They have decided that it is too warm and they predict, based on computer models, that it is going to get even hotter. Soon!

The weather forecast that we are all addicted to is able to predict to a fair degree of certainty, not completely certain, the weather for the coming days. The models used for the prediction provide the foundation of the weather forecast. The models use an analysis of the current weather as a starting point and then project the state of the atmosphere in the future. Okay, here is how it works.

> "Each day, the Met Office receives around half a million observations of temperature; pressure; wind speed and direction; humidity, and many other atmospheric variables. However, there are large areas of ocean, inaccessible regions on land and remote levels in the atmosphere where we have very few, or no, observations. To fill in the 'gaps' we can combine what observations we do have with forecasts of what we expect the conditions in between to be. This is a process called data assimilation and is the first step for the supercomputer."

Currently, well over 10,000 manned and automatic surface weather stations, 1,000 upper-air stations, 7,000 ships, 100 moored and 1,000 drifting buoys, hundreds of weather radars and 3,000 specially equipped commercial aircraft measure key parameters of the atmosphere, land and ocean surface every day. All these do not cover the entire surface of the earth. The gaps, places where no information can be obtained from, will be filled in by what 'they' believe to be happening right there. This is your starting point! This is what goes into the computer as being the 'correct' slate of the weather right now.

> "The next step is to calculate how the current atmosphere will change over time. To do this, the supercomputer uses a

number of complex equations which are repeated many times. Each time the forecast is stepped a few minutes further into the future, and this enables us to produce forecasts from just a few hours ahead, to a climate prediction for the coming 100 years."

The input data contains measured data plus likely probability suggestions. Science tells us that there does not exist something like 'objective' data as all measurements are also influenced by how the measurement is taken. Hence, the data from their observation stations isn't *as clean* as they make it out to be. Then they add 'observations' they had a guess at. With this as their baseline they are going *to calculate* what is going to happen to that data. The way they calculate this, the way they have setup the computer programme, determines the kind of result it is going to give you. The process is already filled with a large number of variables and selective choices humans have made and we haven't even started.

The calculated results are now presented as what the weather is going to do in the future. The calculation process is being repeated in order to turn a one day forecast into a two day forecast, a week's forecast, a year's forecast. Any small error in the input data will through replication, through multiplication, become very large very quickly. How accurate is the weather forecast?

"The Short Answer: A seven-day forecast can accurately predict the weather about 80 percent of the time and a five-day forecast can accurately predict the weather approximately 90 percent of the time. However, a 10-day—or longer—forecast is only right about half the time."

The accuracy of the weather forecast, by their own admission, drops in five days by almost by half! From 90% to 50%. And yet, they also have said that by repeating the calculation cycle they can predict the climate 100 years ahead. Which one of those two statements is definitely false? Either they can tell us exactly what the climate is going to be in a hundred years from now by repeating the calculation cycle over and over again, or the reduction in accuracy between a five and a ten day forecast is 0,00001% and not nearly 50%. It can't be both! When you keep using the same formula to calculate the next few days' weather, any mistakes will be taken further down the line, which will increase the inaccuracy rapidly. Admitting that your 10 day forecast is only 50% of the time correct and then the statement that your 100 year forecast is also 50% correct must be an outright lie. Your computer is only half right in its projection of the weather model in ten days' time. It is completely unreliable to predict the weather in ten years' time.

My guess is that if the drop between a five and a ten day forecast was negligible they would boost about it. You and I would have been notified of their tremendous success. I will go with the second option, which is that there is no way of predicting what the climate will do over the next one hundred years, over the next ten years, or even over the next year. It is pure speculation hidden behind a computer programme and presented in the media as a certainty. And when you start observing this daily process of predicting the weather you will notice the sleight of hand tricks that are being used. Remember the seven day prediction on a Monday and compare this with the prediction made on the following Saturday for the next day. Compare what they said the weather on Sunday would be with what they say on Saturday the weather on Sunday will be. Also, take note of the details of the weather prediction for the next two days, notice how different it turns out to be and how as-a-matter-of-fact it is brushed over the following day when they talk about what the weather has been. It almost sounds as if that was they had predicted.

Bullet points to remember:

• Short term weather predictions are not statements of facts. They do have a failure rating.

- Long term weather predictions are completely unreliable as the accuracy of the prediction drops off at an alarming rate.

But none of the above seems to have any relevancy as far as our climate activists are concerned. They are on a mission, a mission to save the planet, as the poor thing doesn't know how to do that itself. They have decided it is all the fault of the human race. We are emitting gases into the atmosphere that are responsible for the heating up of the entire globe.

> "The earth's greenhouse gases trap heat in the atmosphere and warm the planet. The main gases responsible for the greenhouse effect include carbon dioxide, methane, nitrous oxide, and water vapour. In addition to these natural compounds, synthetic fluorinated gases also function as greenhouse gases."

Why do we do this? Especially if it causes so much damage and even endangers our own survival. How stupid can we be! Let's take a look at what the various sources are of these gases.
Carbon dioxide enters the atmosphere through burning alleged fossil fuels (coal, natural gas, and oil), solid waste, trees and other biological materials, and also as a result of certain chemical reactions (e.g., cement production). Cows, pigs and other farm livestock in Europe are producing more greenhouse gases every year than all of the bloc's cars and vans put together, when the impact of their feed is taken into account, according to a new analysis by Greenpeace. It turns out that CO2 is a waste gas emitted by almost all living creatures. It, therefore, must be seen as part of a natural cycle. In nature nothing gets wasted. Everything has a purpose. Carbon dioxide is removed from the atmosphere (or "sequestered") when it is absorbed by plants as part of the biological carbon cycle. Green leaf plants absorb carbon dioxide and release oxygen in the process. Adding large quantities of carbon dioxide to the atmosphere is used in commercial greenhouses to enhance plant growth and crop yield. The greater the CO2 atmospheric content the more and

stronger plant growth will become, resulting in an increased oxygen production. In short, the more carbon dioxide in the atmosphere the more oxygen the atmosphere will contain. But I suppose that is not such a good idea, is it?

Methane is emitted during the production and transport of coal, natural gas, and oil. Methane emissions also result from livestock and other agricultural practices, land use, and by the decay of organic waste. Methane is naturally destroyed by both chemical and biological processes, including reaction with atmospheric hydroxyl [OH] and chlorine, and by methane-consuming bacteria (methanotrophs) in soil and water. The primary natural sink for methane is the atmosphere itself, as methane reacts readily with the hydroxyl radical (OH−) within the troposphere to form CO_2 and water vapour (H_2O). When methane (CH_4) reaches the stratosphere, it is destroyed. Another natural sink is soil, where methane is oxidized by bacteria. Methane increases the amount of ozone in the troposphere and the stratosphere. Wouldn't that be a solution for the problem that fifty years ago was going to destroy life on earth: big holes in the ozone layer?

Nitrous oxide is emitted during agricultural, land use, and industrial activities; combustion of fossil fuels and solid waste, as well as during treatment of wastewater. Of course, nitrogen fertilisers have been recommended by governments and agricultural authorities to increase crop yields over many decades. More than two-thirds of the nitrous oxide emissions arise from bacterial and fungal denitrification and nitrification processes in soils, largely as a result of the application of nitrogenous fertilizers. Now one of the greatest contributor to the nitrous oxide gases in the atmosphere is the agricultural soil. So it's the farmer's fault! Nitrogen dilutes oxygen and prevents rapid or instantaneous burning at the earth's surface, as oxygen gas is a necessary reactant of the combustion process. Nitrogen is also needed and used by living things to make proteins. The first important step of the fixation of nitrogen in various forms that can be used by plants happens in the atmosphere. The enormous energy of lightning breaks nitrogen molecules and enables their atoms to combine with oxygen in the air forming nitrogen oxides. These dissolve In rain, forming nitrates that are carried to the earth, where it stimulates plant growth.

Water vapour is the most abundant greenhouse gas in the atmosphere, both by weight and by volume. Water vapour is also an effective greenhouse gas, as it does absorb longwave radiation and radiates it back to the surface, thus contributing to warming. The addition of water vapour to the atmosphere, for the most part, cannot be directly attributed to human generated activities. Increased water vapour content in the atmosphere is referred to as a feedback process. Warmer air is able to hold more moisture. As the climate warms, air temperatures rise, more evaporation from water sources and land occurs, thus increasing the atmospheric moisture content. In other words, the earth must already be warming up and then the changes within the atmosphere itself will enhance that process. Excess water vapour is the result of more evaporation of moisture into the atmosphere. It is not the cause of it.

And then there are the synthetic fluorinated gases. Hydrofluorocarbons, perfluorocarbons, sulphur hexafluoride, and nitrogen trifluoride are synthetic, powerful greenhouse gases that are emitted from a variety of household, commercial, and industrial applications and processes. Fluorinated greenhouse gases (F-gases) are man-made gases used in industry and they have a high global warming potential, often several thousand times stronger than CO2. Fluorinated gases are used inside of products like refrigerators, air-conditioners, foams and aerosol cans. Emissions from these products are caused by gas leakage during the manufacturing process as well as throughout the product's life. Fluorinated gases are also used for the production of metals and semiconductors. For a long time now human activities have been creating fluorinated gas emissions much more rapidly than the earth can remove them, increasing global levels. Hydrofluorocarbons (HFCs) are the largest source of fluorinated gas emissions. They are also the fastest growing source of greenhouse gas emissions. I make this the fault of the industry,

370

not mine!

It looks as if all the greenhouse gases, except the manmade fluorinated gases, are part of a natural phenomenon. They have always existed. The fact that mankind is now adding to some of these natural substances, bearing in mind that this addition is miniscule in comparison to the combined natural sources, only encourages the recycling of these elements to speed up a bit. In the case of carbon dioxide it delivers more oxygen. In the case of methane it delivers more water and more carbon dioxide, which will give us more oxygen. In the case of nitrous oxide it delivers more nitrates to the bacteria and plants, so more proteins can be built. In the case of water vapour it might be a good idea to be glad that the atmosphere is holding that extra water when on the surface of the earth it has become a bit too warm for the moment. At least the water has not been lost and we will get it back sooner or later.

So what's the real problem?

The real problem is pollution. An increase in natural products results in a response from nature to remove the excess and bring it all back to its easy balance point. The real problem is the industry. It produces greenhouses gases that are not part of a natural recycling process and that are difficult for nature to break down. It has produced and encouraged nitrogen as a fertiliser, destroying the natural balance of the soil. Lured by a short term gain of more yield and more profit from the same land, the farmers and the rest of us (happy with the reduce cost of agricultural food items) are now reaping benefits like poor quality agricultural land, toxification of soil and groundwater and, so we are told, global warming. The industry keeps producing gases the atmosphere has no effective natural pathway to breakdown and recycle. These gases then interfere with normal natural processes and they disrupt the natural balance of the system.

The earth is rapidly heating up, ice caps are melting at a rate never seen before and the water level of the seas are rising alarmingly quickly. So they keep telling me! However, it is not so easy to maintain the narrative amidst news that early in the winter Madrid is covered in snow for over a week, totally disrupting city life. That is not very warm for Spain, is it? It is difficult to maintain the narrative when at the end of the winter in 2023 the canals in Venice are dry. Or did the sea level rise somewhere else and not in Venice? It is difficult to maintain the narrative when the Maldives are consistently gaining land as a result of the sea retreating. Since 2000, the Maldives have added 37.50 km2 of land area, while 16.57 km2 of new islands have appeared within the South China Seas Spratly and Paracel chains. Augh, not good!

Let's change the mantra from 'global warming' to 'climate change'. When it is warm, as happens in the summer, we can still bang on about global warming. But the added advantage of the climate change mantra is that we can name any extreme event, be it the weather, volcanic eruptions, forest fires, floods, drought, and so on, as a result of the climate becoming *more extreme*. The climate is changing! And then I read study and research papers from eminent professors and researchers saying that there are globally now less forest fires than twenty years ago and that a smaller area is burned each year. I keep asking climate activists to tell me how much CO2 is being released every year by forest fires and volcanic eruptions compared to what my car has produced in that year. I am still waiting. Other papers clearly state that the ocean's water levels haven't risen by any amount that is worth mentioning (millimetres in years!). I am also still waiting for an explanation for those planes that, high up in the sky, produce a checkerboard pattern of persisting clouds, which don't dissolve. They spread out and block the sunlight. What does that white stuff consists off? And if, as the authorities say, these are ordinary line flights why has nobody ever bothered, in response to persistent questioning, to publish the relevant flight plans?

Climate changes, that is a certainty. It is a natural phenomenon. Whether or not it has been speeding up a bit over the last thirty years, who can tell? You can't measure these things. Playing with molecules is not scientific proof of anything. Using computer models to project life into the future may work well for human projects but it certainly is a waste of time for nature. In order to have a pretty good idea about the future, one needs to know the process very well. The truth is that we don't know nature. And I think that 'they' don't want you to learn more about nature as it would quickly reveal how manipulative their information control really is.

Nature has warm summers and it has cool summers. For nature to turn all summers consistently into much warmer summers it takes a thousand years. Look at how long ice ages lasted. It did not change from warm to freezing cold in fifty years. There is no linear progression within nature. There is movement between low tide and high tide, and if the water level is rising it will also do this in a movement between a higher level and a lower level, gradually over many centuries raising the level. Nature takes its time. It's not in a hurry. It moves in a balanced way.

Human beings are time short-sighted.

Human beings are prisoners of their past.

Human beings are projectionists of an illusionary future.

Human beings like to be scared. It is the one emotion they are freely allowed to have, to talk about, to display. Well, let's do that then, shall we? Ignorance leads to fear. And we embrace our ignorance. We don't want to know more. We want others to shut up so we don't need to hear the reasons why climate change is not a major emergency.

And 'they' need you to be scared. 'They' need you to be ignorant. 'They' don't want you to see that industry is a major emergency, destroying life rapidly. So 'they' make you scared of life itself. And you kiss their feet, put money in their collection boxes and attend their ceremonies.

A ONCE CARING PROFESSION

My own personal experiences with the NHS and the medical profession started as a very young boy, maybe four years old, with breathing issues or asthma. Putting the allopathic treatment aside, which I feel now led to more severe breathing issues, eczema and allergies, I have to say I have vague memories of being well cared for. I remember spending at least a week in hospital over one Christmas; I must have been about seven. I spent most of the time in bed with an oxygen tent around me. My mother came in on Christmas day with presents, one being a toy bow and arrow set that had rubber suckers on the end to stick to walls. I have a memory of laughing watching the doctors and nurses laughing and smiling whilst playing with the toys, I even think one doctor fired an arrow and it got stuck on the ceiling. I may have been ill but that did not stop us from having a good time, something I now know is so important for children when going through an illness process. This was in the mid 1970's when I would say the main focus of the doctors and nurses in the NHS was to care for the patient. I certainly never felt afraid whilst in hospital.

My own GP practice was a house in the council estate I lived on, Wythenshawe in Manchester. It was a large house converted to a doctor's medical practice with about three doctors working from there. When I had an appointment regarding my ailments the doctor was actually attentive and listened and not always too quick just to give a prescription and rush me out. As I had a regular doctor he actually knew me, my mother, brother and grandparents, it was a real local practice providing a real local service for the people in the community. These various small medical practices around the council estate were eventually taken over by one mega centre that covers the whole area and where people now have been reduced to numbers.

I myself never allowed my health issues to hold me back and was always out playing football, cricket, cycling and generally being an active outdoor kid and eventually I 'grew out' of my asthma and I took myself of the inhalers at around eleven years old or less.

In 2000 I was married and in 2001 our first child came along, Isabella. I had spent two years wandering around the Americas and had seen the power and control of big corporations, which had started to open my eyes up to the fact the world was possibly not as it was presented to us by the media and politicians. However, I was still a way off figuring out how it was actually run. I was totally ignorant of health, disease and how the medical profession worked.

Though I could not understand it at the time it did seem strange that just the fact of my wife being pregnant was being treated as a medical condition. We just went along with it all, vaccines included, and it was only when looking back that we could clearly see how the medical professionals took control of something as natural as giving birth. It is clear to me now that being pregnant is not a medical condition, and giving birth is not a medical procedure.

With our second child in 2010, Alejandro, I clearly remember having lots of meetings and check-ups with lots of questions and forms to be filled in with many personal questions. I now know that we were being interrogated by the state to see if we were fit, or compliant, enough to look after what they deem to be their property. I remember one health visitor talking to us about the MMR vaccine and reassuring us it was safe and to ignore the false science of Dr Andrew Wakefield and that we were not to worry as "we got him" so he is not a threat anymore. Though I believed in vaccines at the time, it still felt like a strange comment to make.

It was not until early 2011 I came across the book 'The Science of Health and Healing' by Trevor Gunn that in one reading opened me up to all the lies we had been fed regarding the nature of illness and disease. I had already figured how the bankers had taken over the whole political system and had most of the pieces of the control system in front of me. This new piece was to become a huge piece for me personally, forcing me to understand the human condition and the nature of reality so as to get a better understanding regarding the full extent of the control of humanity.

In October 2011 my youngest came along, Rosalia, and I had now gained a decent understanding of health and disease in a short period of time, simply because I felt I had to. I knew what to expect and how 'they', the medical professionals, would try to take control of everything and push the Vit K jab onto my new baby. I prepared my mind for the onslaught and they did not disappoint. Literally a few minutes after the birth, with my wife totally exhausted and a naked baby on her chest, we were asked if they could go ahead with the Vit K jab. I calmly declined, took a deep breath and waited for the reply. The reply was "oh I'll have to get the paediatrician in then". Moments later, with me still trying to comfort my wife, a lady came in and bombarded me with psychological attacks, one after the other, stating how I was putting the life of my baby at risk, how she was not accusing me of ,'neglect', but! And it went on. I just wanted to comfort my wife and embrace our new arrival into this world and enjoy the moment but that was not of any importance to the paediatrician. At one moment, whilst the next psychological attack was under way, I felt myself for half a second starting to cave. I just wanted to comfort my wife and be left alone. After literally about half a second, in fact as soon as I became conscious of my momentary weak state, I took a deep breath and looked at the paediatrician and gave her one simple request. "I will discuss this further after you have brought me the insert with the ingredients". She left the room and thankfully never came back. As soon as my wife was fit enough to go home, about an hour later, we got into the car and headed home to the comfort, and safety, of our own home.

A week or so later we had a health check at the doctor's surgery undertaken by a doctor we had known for about ten years. She offered us the vaccine schedule which I calmly declined and again waited for the reply. She began to tell me of her experience working in Africa and the damage childhood illnesses were doing there and felt it was best to protect our baby from this threat. I mentioned to her I had researched this subject and that children in Africa were having complications to childhood illnesses due to the unhealthy environment they were living in and due to malnutrition. She stopped and took a long, almost shocked, look at me as though she had been hit with a truth bomb. We never discussed our decision not to vaccinate again and that now our other children would no longer be continuing with the vaccine schedule. My youngest is now nearly twelve, vaccine free, medicine free, doctor free and illness free. She has had all the normal coughs and colds and all three have had chicken pox with no complications at all.

I could clearly see a change over the years in the attitudes of the people working in the medical profession. Fortunately, for many years, since the day I read Trevor Gunn's book, we have not felt the need for medical doctors. With my new knowledge of the true nature of disease and illness, backed up by what I could see was a clear global agenda to control humanity via fear, it became clear how medical science and its self-proclaimed 'experts' could be manipulated to become tyrannical in a way that suited the global agenda of control.

In 2009/10 I came across the research of Brian Gerrish, former Navy Officer and now co-presenter of UKColumn News. I highly recommend viewing this interview with Brian from 2011 when he had already been exposing Common Purpose for many years. https://www.dailymotion.com/video/xjl2ej

I also recommend buying the book 'Beyond Authority: Leadership in a Changing World' Julia Middleton, founder of 'Common Purpose'. The title of the book is very revealing and without understanding this piece of the puzzle nothing will make sense, which is how 'they' want it. The insanity and madness we are seeing in the world is controlled insanity and madness. To answer the question "but how could they get away with that?" it is a must to understand this topic and reflect on the chapter on perception to see the whole puzzle before your eyes. Just look at all the global, national and local organisations that promote 'leadership programmes' and all the rich billionaires with their foundations also funding new 'leaders' using 'useful idiots', which is all intended to promote, sell and control the world global control agenda. Many, if not most, of these leaders are not even aware of the agenda they are pushing. Brian Gerrish has stated that organisations like Common Purpose are using a technique called Neuro-linguistic programming (NLP) which can "change people's beliefs and behaviour without them knowing".

Sounds like a secret society? Well it certainly functions as one,

Common Purpose

Here are two articles from Brian published on his website https://www.cpexposed.com/

Understanding Common Purpose 17 November 2013

Many people are now aware of the British political charity Common Purpose and its work to create a network of common purpose across politics, public and private sectors, and throughout society. Many people now understand the sinister role CP played in creating the furore to drive the Leveson Inquiry into the press, using their own Media Standards Trust and the Hacked Off Campaign. Their ultimate goal has been to assist the British State to take control of the Mainstream Press using a Royal Charter with the power to impose draconian penalties should the press fail to live up to State imposed guidelines. We should remember that CP is a secretive and duplicitous organisation that has already been caught breaking the Data Protection laws by collecting data on individuals lawfully asking questions about CP by means of the Freedom of Information Act. CP is terrified of the public gaze and discovery of its real work to undermine democracy and impose a quasi-secret network of state control by means of a network of CP graduates in positions of power and influence. The plan is for a communitarian dictatorship and a controlled press and media is essential to this.

In this short post I would like to help people also understand that the charity Common Purpose is not the all-powerful be all and end all organisation. We can be confident that the charity CP was designed to be the Trojan Horse in British Society with the primary objective of getting the first CP 'future leaders' into place, from where they could open many doors to many more of their own. But alongside infiltration by the political charity CP comes the wider socio political agenda of common purpose; an agenda which is being promoted by a host of different organisations and initiatives. These include Diversity Courses, Community Empowerment, Leadership, Visioning, Community Activism, Social Entrepreneurs and Disrupters - in fact there is now a vast web of these 'vehicles' which are primarily working to promote the change agenda to destabilise our historic organised society. The turbulence of deliberately created change allows the new intended socio political agenda to be established more softly than if there was a sudden onslaught of the new politics in a quiet orderly and stable society. Alongside the common purpose 'vehicles' I have just mentioned comes another 'change agent' web using networks of Neuro Linguistic Programming NLP. Via a myriad of different consultancies boasting everything from self-empowerment to powerful management change in global corporations, NLP practitioners are creating a mass of 'reframed individuals' with boosted belief in their own ability as change agents and leaders, and a low-empathy view of those simple individuals who are left to rely on the 'inferior' mind that God gave them.

Within the NLP networks the anchor of the need for 'change' and 'transformation' into a future utopian society is the common theme or purpose used to destroy people's identity, common sense and their ability to enjoy living in the 'now', albeit having to deal with the day to day ups and downs that life has always delivered. Whilst recognising that many NLP practitioners practice in their desire to help people overcome problems, the real danger comes from NLP practitioners who are now themselves changed as a result of the experiential nature of their original NLP training - that is, they were NLP'd as part of their training. This now leads to the position whereby individuals themselves changed or reframed by NLP are changing and reframing others into mind-sets which interface with the government's own Applied Behavioural Psychology programme - a central programme of David Cameron's Saul Alinsky based Big Society. It's agenda? To create a docile subservient public where the only views that are accepted are the government's specified norms. Believing in different and speaking out will not be tolerated. Hence we return to the common purpose agenda to help install state control of the mainstream press and media as soon as possible.

I have written this post spurred on by the increasing number of emails I have been receiving from those who have experienced problems at the hands of NLP practitioners or who have friends or relations who have suffered. What have they experienced? Personality changes, depression and anxiety for example. These victims are the immediate casualties of the NLP cancer that is now invading our society. However those reframed and now already living blissfully unaware of reality in their new future leader empowered utopia of an NLP restructured mind are also destined to be crushed within the emerging hive mind dictatorship. As the government's own document 'Mindspace' says..."Either people will not know they have been changed or they may realise they have been changed but not know how." Impossible? Google UK Government document 'Mindspace'. You might also consider that this behavioural change programme has been so successful the British government has sold the 'technology' to Australia and USA. Of course Common Purpose has used NLP from the start.

Common Purpose is a political charity using Behavioural Modification

Common Purpose (CP) is a Charity, based in Great Britain, which creates 'Future Leaders' of society. CP selects individuals and 'trains' them to learn how society works, who 'pulls the levers of power' and how CP 'graduates' can use this knowledge to lead 'Outside Authority'.

Children, teenagers and adults have their prejudices removed. Graduates are 'empowered' to become 'Leaders' and work in 'partnership' with other CP graduates. CP claims to have trained some 30,000 adult graduates in UK and changed the lives of some 80,000 people, including schoolchildren and young people.
But evidence shows that Common Purpose is rather more than a Charity 'empowering' people and communities'. In fact, CP is an elitest pro-EU political organisation helping to replace democracy in UK, and worldwide, with CP chosen 'elite' leaders. In truth, their hidden networks and political objectives are undermining and destroying our democratic society and are threatening 'free will' in adults, teenagers and children. Their work is funded by public money and big business, including international banks.

It is important for researchers on this site to realise that the majority of Common Purpose 'graduates' are victims, who have little if any understanding of the wider role of Common Purpose within UK society, nor of its connections to higher government and the European Union. Drawn into CP training by a flattering invitation, or selected by their company or organisation, this recruitment is normally carried out by a previously trained CP person - now recruiting for the cause. Candidates are screened and selected (or rejected) by CP Advisory Board members in their area.

Both candidates and 'trained graduates' will have no real understanding of Common Purpose's wider role to help achieve a political and social paradigm shift in the UK. The real objective, would appear to be to replace our traditional UK democracy with the new regime of the EU superstate.

By blurring the boundaries between people, professions, public and private sectors, responsibility and accountability, CP encourages graduates to believe that as new selected leaders, CP graduates can work together, outside of the established political and social structures, to achieve this paradigm shift or CHANGE. The so called "Leading Outside Authority". In doing so, the allegiance of the individual becomes 're-framed' on CP colleagues and their NETWORK.

Using behavioural and experiential learning techniques, the views of graduates can be remoulded to conform to the new Common Purpose. Most will not be aware this has happened, but we are given immediate clues in descriptions by graduates that Common Purpose training is 'life changing', 'disturbing, or 'unsettling'. Trained and operating under the Chatham House rules of secrecy (details of discussion, those present and location are not disclosed), CP graduates come to operate in 'their world' of Common Purpose. Please go to Document Library ....Category.........Mind Control Background on this site for historical information regarding manipulation of people's free will and behaviour.

The term 'GRADUATE' is used deliberately so as to prevent disclosure of involvement with Common Purpose. As 'MEMBERS' of CP, which is more appropriate, individuals in the public sector would have to declare their interests. So strong is the Common Purpose bond, that some individuals will lie to hide information and documents considered 'dangerous' to the CP cause. People challenging CP colleagues have been victimised and forced out of their positions.

Common Purpose is linked to a host of other suspect trusts, foundations, think-tanks, quangos and so called charities. DEMOS is a key example. These organisations funnel political and social CHANGE policy through CP, to re-frame graduates. Examples range from promotion of Diversity in every company and organisation, to Curfews for young people.

Common Purpose promotes the 'empowerment of individuals', except where individuals challenge the activities of CP, and public spending on CP. These people are branded vexatious, extremist, right wing or mentally unsound. Mrs Julia Middleton, the Chief Executive of Common Purpose, praises the work of German bankers. Deutsche Bank is, of course, a major power behind Common Purpose. Mrs Middleton, earning circa £80,000 p.a. from her charity, is also very happy to promote the term 'USEFUL IDIOTS' in her book 'Beyond Authority'. Are we the General Public the USEFUL IDIOTS, or are the Elitest Common Purpose Graduates? You must decide.

So what has happened over many years is that various leadership programmes have 'educated' its graduates to infiltrate all areas of society, especially public institutions. They have been put in to push an agenda, one they undoubtedly know nothing about, and 'change' society. In the political arena it must be clear now we have leaders and not public servants. The police are now working for the government and enforcing whatever rule and not serving the people and upholding the common law and just keeping the peace. We now have political policing meaning we live in a police state. Education has been transformed so much that talking about objective truth and independent investigation and looking at all opinions is seen as extremist behaviour. The NHS is now run by managers who have the final word over doctors. Yes, there is still the issue of doctors being trained in allopathic medicine, but at least years back they had the power of decision making and were allowed to use their own common sense, but now the doctors job is not to think but to do the will of the people running the hospitals and follow protocols regardless of how harmful these policies are.

I will give you here one clear example of this manipulation of consciousness that this training in public service is doing to the minds, hearts and humanity of the people 'in whom we trust'.

During the after math of the first lockdown I was talking to a policeman in the street. I was talking to him about the lockdown policies and how they affected the people and the NHS. I explained to him many people had died at home who were in need of emergency care but were too afraid to phone for an ambulance, they were too afraid to go into hospital. I had pointed out that the government were using a team of psychologists that were working to use fear to control public behaviour which then resulted in many of the deaths I have just spoke of, people afraid to go to hospital when in need of emergency care, His reply was very clear and cold and sadly exactly what I expected "well it's their own fault then ". This is what the mental re-framing has done to almost all of our public servants and almost anyone who has a badge, a clipboard, a uniform or an illusionary position of authority.

When Patrick Quanten left the medical profession he made this public statement on his website (2001). I'll leave Patrick himself to explain the rest.

Personal Statement
Today is a sad day for me.

I became a doctor with the firm intention of wanting to help people, wanting them to "heal". My initial disappointment when I experienced that this was not happening, turned into great excitement when I learned that there were other things one could do, outside the medical textbooks. I even ignored the opposition I encountered. Soon my new found enthusiasm started to wane too, because although everything seemed to have its uses, nothing was definitive.

Looking for the answers to health and illness, using my knowledge and the science available, slowly became a crusade. Mathematics, Physics, Chemistry, Astrology, as well as Ancient Medical systems, it was all explored in search of more complete answers.

More and more compelling evidence appeared, and eventually the camel's back broke. Being confronted with the fact - no more excuses available - that my way of helping people, that my medicine - the truth beyond a shadow of a doubt - was not only preventing people from recovering from illness, but was actually introducing illness, more illness and suffering than ever before in the whole history of humanity. That shocked me to the core. The realisation of all the damage I personally have caused in the name of "making people better" is sickening me.

Today is a sad day for me.

I worked hard because I was convinced that Western Medicine could change. Now I know it can't. The change involved is a complete U-turn; the truth lies in the direction totally opposite to the one in which Western Medicine is going. As a direct result of that realisation I have to get of this wagon here and now. I can no longer justify being a member of this sect and I hereby resign my post as a medical doctor.
Dr Patrick Quanten MD

I truthfully thought medicine was science. And science, as I understood it, was questioning things. I thought that if and when an answer we provided did not solve the problem I, as a medical doctor, was obliged to search for the answer that would solve that problem. But when I did, it was quickly made clear to me that that wasn't the done thing. The profession, as it was made clear to me, already provided the best possible answer and I was simply to hand that to the patients. They, the profession, were continuously looking to expand their knowledge of disease and as soon as they had a 'better' answer they were sure to let me know. So far so good!

I came across some very promising answers to a great variety of health problems but none of these seemed to be worth investigating as far as the medical authorities were concerned. I did not understand that attitude, as medicine is science and science is questioning everything. The exclusion of these other routes with potential for improving the state ill people were in shocked me. So I did my own research, and I found answers. Not so much about absolute cures for diseases, but about the direction the medical profession was heading in. They had boarded the train, destination 'diseases'. They were not even trying to move people towards health. Even worse, they did not know what health was. Now I remembered that at university we were never instructed anything about health, only about 'curing' and 'preventing' diseases. I now realized that, as a GP, I had been a foot soldier in the medical army, fighting diseases but, more importantly, conquering the world. We were spreading the one 'scientific' answer without being scientific. I deserted, narrowly escaping a court martial.

Now I can see that there is nothing to be gained from arguing with anything the medical profession claims, says or does, because their train is heading in the opposite direction. They want, they need, people to be ill. What reason can they possibly have? Which one do you like best? Huge eternal profits. Total population control by the power invested in me, by me. They will decide, and they are deciding, who is allowed, capable in their eyes, to do what, to go where, to know what.

The medical profession already decides who needs to work and who doesn't. They decide the traffic rules, to reduce major accidents happening, or so they say. They decide what is good for you and what is bad, as far as your behaviour is concerned, not just your eating habits. They decide who lives and who dies. They decide what 'cures' are good and which ones are bad, in fact they decide what a cure is. They decide what profession you are allowed to have and how you must conduct yourself. For example, a farmer is only a good profession, sustained by government subsidies, if you do not possess livestock and you don't grow crops. Farming is good if it is an industry, not a farm.

If you want to lead a healthy life you need to turn away completely from the medical profession as they are heading in the direction of diseases, ailments and professional dependency. The truth is that your health is solely dependent upon nature, the very force that created you, that keeps you alive in spite of your ignorance and even more so in spite of your stubborn insistence of trying to do the opposite. In no small portion are we helped in this by the medical profession, who has managed to make us all believe that they know more than science does, that they are more right than science is.

Here is the difference in a nutshell:

But everybody knows!
In science, nobody knows.

It is a hard truth to be confronted with. Who are you telling? I know. I have been there too. However, it doesn't make it less of a truth. Shouting your innocence of the rooftops, accusing everybody else of inappropriateness whilst behaving in a destructive, uncaring, calculated manner does not make you an acquaintance of mine. I don't know you. You don't exist to me.

"We have no choice to be in the world. The only choice we have is how we respond to the fact that we live in the world."

-    Yolande Norris-Clark

WHAT NEXT?

"It is no measure of health to be well adjusted to a profoundly sick society."

– J Krishnamurti

Humanity is now at a crossroads, and this sure does seem the time for the final battle of Good vs Evil, Truth vs Ignorance, Living conscious lives vs Living unconscious lives, Taking responsibility vs Being a victim or simply, Freedom vs Slavery. The true battle is a battle for our minds, for our beliefs, for it is those beliefs that will control our behaviour, along with another arch enemy, Fear.The real battle then is on consciousness. For if we are being controlled by beliefs we have no conscious knowledge of, then how can we free ourselves? Becoming conscious is the first step.

Yes, we live in a 'profoundly sick society', all of us. A sickness that has infected all nations, all cultures and all people. We, humanity, are out of balance. To restore balance individually and collectively we need to become conscious, conscious of who we are, of our actions and how they affect ourselves and how they affect others. Most of the world are living semi-conscious or unconscious lives, indoctrinated to act or think a certain way by a system that isn't even real and controlled by belief systems that serve to imprison the spirit of humanity. Most of all we believe in the authority and legitimacy of government and being governed.

What we are, all are, are sovereign human beings, we have just forgotten, helped by our controllers who want us to forget. True balance is expressing the fullness of who you are, your true self, in harmony with your surroundings and respecting every other expression of self under the universal law of 'do no harm', at least not deliberately. When you cannot be yourself, whether it is because of indoctrinated belief systems, oppressive regulations of society or fear of being different, then you cannot truly be in a state of balance, or free.

Fearful, indoctrinated minds create a 'survival of the fittest' mentality leading to wars and violent behaviour, and just in case people start to 'wake up', we have the endless distractions to divert our attention.

Rigid belief systems must go as they create limitations. A realisation that no man/woman has authority over another is a must. Understand that we are all different expressions of self; there is no one-size-fits-all, and look to nature to guide you as nature always looks to be in balance. And also when accepting that our life is our own then we cannot expect, or insist, that everyone else has to 'wake up' too. The only person that needs to change is YOU, as you have authority over yourself and no-one else.

We are spiritual beings having a human experience, **that is it**, It is an opportunity to experience this life, this reality, in our own individual way and then express our true self. As far as we know we have one shot at this life and we are just throwing it away obeying orders from psychopaths and morons in nice clothes.

By taking control of our thoughts and beliefs, understanding our own God given sovereignty, accepting responsibility for our own lives, being our own leaders, being reasonable, making compromises, not conforming, using common sense, learning to say NO and accepting that your idea of what is right for you may not be right for others, we may start to make progress on the road to freedom.

Lose the fear of authority. *"And fear not them which kill the body, but are not able to kill the soul: but rather fear him which is able to destroy both soul and body in hell."* – Matthew 10:28.

We are all energy. Energy cannot be destroyed; the body is our vehicle for this experience and it has a life span and is going back to dust anyway. We have a choice. We can live a long life in fear and with our heads bowed down and then die having not really lived, or we can stand up straight and look them all in the eye and live life as we see fit, regardless of how long we have.

As Bill Hicks says, *"it's just a ride"*.

"The meaning of life is just to be alive. It is so plain and so obvious and so simple. And yet, everyone rushes round in a great panic as it were necessary to achieve something beyond themselves."

   – Alan Watts

We still have one question to answer. **Do you want to be free?**

If we are all free to choose, whether we choose to be afraid and obey self-proclaimed government authority, or choose to just get on with life doing as we see fit and best for ourselves, to choose a vaccine or not, to choose to wear a mask or not, it has to come from us. The system does not provide a choice. We have to start to learn to live outside of the system if we cannot change it.

Positive thinking may open doors of opportunity but only positive action walks through them. With our backs now against the wall and nowhere to go, it's time to stand up and face what is in front of us.

The world has been filled with darkness for a very long time; there is no saviour outside of yourself. As the Hopi Indians have stated,

   "We are the ones we've been waiting for",

Or as Patrick Quanten says,

   "The only light at the end of the tunnel or in it is the light you shine yourself".

Patrick Quanten in his search of true health and understanding of disease eventually brought everything down to one simple thing, 'Self-Empowerment'.

Take a deep breath, connect to whatever creation is, be guided and remember, positive thinking has to be backed up by positive action.

Hold tight, start shining, it's gonna be a bumpy ride.

SELF-EMPOWERMENT AND SOCIETY

Patrcik Quanten MD

What gives you life and what sustains your life is a natural power that originates within the universal power, within the evolution of nature. It is an energetic force that forms and runs through the physical shape of the human being. Each specimen is unique in its combination of frequency bands from the entire energetic spectrum that covers the range of possibilities of human expression. Each of these unique specimens has, therefore, a unique energy balance, which means that each one requires a different combination in energy flow in order to sustain life easily, without losing too much energy. The greater the obstruction to the flow of this individual energy is, the more power the individual has to generate, the more energy he needs to burn, in order to live. The energy balance of the individual is called the Self.

There is the innate power of every individual, which sustains his life, and that life is sustained within the environment the individual lives in. His living conditions are generated by two different forces: nature and society. Every living creature, including human beings, lives within the boundaries of nature and is therefore subject to natural law. Every human being also lives in a social structure, created by mankind, and is therefore subject to the laws of that society.

The way nature functions is something we as human beings can't change. We are part of it, created by it, and we follow unwittingly and naturally, governed by our unconsciousness, the same rules. We are constructed in such a way that those rules can be followed and we have been given the tools to do so. In fact, it is to the benefit of our creator, nature, that we can follow the path it is following itself. There is no conflict between human life and nature, between human life and natural law.

The first definition of a society is a voluntary association of individuals for common ends. Individuals with a common interest join together voluntarily to pursue that interest, to share their knowledge and skills, to enhance their power with regards to their interest. But the same word gets used in different ways and modern times defines society as a large group of interacting people in a defined territory, sharing a common culture. Notice the differences:

- No mention of voluntary anymore
- The introduction of a specific living space, a territory
- The introduction of culture to replace common ends

This is by no means the same definition anymore! You are now part of a society when you live in the same area, not because you are choosing to belong to that society, out of personal interest and personal benefit. You are now part of a society when you have the same culture, not because you have the same goals in life. We have introduced a new concept in our definition of society and that is the concept of culture. Now we have to ask the question: what is culture?

Culture is the sum of attitudes, customs, and beliefs that distinguishes one group of people from another. So culture refers to a group of people that have come together around specific attitudes, customs and beliefs, which is basically how we defined society itself, bearing in mind that the definition of culture doesn't involve a voluntary choice. This means that the last part of the modern definition of a society, 'sharing a common culture', in fact means sharing a common society. This renders these words in this context completely pointless. The mention of culture within this definition of society does not alter the meaning. So now the modern definition of a society reads as a large group of interacting people in a defined territory. In short, if you live in a certain area you are said to belong to a certain society. Or in different words, lines on a map define the group, the society, you belong to, not your choice, not your common interest.

In practical, everyday terms, societies consist of various types of institutional constraint and coordination exercised over our choices and actions, because societies are no longer a matter of choice for the individual. The type of society we live in determines the nature of these types of constraint and coordination, enforced by people who have determined the kind of society we live in, by people who have decided we belong to the same culture. The nature of our social institutions, the type of work we do, the way we think about ourselves and the structures of power and social inequality that order our life chances are all products of the type of society we live in. Modern societies are entities that we have been forced to be part of and that are subsequently ruling us, governing us. This no longer is about individuals choosing to come together to expand their knowledge and skills on a particular interest they share. The shared interest of a modern society is one of the creators of such a society. They create all aspects of living the way they want to, the way it benefits them. Modern society is about the few who rule and decide. It is not about the individual. It is not a society formed by individuals coming together on shared views, interests and rules commonly agreed upon.

And yet, life is about the individual in the first place. Without individuals there could not be a society. And here is the problem. If society is a mix of people with different needs, different ideas, different talents and skills, wrestling with different problems in their lives, and yet society orders them, forces them, to all need the same, believe the same, act the same and judge things in the same way, then an individual is not going to be supported by such a society but rather will be obstructed by it. He will have to fight harder to survive within his 'own' society, burn more energy, lose strength more quickly. Society has become his worst enemy. Society has created a toxic living environment for the individual.

The only recourse open to the individual in his plight to survive the onslaught on his existence is to separate from the society he was lured into. Only by empowering his Self will he be able to live in peace, without having to fight battles all the time. His inner Self, his natural Self, knows how to live. It knows what the individual requires at any given moment in time. Nature has created the path your life is on, so it also knows where it is heading. The creators of the modern societies do not and are not interested. All they know is where they would like to go.

Separating yourself from the society you belong to, empowering the Self, involves cutting yourself loose from all institutions of that society, from all habits and benefits. This means education, health, finances, essential living requirements, governments, land, nations, information channels, … Take your time. It is impossible to do it all at once. It is impossible to it all by yourself.

By focussing your life on your personal needs and disregarding what society wants you, needs you, to be you will strengthen your inner power, the power that gives you life and that sustains your life. Individuals that no longer cooperate with society, that no longer subscribe to the rules of that society, that no longer empower that society, are beginning to empower themselves. From such an individual basis, from a point of freedom of choice, people can decide who they want to attach themselves to. They can voluntarily join together. These are the first steps towards building a different society, separate from the existing one. People voluntarily join together for common ends. Have the same ideas and find ways to work those out, together. The two main principles of this revolution are: freedom of choice and mutual benefit. Start locally. Building a society is about people finding each other, in other words, locally. Only deal with people you are able to communicate with, are able to talk to and in the first place are able to listen to. You need to be fed and surrounded by people who offer you ideas and solutions that work for you.

Be patient.

Be alert for humans that try and force you.

Be alert for where nature wants to take you.

Life is a school. It educates human beings. You have just entered a crucial educational level. Pass this exam and you will be moved up to the next level.

September 2023

THE BEST CHICKEN SOUP EVER!

End of summer 1998. Mission: fly to New York and somehow, some way, get to Rio for the millennium. Just a few hundred quid, a dream and knowing it was now or never. I was gonna eat the best food, drink the best beer and have all the adventures along the way, yes, and with just that few hundred quid. How was I gonna do it? I didn't know. Was I gonna survive? I didn't care. It just had to be done, man against the world.

New York, Miami, Texas and all in between; great times, great people but now to cross the border into strange lands and unknown possibilities. Crossing the border into Mexico at midnight, the only white man on the bus, I was stopped by the American police. *What is this little white English guy doing here?* they must have thought. After pulling me to one side and making sure I wasn't a mass murderer on the run they let me pass. Now I was here, over the border into new territory.

Two men approach and ask me if I need a hotel. One a taxi driver, one a policeman. I roll the dice and go with the policeman; at least he said he was gonna take me round the corner. The taxi driver, well, who knows where he would have taken me? I pulled out my main form of protection, a Manchester United souvenir, a scarf. We talked about David Beckham, made friends and ten minutes later I was in a hotel, door shut, locked and safe.

The next morning in the light I walked out into this strange new land and the real adventure started now. Six weeks later I left Mexico, after eating maybe the best street food on Earth, some nice cold beers with lime in them – come to think of it most things were served with limes.

Now it was Venezuela for the South American tour. After a few days in Caracas I met up with Andy, another lad from northern England who I had met in Miami. We had arranged to keep in touch and we met up in Caracas so he could join in the adventure. Just a few days later on a ship to a Caribbean island we met Dave from Australia, later to become Crocadili Dave, at the bar of course, and over a couple of beers he was sold. We had a new recruit; we were now the "Three Amigos".

We ate all the food and washed it down with all the beer. We walked and slept on the ground through savanna land with snakes and scorpions for company. We climbed mountains, swam in piranha-infested waters and met all the weird and wonderful people along the way. We got stuck in Manaus in the heart of the Amazon, part by choice and part because we couldn't get a boat to get us out, always "we sail tomorrow", so another night on the beer then, another day of eating "meat-like" burgers. You could get it all – crocodile burger, piranha soup, turtle soup, insect and grubs on a stick, but no bat soup so far.

Then eventually we sadly said goodbye to Manaus, in a village river boat for four nights down the Rio Madeira. The boat was crammed, animals and helpers below and the rest of us on deck. Sardines in a can when all the hammocks were out at night. Eating rice and beans twice a day after a breakfast of tea and bread, the cooking water coming straight out of the murky river below and showering in the same water – the same water the sewage just went into.

On the first day Andy got the fever, the Latin lady eye fever; one look and he was gone like Mowgli walking into the man village, and four more nights crammed up in a hammock under the romantic Amazon moon and we knew we had lost him.

We got off after four days and then after a 36-hour bus journey through the Brazilian Amazon we got off in a town somewhere. I am not sure where exactly but I am sure it was somewhere, it must have been somewhere because we were there. We stayed the night and after a meal and another few beers and a good night's sleep we left Andy with his eyes still hypnotised and fully infected.

So now there were two.

A few days later we made it to Rio, New Year's Eve morning. Copacabana was too expensive for us, millennium prices, so we took two buses four hours out of town to a beach camping ground then four hours back to the Copacabana. We made it, just two hours to go before the midnight celebrations but somehow, some way, we were there and ten minutes later Andy arrived too. He said he would be there and he was good to his word. One last fling with boys to finish what we had started, together.

Champagne and many beers later and well into the next morning, we were all lost, split up and in different parts of Rio. I got back to the tent somehow about seven in the morning, David a couple of hours behind, Andy, well, he never made it back and that was the last we saw of him, he had Latin love on his mind. So it was me and Dave again.

Many places, adventures, rivers, mountains, deserts and even an illegal Bolivian prison tour later we were in La Paz, the cheapest place so far on our trip. We were planning more trips and more street food and much more beer for our next leg up to the north to cross the Atacama into Peru.

After all the plans were set, we were set to leave La Paz for the next leg. There we were outside a bus station, life everywhere, sitting on the floor, wild dogs looking for scraps – they probably peed where we were just sitting, diesel fumes everywhere from buses, taxis and wagons. The noise, the life, the culture, the dirt, and the middle-aged plump Bolivian lady in her traditional dress of layered skirts, cardigan and bowler hat, her hands as rough and as dirty as mine. On the floor was a big pot with steam coming out, her tin bowls and a big pot of murky soapy water to 'clean' the dishes and some homemade 'juice' in a plastic jug, no hand sanitiser in sight. We couldn't resist. We'd had a few beers the night before, well, that's how we made our plans, and had a long bus ride ahead. Two bowls of that hot chicken soup were ordered and a glass of that 'juice'. She served it while her baby boy was suckling on her breast, breast milk even pouring out of his nose as he couldn't get it down quick enough. We got stuck in; hot soup fresh made, where I don't know but I'm sure it was fresh where she made it. Incredible flavour and all natural ingredients, even had a hint of cream, or was it some breast milk that had slipped from the little boy's nose and into the bowl? Well, who cares? It tasted great and after a night on the beer was just what we needed to set us on our way for the next adventure.

We drank all the beer, the jungle juice too, all the street food, the good, the bad, and the ugly, and met some crazy people on the way. Some dodgy toilets, some without even toilet roll so we used our imagination, sometimes the odd bush, but we did it and we knew what it was like to be free, to experience the roller-coaster ride of life, but as we wanted.

And twenty years later we are all still here to tell the tale. Apart from a few times when we had to run to the toilet – well, even our bodies had their limits – we lived through it and were alive, strong and well until I too got 'infected' in Peru and left Dave to go on alone.

How on earth did we survive?

Danger everywhere, dodgy food and dodgy beer, in dodgy bars, sleeping in dodgy hotels. Not that South America is all like that but those were the places we chose to frequent. We wanted to see and experience the real life of the real people. To live surrounded by dirt and disease, dodgy toilets, 'meat-like' burgers, and real working people full of life and life's struggles. The hard life in South America means most people live for the day, whereas most westerners only strive to be in 'the now' but never seem to get there. To be free, to experience life, the now is all most of them have.

We survived all that and lived to tell the tale. Apart from the odd day rushing to the toilet, or the odd bush, we survived. We survived because we were three young men on an adventure, we were just passing through, we came into their world with all their dangers but we were just visiting. We didn't have to live the life there, the social, economic, cultural and political life that was making many of them poor and ill. The polluted environment for them became an extra burden they couldn't take; we just seemed to shrug it off. We didn't succumb to their diseases, just the odd day running to the toilet. We ate the 'meat-like' burgers and we never set off a global pandemic. We didn't eat bat soup, not that we know of, but we survived and the world survived too.

As for Andy, well, his 'infection' wore off, they sometimes do.

Dave, well, he got 'bitten' somewhere in Asia.

As for me, well, twenty years and three kids later, let's face it, it's terminal.

There is more to life than the system, and there is more to disease than dirt and germs. Life is a balance of all and more than everything an adventure to be lived. More should have our adventures and know real freedom, if only for a while, then maybe what is really making us sick in this world will become more obvious.

I thank Nature, or God, for all the adventures I had, for the people I met, and the lessons I learnt.

But most of all I thank God for that woman outside the Bolivian bus station (and her son) for just when we needed it most, serving up the best chicken soup, EVER.

Rob Ryder
May 2021

References

Books

'Debt Slavery – The Economics of a Banking Mafia'
– Rob Ryder

'Awareness and Well-being Guided Journal -
And the truth shall set you free!'
– Rob Ryder

'Medical Fascism– How Coronavirus Policy Took Away Our Freedoms And How To Get Them Back'
– Rob Ryder

'A Conscious Humanity: Morality, Freedom & Natural Law'
– Rob Ryder & Patrick Quanten

'Little Miracle Baby: The Perfect Life of Kennedy Jack'
– Patrcik Quanten MD

'Why me?: Science and Spirituality as inevitable bed partners'
– Dr. Patrick Quanten & Erik Bualda

Patrcik QuantenWebsites

https://pqliar.net/

 - Self Empowerment

https://activehealthcare.co.uk/

- Health, Science and Spirituality

https://www.quantics.org/

 - The Science of Nature

Researcher Tracy Northern website

https://northerntracey213875959.wordpress.com/

YOUTUBE

https://www.youtube.com/@robryder3505/featured

- Rob Ryder channel

https://www.youtube.com/watch?v=xa4dK-RV2aI

- 'UKColumn Live - Interview with Dr Patrick Quanten' regarding the nature of infections and safety and effectiveness of vaccination

Rumble

https://rumble.com/user/robryder

- Rob Ryder Rumble channel including interview that was deleted by YOUTUBE with Patrcik Quanten 'Modern Medicine – Truth Lies in the History'